SURGICAL TREATMENT OF ANAL INCONTINENCE

Springer-Verlag London Ltd.

Charles V. Mann • Richard E. Glass

SURGICAL TREATMENT OF ANAL INCONTINENCE

Second Edition

Illustrations by B. Hyams, R. Lane and G. Oliver

With 173 Figures

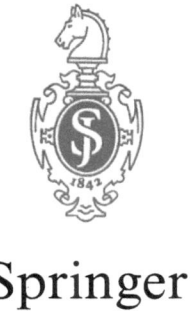

Springer

Charles V. Mann, MCh, FRCS
Emeritus Surgeon, Northwick Park and St Marks Hospital Trust, Harrow and Emeritus
Surgeon, The Royal London Hospital Trust, London

Richard E. Glass, MS, FRCS
Consultant Surgeon, Princess Margaret Hospital, Swindon SN1 4JU, UK

The illustration on the front cover is Figure 3.7. (page 32)

British Library Cataloguing in Publication Data
Mann, Charles V. (Charles Victor)
    Surgical treatment of anal incontinence.
    1. Mann. Anus & rectum. Surgery
    I. Title II. Glass, Richard E.
    617.555

Library of Congress Cataloging-in-Publication Data
Mann, Charles V.
    Surgical treatment of anal incontinence/Charles V. Mann and Richard E. Glass.
        p.   cm.

    ISBN 978-1-4471-1239-6   ISBN 978-1-4471-0935-8 (eBook)
    DOI 10.1007/978-1-4471-0935-8

    1. Fecal incontinence – Surgery. 2. Rectum–Surgery. 3. Perineum Surgery. I. Glass, Richard 1948–
    II. Title
    [DNLM: Fecal Incontinence–surgery. WI 650 M281s]
    RD544.M36 1990
    617.5′55–dc20
    DNLM/DLC
    for Library of Congress   90–10037

Typeset by EXPO Holdings, Malaysia

28/3830-543210 Printed on acid-free paper

*To those unfortunate patients with anal incontinence
and to their surgeons*

PREFACE TO THE FIRST EDITION

It is only in the last 25 years that the treatment of anal incontinence has become an important surgical discipline. This is not only because our understanding of the disorder has been greatly augmented by new investigative methods. It is also because the hydrocarbon industry has provided us with suitable materials with which to carry out the complex repairs that are now possible.

Like most new areas of therapy, initial enthusiasm has been modified by experience. Some techniques have been amended or abandoned. Others have been shown to have very specific indications and to be unsuitable for general use. But the total of cases treated by surgical means continues to grow, and as the field widens it is apparent that large numbers of people are still suffering from anal incontinence silently and unheard, and have been abandoned to their misery by society at large. For some of these unfortunates, the consequences are appalling: they become outcasts even within their own families; in some communities they are unable to practise their religion. They are truly regarded as "dirty", and are shunned.

Because a large body of surgical experience has accrued, nowadays many of these cases can be cured, and most of them substantially alleviated. But a mis-applied or badly performed operation can be a disaster for both the patient and the surgeon.

For these reasons, we have decided that the time is ripe for a book specifically directed at the techniques of procedures developed for the treatment of anal incontinence. This book is unashamedly concerned with surgical craftsmanship. We hope that by careful selection and application of these techniques, surgeons who need to perform these operations will obtain the best results possible.

Because matching the patient's needs to the best available procedure must be based on sound judgement, we give guidance from our own experience as to "what" should be offered to "whom", and include advice on pre- and post-operative care which can make the difference between success and failure.

Above all, we hope that readers enjoy the book and are stimulated to participate actively in the development of this new and growing field of surgery. There is still much to be done, and so many patients need your help.

London   Charles V. Mann
January 1991   Richard E. Glass

PREFACE TO THE SECOND EDITION

Since the first edition, there have been further developments in surgical techniques for the treatment of faecal incontinence of anal origin, most notably the stimulated graciloplasty procedure. The laparoscopic approach for abdominal surgery has also established itself and laparoscopic rectopexy is accepted as an option for managing elderly infirm patients with rectal prolapse. The results achieved by surgery can be improved by employing drugs to modify colo-rectal motor functions and to alter stool consistency, while there still remains a small number of patients for whom surgical treatment is inappropriate or unsuccessful. The authors believe that the advances justify a new edition of this book which incorporates the latest information on these aspects of surgical treatment for anal incontinence and are optimistic that professional acceptance of the second edition will be as favourable as it was for the first.

London
August 1996

Charles V. Mann
Richard E. Glass

CONTENTS

CHAPTER 1
Essential Anatomy of Anal Continence

General Introduction

It is customary to divide the lower intestine into three constituent parts – colon, rectum and anus. While the colon is intimately linked in functional terms to the control of continence, it has no relevance to the structural factors that govern the control of anal continence. However, the same is not true for the rectum and anus: both are vital to the structural basis by which the body governs defaecation. Because of this strong interrelationship between the rectum and anus it is best that the anatomy and the physiology of the continence mechanism are regarded as belonging to one unit – the ano-rectum.

Topographical anatomy remains the basis of surgical handicraft. No procedure can be developed without attention to the structure of the organs concerned, and nothing of lasting surgical value grows out of concepts that are not anatomically sound. However, the viewpoint of the topographical anatomist, who describes structure as a rigid framework, differs from that of the surgeon, who sees anatomy as something mobile to be moulded and changed for the patient's benefit. Therefore, this chapter is divided into two parts: one devoted to the basic anatomical construction of the ano-rectum and the other concerned with those aspects of the structure of the ano-rectum that can be modified by surgical techniques.

In subsequent chapters concerned with individual operative techniques, it will be seen that in some cases the effectiveness of an operation is limited by the harsh realities imposed by the anatomy of the organ that is being worked upon. From this it follows that newly devised operations demand accurate knowledge of the fundamental structure and function of the ano-rectal organ. It is for this reason that modern surgical techniques have frequently developed as a result of multidisciplinary co-operation by surgeon, physiologist and neurohistologist, with each making vital contributions. But the bedrock remains the anatomical structure of the ano-rectal organ.

Because surgeons need to compare the results that can be achieved by different incontinence procedures it is useful to have a baseline measurement of the severity of incontinence. For this reason an 'incontinence score' system has been devised by Miller et al. (Table 1.1) which can be recommended for general use.

Table 1.1   Incontinence score

Grade	Flatus	Fluid	Solid
I	1	4	7
II	2	5	8
III	3	6	9

Key: Grade I = incontinence < 1 episode per month
Grade II = incontinence between once a week and once a month
Grade III = incontinence > once per week

The table is based on the scoring system originally devised by Miller et al. (British Journal of Surgery. 1988). The higher the number scored by the patient, the greater the degree of incontinence. At the Royal London Hospital, faecal incontinence is graded as *major* (loss of control for solid faeces several times weekly or daily for liquid faeces) *intermediate* (loss of control for solid faeces several times monthly or several times weekly for liquid faeces) or *minor* (no loss of control for solid faeces but loss of control of liquid faeces once a month or during episodes of diarrhoea).

Structural Anatomy

Development [1,6,7]

The ano-rectal organ derives from two sources: (1) *the hindgut* and (2) the surface (dermis), the *proctodaeum* [6].

The hindgut portion which forms the rectum proper is split off from the original common cloaca by the uro-rectal septum, but it retains the nerves and blood vessels that supplied the part of the cloaca from which it was derived. This means that the anterior derivatives of the cloaca that develop from the uro-genital sinus share the origins of the nerves and blood vessels to the rectum and anus.

The anus itself develops in the upper part of the uro-rectal septum, and migrates downwards towards the perineum during the process of absorption of the tail-gut. Many anatomists believe that ridges of tissue derived from the lateral parts of the uro-rectal septum also contribute to the developing anus: this accounts both anatomically and physiologically for the close association between the muscle of the pub-orectalis portion of the levator ani muscle and the deep part of the external anal sphincter [23].

The lowest portion of the anus is developed by an initial indentation of the perineal skin ("perineal sinus") which is deepened by enlargement of the genital folds. Because of this, it can be no surprise that occasionally the anal and genital structures are not correctly aligned and ectopic anal openings are formed. At the deepest posterior aspect of the perineal sinus (which is now known as the proctodaeum) the bridging layer of skin is stretched over the developing hindgut and is termed the cloacal membrane. This membrane, which separates the future anal opening from the hindgut and anal bud, thins and gives way prior to birth, forming a conjoined ano-rectal tube. If the membrane does not fenestrate, a "covered anus" deformity results, but the anus and its surrounding muscles, although buried, are substantially normal. Because of the dermal origin of the lowest (proctodaeal) part of the anus, the anal canal is lined in its lower half by squamous epithelium and in its upper half by epithelium of "gut" type (cubical): these two epithelial types meet at the dentate line, and are each supplied by nerves and blood vessels that reflect their origins (Fig. 1.1).

If the rectum fails to develop by a normal and complete separation from the cloaca by the uro-rectal septum, it is usual for the pelvic floor muscles and anal sphincters to be maldeveloped as well [15] (Fig. 1.2). Therefore, a *high* failure of development not only leads to persistence of (cloacal-type) connections between the rectum and the bladder and urethra, but also to partial or complete absence of anal sphincters. In such

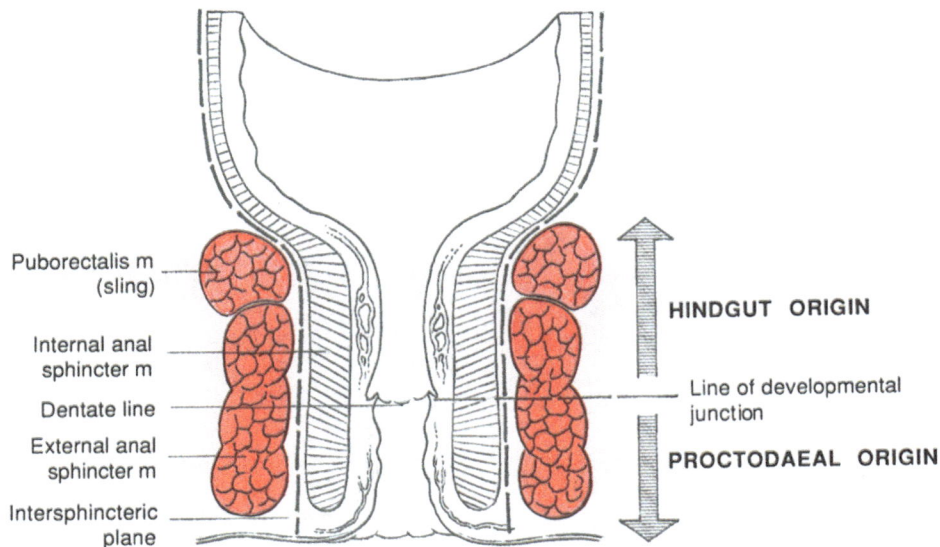

Puborectalis m
(sling)

Internal anal
sphincter m

Dentate line

External anal
sphincter m

Intersphincteric
plane

HINDGUT ORIGIN

Line of developmental
junction

PROCTODAEAL ORIGIN

Fig. 1.1. The line of developmental junction between hindgut (above) and proctodaeum (below) is shown clinically by the wavy mucosal junction ("dentate line") between the cubical epithelium above and the squamous stratified epithelium below. Above the dentate line, the nerve supply of the mucosa is autonomic (insensitive to touch and pain) and both the lymphatics and the veins drain towards the abdomen. Below the dentate line, the mucosa is supplied from spinal nerves (sensitive to touch and pain) and the lymphatics drain to the inguinal nodes and the veins join the external iliac system on each side. From the viewpoint of surgical operations for incontinence, the absence of sensibility of the mucosa above the dentate line is partially compensated by afferent impulses arising in the muscles surrounding the ano-rectal junction. Therefore, control of defaecation is still possible even if the lower rectum and the ano-rectal junction are not present.

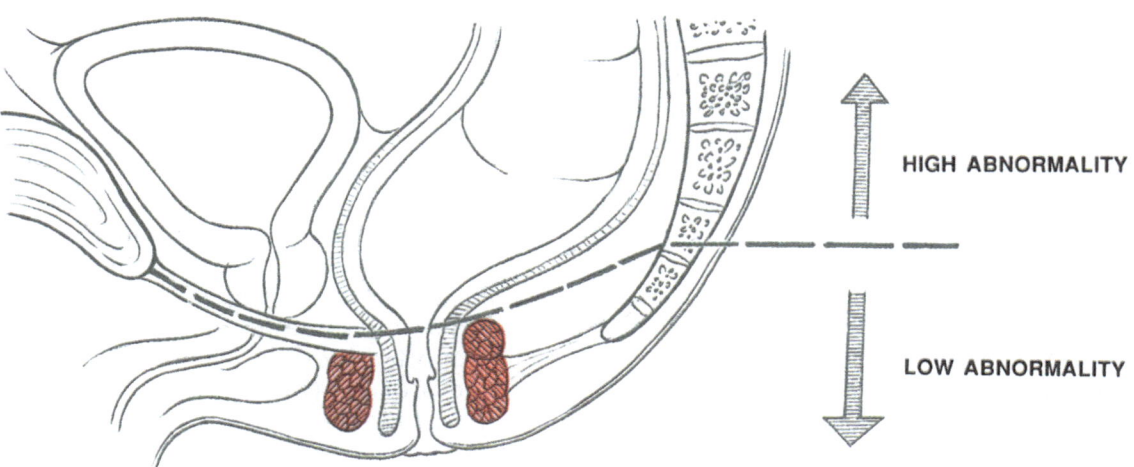

HIGH ABNORMALITY

LOW ABNORMALITY

Fig. 1.2. If the hindgut fails to separate from the cloaca in a normal way, the maldevelopment is usually a "high" one. A high abnormality usually has virtually complete absence of normal ano-rectal musculature, as well as persisting fistulous connections to uro-genital organs. If the hindgut develops normally, but there is failure of proctodaeal tissues to form or meet up with hindgut structures, the maldevelopment is "low". A low abnormality is usually associated with the presence of some ano-rectal muscle, and fistulous connections to bladder or other uro-genital organs are rare. Surgical correction of low abnormalities is usually accompanied by good functional control. The results of operations for high abnormalities depend greatly on the degree to which the pelvic floor muscles can be restored to a correct relationship with the ano-rectal junction.

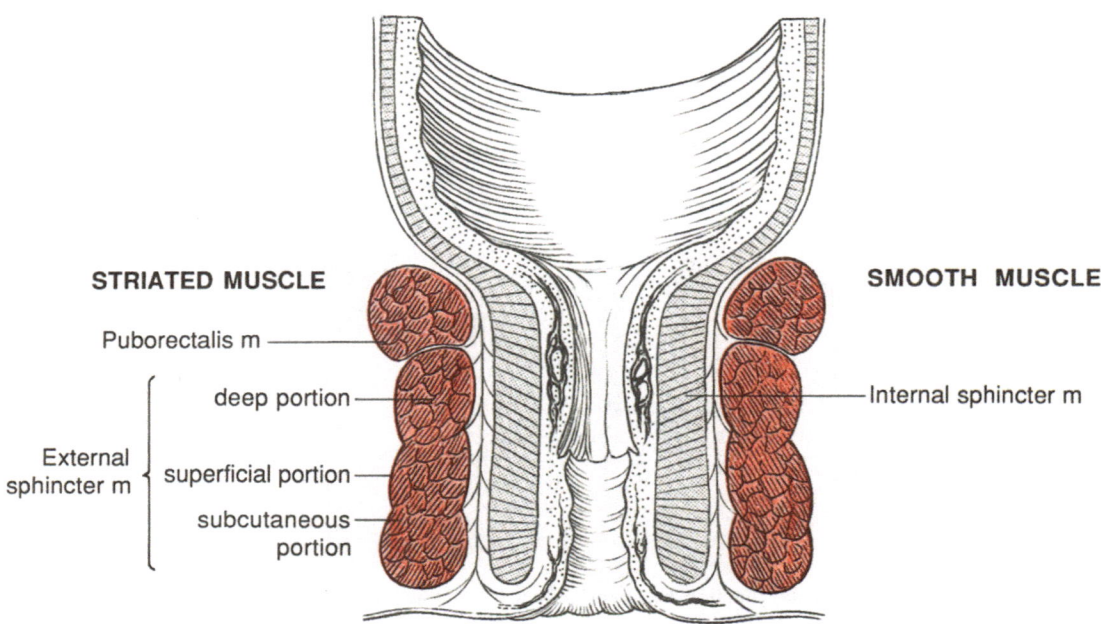

Fig. 1.3. The puborectalis muscle is structurally similar in its organisation and nerve supply to the deep portion of the external sphincter muscle. They can be regarded as forming one functional unit. A plane separates the striated muscle tube from the internal smooth muscle tube (the "intersphincteric plane", see Fig. 1.2). This plane is occupied by loose tissue and fibrous condensations derived from the longitudinal muscle coat of the rectal wall. These condensations can be dense and have been called the "levator plate" (Shafik). The internal sphincter muscle is formed by thickening of the inner circular smooth muscle coat of the intestine. In normal subjects the lower end of the internal anal sphincter is found near to the anal verge, and the entire length of the anal canal has a complete surround of external and internal sphincter muscle.

cases, before a surgical reconstruction can be carried out the presence (or absence) of anal sphincter muscle must be established. In the female, ectopic anal tissue (and orifices) may occur in the vagina. If, however, a substantial degree of normal hindgut development takes place, and the deformity can be regarded as *low*, in most cases a fistulous track is not present between the rectum and the uro-genital organs and some anal sphincter muscle can be identified. These cases are very suitable for surgical correction. Patients who are incontinent from an ectopically positioned but low anal orifice (e.g. in the vagina or abnormally far forward on the perineum) can be made continent by a correct repositioning which takes care to align (and/or reposition) the anal sphincter muscle around the anal orifice. The "covered anus" type of deformity needs only the surgeon's knife to complete the fenestration of the cloacal membrane (the site for the insertion

of the knife is betrayed by an anal dimple), followed in some cases by subsequent regular anal dilation [1].

Anal Muscles (Fig. 1.3)

Immediately beneath the skin is a thin, unimportant layer of involuntary muscle – the corrugator cutis ani. Continence depends upon two much larger muscle groups – the external and internal anal sphincter muscles – supported by the pubo-rectalis portion of the levator ani (Fig. 1.3).

The organisation of the *external anal sphincter* is still debated but all recent authorities agree that it is (1) composed of striated muscle, (2) forms a circular tube around the outer circumference of the anal canal approximately 3–5 cm long and (3) is composed of three aggregations which function as an integrated unit (Figs. 1.4, 1.5). The three aggregations are most easily

Fig. 1.4. The three parts of the external sphincter muscle, emphasising the close relation between the deep portion of the external sphincter and the puborectalis sling, which can be regarded as one functional unit.

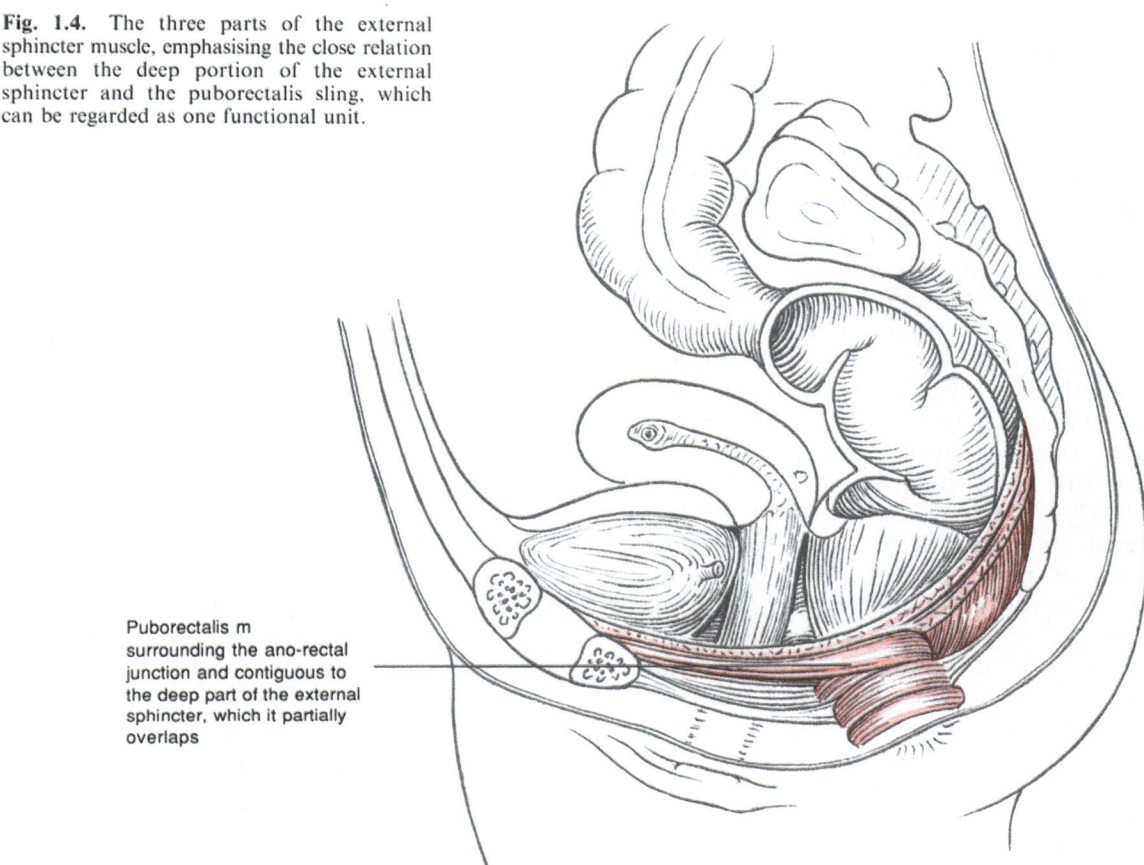

Puborectalis m surrounding the ano-rectal junction and contiguous to the deep part of the external sphincter, which it partially overlaps

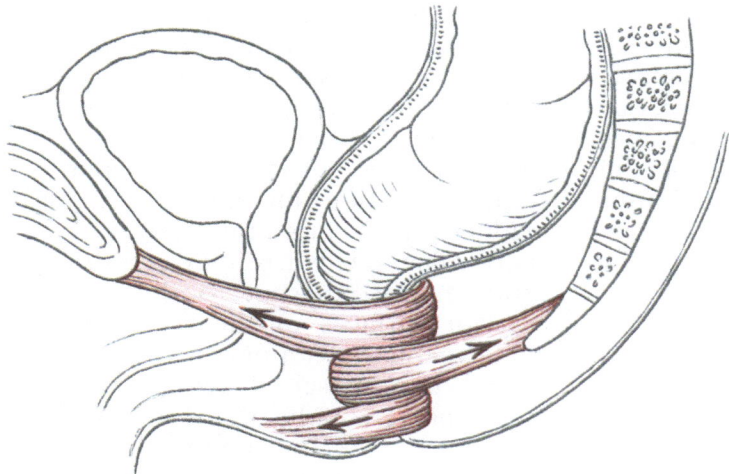

Fig. 1.5. Attachments of the puborectalis muscle and the external sphincter are responsible for differential forces acting on the anal canal. These pulls (described by Shafik as a "triple-loop" system [18]) act to angulate the ano-rectal junction and compress the anal canal, and so to assist the circular tonus of the sphincter muscle rings to maintain continence.

recognisable in the posterior aspect of the anal circumference and are less obvious in the lateral and anterior quadrants. The aggregations are commonly called respectively the *subcutaneous, superficial* and *deep* parts of the external sphincter. The external sphincter has attachments behind to the coccyx and anteriorly to the pubis (in men) and perineal body (in women). The lowest part of the levator ani muscle – the puborectalis muscle – forms a sling around the top postero-lateral aspects of the anal canal and reinforces the external sphincter at these points. There is considerable overlapping of these various muscles, and in the female the external sphincter is quite thin anteriorly. There is histological similarity between the microstructure of the muscle bundles of puborectalis and the deep part of the external sphincter, which function as one unit [13,24]. The *internal anal sphincter* is composed of unstriated muscle and is separate from the external sphincter (although some fibres of the two muscles may intermingle across the intervening plane of loose connective tissue).

Some authors [18,19,20] have published material that has demonstrated longitudinal muscle [12], as well as strong fascial condensations, between the circular internal and external sphincter muscle groups.

Blood Supply

The ano-rectal organ derives its arterial supply from three sources. The principal source is from the inferior mesenteric artery, which is continued as the *superior rectal/haemorrhoidal artery*. This vessel comes into close contact with the back of the rectum just below the pelvic brim, and after this point it lies within the connective-tissue-filled space that surrounds the lower rectum, which is itself contained by the rectal "fascia". Opposite the lower third of the rectum the superior haemorrhoidal artery forms a variable number of smaller branches that continue the arterial supply to the upper half of the anal canal. The *middle rectal/haemorrhoidal artery* is a branch of the internal iliac artery that approaches the rectum from each side of the mid-pelvis in the lateral connective-tissue condensations ("ligaments") of the rectum: it usually breaks up into a leash of vessels just short of the rectal wall. The *inferior rectal/haemorrhoidal artery* comes from the internal pudic artery and crosses medially near the roof of each ischiorectal fossa to enter the anal canal in its upper part. There is free communication between the terminal branches of all three arteries, and the surgeon does not have to fear ischaemia as a rule, even after the most complex anal procedures.

Venous Drainage

In general, this follows the arterial pattern and is not an important element of operative detail.

Nerve Supply [3,7,8,10]

The rectal wall has an autonomic nerve supply from both the sympathetic and parasympathetic systems. The sympathetic supply comes from the first three lumbar segments. The sympathetics are distributed mainly via the hypogastric plexus, which bifurcates at the brim of the pelvis into two lateral portions – the pelvic plexuses – as well as other nerves which accompany the blood vessels. The hypogastric and pelvic plexuses also distribute parasympathetic fibres. The parasympathetic supply to the rectum comes from sacral segments S2, 3 and 4 and is distributed through the nervi erigentes. These also contain afferent nerves from the rectum and anal canal (and the bladder). The autonomic nerves are especially vulnerable where they cross the pelvic brim, or are adjacent to the lateral and anterior surfaces of the rectal wall. The anal canal has a complex nerve supply. The puborectalis muscle shares in the double motor nerve supply of the rest of levator ani muscle from both the 4th sacral and pudic nerves (usually the inferior haemorrhoidal division of the latter). There is some evidence after rectal excision that there is transmission of afferent stimuli by these nerves (or from end-organs in the pelvic floor muscles) because these patients can still appreciate the need to defaecate even when there is direct anastomosis of colon to anal canal [9]. The external anal sphincter has a multiple nerve supply from the inferior haemorrhoidal nerve (subcutaneous part), the 4th sacral nerve (superficial part) and from branches of the pudic nerve (deep part). The internal anal sphincter has the same autonomic nerve supply as the rectum. Afferent sensibility in the anal canal is somatic in type below the dentate line but above this the mucosal lining is insensitive to pain. More detail concerning the nervous regulation of anal function is given in Chapter 2, but it is relevant to note that the arrangement of the puborectalis muscle fibres (horizontal loops) is not only very similar to that of the deep part of the external sphincter muscle (see earlier) but that they also share the same nerve supply (inferior haemorrhoidal nerve) which enters both of them from the perineal aspect.

Surgical Anatomy
[12,18,19,20,21,22,24]

Drawings of the anatomy of the ano-rectum do not convey the flexibility and variability of the organ observed by surgeons.

The Rectum

The normal rectum is not full of faeces, and indeed may be empty for most of the 24 hours, except immediately prior to and during the act of defaecation. However, because man is by origin a hunter and in civilised society needs to control the timing of the defaecatory act, the rectum must also have a reservoir function. There is some evidence that filling of the rectum

may be also partially regulated by the recto-sigmoid junction [11], which is not only narrower than the sigmoid colon above and the rectum below but has other characteristics well appreciated by the surgeon. These are:

1. It is frequently angled sharply
2. It is the region through which a rectoscope can often be most difficult to pass
3. It is the area which can be "relaxed" (e.g. by deep breathing, anti-cholinergic drugs or by air-insufflation)
4. It is the part which can release accumulations of faeces and fluid after it has opened up (to the discomfiture of the endoscopist)

The surgeon should be aware that left-sided colon resections that abolish the recto-sigmoid junction may lead to more rapid and easy transit of the faecal stream into the rectum, and that this may be due, in part, to the effects of straightening and widening the colo-rectal junction [22]. The rectum itself has both antero-posterior and lateral flexureal folds and meets the anus at another sharp bend – the ano-rectal angle [22]. This angle is maintained by the pull of the puborectalis muscle sling (Fig. 1.6). The rectal folds are marked internally by the valves of Houston, and these valves can overlap each other when the rectum is empty: Houston himself thought these values delay the descent of the faeces down the rectum and prevent precipitous urge to defaecate. But probably the greatest contribution the rectum makes to the control of defaecation is by being an expanded, pouch-like organ with pliable muscular walls (that are usually in a state of relaxation) which can accommodate accumulations of faecal material. From this it follows that a straight, inflexible and narrowed rectal tube (such as may be created by wrapping the rectum in prosthetic material) may contribute significantly to problems of defaecatory control by loss of reservoir capacity. In both sexes, an excessively floppy or distorted rectum can create mechanical factors promoting rectal faecal

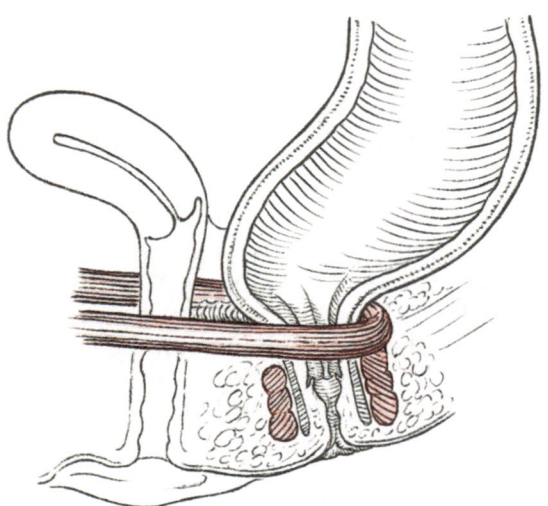

Fig. 1.6. The normal angulation of the ano-rectal junction which is maintained by the pull of the puborectalis muscle. The normal anal canal in the adult is a closed tube 3.5 to 4.5 cm long surrounded throughout its length by both external and internal sphincter muscles. The normal anal angle is between 80°–120° at rest (mean 90°) but the measurements depend on the technique used (Table 1.2)

may be so floppy that it balloons down during episodes of raised abdominal pressure, typified by straining defaecation ("perineal descent") [8,14,17]. In the female, stretching of the recto-vaginal septum is common during childbirth, and may lead to protrusion and herniation of the anterior rectal wall either forwards into the vagina or backwards into the rectum itself ("anterior mucosal prolapse"). All these clinical syndromes are associated with problems of constipation and incontinence of varying degrees which result from loss of normal rectal anatomical integrity.

retention and constipation. Absence of anterior buttressing of the rectal wall may result in an out-pouching ("rectocele") which can act as an acquired diverticulum to divert or retain a faecal bolus. In both sexes the pelvic muscular floor may become weak as a result of old age or disease, allowing descent with eventration and intussusception of the rectum ("rectal prolapse"). In some patients the pelvic floor

The Anus [2,16]

The anus joins the rectum at an acute angle (range 80°–120°) with the patient standing, reduced on full flexion of the hip joints (as in squatting). This angle (Table 1.2) has been thought important for creating a "flutter" ("shutter") valve effect which can aggravate constipation by being closed too tightly by abdominal straining, or alternatively can promote incontinence if it is absent or reduced (Fig. 1.7). The angle is not considered an important contributor to continence at present. The forward pull of the puborectalis sling around the ano-rectal neck is a prime factor in maintaining the ano-rectal angle (Fig. 1.6) [19]. The ano-rectal junction (like the oesophagogastric junction) passes through a muscular

Table 1.2 The ano-rectal angle

Reference	Angle		
Womack N.R. et al. *1985*	Normal (rest)	92° (range 80°–100°)	
Brit. J. Surg. 72. 994–998	Straining	130° (range 120°–150°)	
Bartram C.I. et al. *1987*	Normal (rest)	94° (±19°)	
Gastroint. Radiol. 13. 72–80	Straining	113° (±16°)	
Goeti. R. et al. *1989*	Normal (rest)	females	112° (±23°)
		males	104° (±25°)
	Voluntary squeeze	females	86° (±20°)
		males	81° (±23°)
	Straining	females	129° (±11°)
		males	122° (±22°)

The ano-rectal angle is measured by defaecography with reference to lines drawn either between the ischial tuberosities (the *bi-ischiatic line*) or from the pubis to the tip of the coccyx (the *pubo-coccygeal line*). Cineradiography has been replaced by video-recording of the events as this greatly lowers the radiation dose. In the table, the normal values represent resting measurements (rest).

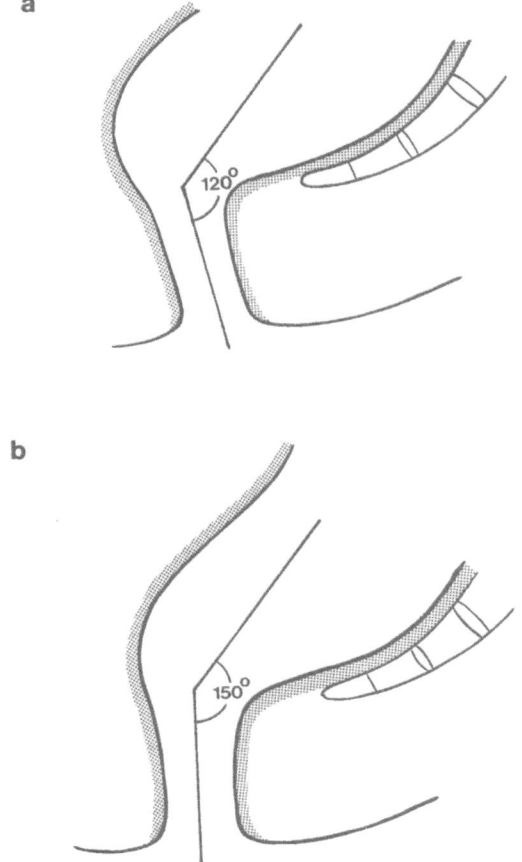

Fig. 1.7. **(a)** Normal ano-rectal angle (120°) **(b)** Straightening of the ano-rectal angle can promote incontinence. The angle is normally straightened during *evacuation* and by *straining* (mean 130° range 120°–150°) and is sharpened by voluntary *anal squeezing* (mean 80°; range 75°–104°). (Womack et al. 1985 (9)).

diaphragm (the levator ani muscle) in which there is an opening (hiatus). The mechanical arrangement of the hiatal orifice can affect continence. In a normal subject the levator floor hiatus is an antero-posterior slit which is 3.5–4.5 cm long and 2.5–3 cm across. The intra-hiatal structures are held to the edges of the opening by condensed fibrous tissue ("fascia") which has been called the hiatal "ligament" [19]. This fascia not only controls the position and angle of the ano-rectal junction, but is able to transmit defaecatory opening and closing efforts to the entrance of the anal canal; and if it is weakened it can lead to

incontinence and prolapse in the same manner that weakening of the phreno-oesophageal ligament can allow reflux or the development of a hiatus hernia. The presence of fascial condensations at the ano-rectal junction, and also in the inter-sphincteric groove, is important to the surgeon as it enables his stitches to hold under tension without cutting through.

However, the main anatomical contributions of the anus to continence are by the *length* and *shape* of the anal canal. The normal canal is approximately 3–5 cm long, and is of tubular shape kept closed by the tonic activity of the anal sphincter muscles except during defaecation. In a few patients, the lower anal canal is not kept shut, and the anal canal is effectively closed only in its upper half: this is known as a "funnel-shaped" deformity, with its apex at the top of the anal canal. Such patients are abnormally dependent on the anatomical and functional integrity of the muscles of the ano-rectal ring for maintaining continence (Fig. 1.8a). In some patients the anal canal is shorter than normal (Fig. 1.8b); at the extremes of life the anus is naturally shorter as well as weaker than in the adult, and at both ages any reduction in muscle tone can lead to faecal leakage. Because of the angulation of the anus, with a posteriorly directed opening, the anal canal is slightly shorter anteriorly than posteriorly. In females the anal sphincter muscles are often thinner, shorter and more fused than in the male. If the normal tubular shape of the closed anal canal is lost (e.g. by trauma to the anal muscles), various degrees of incontinence can result:

1. If the anal muscular framework is completely divided, total faecal incontinence is caused
2. If the muscles of the lower two-thirds of the anal canal are cut, and the edges of the sphincter retract, a grooved or "gutter" deformation occurs which can allow fluid faeces or mucus to filter onto the perianal skin
3. If the internal anal sphincter only is divided in its lower part (as after inter-

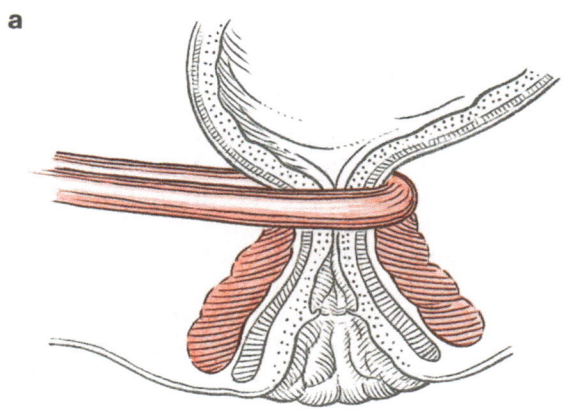

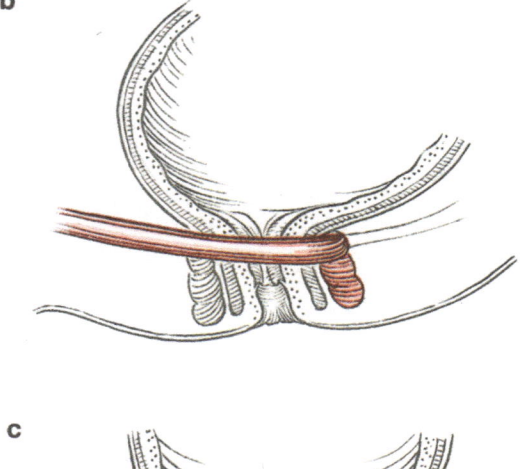

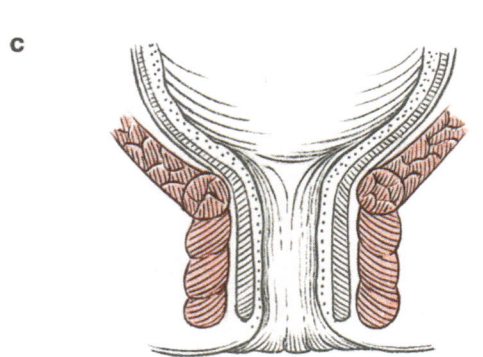

Fig. 1.8. **a** The "funnel" deformity of the anus, which leaves the patient entirely dependent on closure of the top end of the anal canal for continence. Anal dilatation, sphincterotomy procedures, operations for fistula-in-ano or simply diminished anal sphincter tonus can all lead to incontinence when allied to this abnormality. **b** The shorter anal canal found at the extremes of life can promote incontinence, especially if sphincter tonus is diminished. **c** If the mucosal lining of the anal canal becomes smooth and atrophic (e.g. oestrogen deficiency, postradiotherapy) mucus and faecal leakage frequently results.

nal anal sphincterotomy) the anus retains both its shape and length and there should be no loss of control other than minimally to flatus during muscular exertion

It must be remembered that the mucosal lining of the anal canal, especially above the dentate line, is thrown into prominent folds ("anal cushions") that contribute to a watertight seal of the closed anal sphincter [4]. (We are all familiar with a cloth or flannel blocking the bath-outlet: the anal cushions act in much the same way.) If the anal lining becomes totally smooth (Fig. 1.8c), leakage of flatus, fluid or mucus is promoted, especially if there is any accompanying deformity or weakness of the anal sphincters.

The presence and bulk of the anal sphincter muscles can be demonstrated electromyographically (EMG sphincter mapping) and by ultrasound (anal endosonography)

References and Further Reading

1. Ball CB (1908) The rectum: its diseases and development defects (ed Frowde). Hodder and Stoughton, London
2. Duthie HL (1971) Anal continence. Gut 12: 844
3. Duthie HL, Gairns FW (1960) Sensory nerve endings and sensation in the anal region of man. Br J Surg 47: 585
4. Gibbons CP, Bannister JJ, Trowbridge EA, Read NW (1986) Role of anal cushions in maintaining continence. Lancet i: 886
5. Goligher JC (1984) Surgery of the anus, rectum and colon, 5th edn. Ballière Tindall, London, pp 1–47
6. Miller R, Bartolo DCC, Locke-Edmunds JC and Mortensen NJMcC (1988) Prospective study of conservative and operative treatment for faecal incontinence. Brit. J. Surg. 75: 101
7. Williams PL, Warwick R, Dyson M, Bannister LH (1989) Gray's Anatomy, 37th edn. Churchill Livingstone, London, Chap. 2, pp 231–236
8. Williams PL, Warwick R, Dyson M, Bannister LH (1989) Gray's Anatomy, 37th edn. Churchill Livingstone, London, Chap, 8, p 1373
9. Womack NR, Williams NS Holmfield JHM et al. 1985. New method for dynamic assessment of ano-rectal function in constipation. Brit J Surg 72: 994

10. Henry MM, Parks AG, Swash M (1982) The pelvic floor musculature in the descending perineum syndrome. Br J Surg 69: 470
11. Lane RHS, Parks AG (1977) Function of the anal sphincters following colo-anal anastomosis. Br J Surg 64: 596
12. Lawson J (1981) Motor nerve supply of the pelvic floor. Lancet i: 999
13. Martin E, Burden VG (1927). The surgical significance of the recto-sigmoid sphincter. Ann Surg 86: 86
14. Morgan CN, Thompson HR (1956) Surgical anatomy of the anal canal, with special reference to the surgical importance of the internal sphincter and conjoint longitudinal muscle. Ann R Coll Surg Engl 19: 88
15. Oh C, Kark AE (1972) Anatomy of the external anal sphincter. Br J Surg 59: 717
16. Parks AG, Porter NH, Hardcastle JD (1966) The syndrome of the descending perineum. Proc R Soc Med 59: 477
17. Pena A (1989) Surgical management of ano-rectal malformations. Springer-Verlag, New York
18. Phillips SF, Edwards DAW (1965) Some aspects of anal continence and defaecation. Gut 6: 396
19. Rutter KRP, Riddell RH (1975) The solitary ulcer syndrome of the rectum. Clin Gastroenterol 4: 505
20. Shafik A (1975) A new concept of the anatomy of the anal sphincter mechanism and the physiology of defaecation. I. The external anal sphincter. A triple loop system. Invest Urol 12: 412
21. Shafik A (1975) A new concept of the anal sphincter mechanism and the physiology of defaecation. II. Anatomy of the levator ani muscle with special reference to pubo-rectalis. Invest Urol 13: 175
22. Shafik A (1976) A new concept of the anal sphincter mechanism and the physiology of defaecation. III. The longitudinal muscle: anatomy and role in the anal sphincter mechanism. Invest Urol 13: 271
23. Stephens FD, Smith ED (1987) Anatomy and function of the normal rectum and anus in ano-rectal malformations in children. Year Book Medical Publishers. Chicago, pp 14–32
24. Tagart REB (1966) The anal canal and rectum: their varying relationship and its effect on anal continence. Dis Colon Rectum 9: 449
25. Tench EN (1936) Development of the anus in the human embryo. Am J Anat 59: 333
26. Thomas PA, Mann CV (1981) Alimentary sphincters and their disorders. Macmillan, London
27. Thomson WHF (1975) The nature of haemorrhoids. Br J Surg 62: 542

CHAPTER 2

Physiology of Anal Continence

General Introduction

Although the anatomical structure of the ano-rectum provides the *framework* for continence, the interrelated *functions* of the various parts are what determines the continence status of an individual. It is not possible to isolate any constituent organ or part of the distal bowel from its immediate neighbours in regard to the efficiency with which defaecatory control is exercised. An excellent anal sphincter muscle can be totally negated, not only by colonic overactivity (e.g. in severe diarrhoeal states), but also by a sluggish inert rectum that allows faecal impaction to occur. In the same manner, a colon or rectum of impeccable performance are negated by a patulous or damaged anal sphincter.

While the surgeon faced with an incontinent patient may be primarily concerned with the integrity of the anatomical and physiological structure of the ano-rectal organ, he must always remember the complex interdependency of the intricate neuromuscular and reservoir functions of different parts of the alimentary tract; and

both of these must be placed in the context of the whole person. Brilliant ano-rectal surgical procedures are misplaced both in their intent and in their effect in a patient suffering incontinence because of senile dementia.

This section attempts to provide a logical programme for the diagnosis of the causes of incontinence, and the application of the outcome of this process for the management of an individual patient with incontinence. The key to a successful surgical result lies in appropriate matching of the clinical problem with the correct operation. While the surgeon has to be aware that any repair must be carried out with due consideration of the anatomy, the final test of his operation will be physiological, i.e. the completeness (or otherwise) of defaecatory control. Such is the subtlety of ano-rectal function that the surgeon needs to combine physiological knowledge, clinical flexibility and sound judgement with an impeccable surgical technique when he is seeking to alleviate incontinence by surgical operations involving the muscles of the pelvic floor and anal sphincters.

Patho-physiology of Continence
[3,4,5]

Proximal Alimentary Tract

Disorders of the proximal gastro-intestinal tract that may be associated with incontinence are shown in Fig. 2.1a, b. Explosive diarrhoea is the principal underlying factor that is common to all these varied conditions.

Colon [6,11]

It is impossible to consider continence of the ano-rectum without reference to the colon. If the colon transmits loose stools to the rectum in an uncontrolled and/or violent way, normal ano-rectal physiological mechanisms are not invariably able to guarantee continence. To provide crude illustrations of such colon-originated breakdowns of the continence mechanism one can consider the case of the patient with massive diarrhoea (e.g. from dysentery or cholera) who is frequently completely incontinent; similarly surgeons using massive intestinal purgation to effect a clean colon prior to surgery also reproduce the circumstances in which extreme intestinal hurry coupled with watery stools causes incontinence despite a physiologically intact ano-rectum.

Normally the colon works quietly, by low pressure activity occurring in an intermittent manner. This type of activity occurs over short lengths (5.0 cm) and is called "segmentation"; it is responsible for kneading and turning over the faecal content (Fig. 2.2). Excessive segmental contractions can cause slowing of faecal transit, and the extra time spent by the faecal stream in the colon allows increased resorption of water. Such delayed colonic passage results in a type of constipation associated with scybalous small faecal pellets. Such tiny hard faecal "pebbles" are unable to initiate a normal defaecatory response by rectal distention, and the patient frequently responds to this situation by excessive abdominal straining. Every so often segmental activity of the normal colon is replaced by "mass movements" which are now known to be peristaltic in nature: these result in abrupt onward emptying of long (30–45 cm) lengths of colon, and when the contents of the pelvic colon are thus emptied into the rectum by such activity, the sudden rectal distention so produced triggers defaecation. If the colon becomes inert or paralysed (e.g. by excessive use of drugs – the "cathartic colon" syndrome) the rectal wall is not stimulated by the normal rapid stretching that accompanies such emptying of the pelvic colon (and which is a feature of the well-known gastro-colic reflex that commonly occurs at breakfast-time), and a loaded (impacted) rectum that does not empty efficiently can become a cause of "spurious" diarrhoea due to overflow faecal incontinence.

Abnormal constituents appearing in the faeces (e.g. laxative drugs such as senna or bisacodyl; blood; bile) can cause prolonged or excessive peristaltic activity. Certain pharmacological enemas contain material that directly stimulates such hyperactivity (e.g. sodium acid phosphate, sodium picosulphate, oxyphenisatin) which can overwhelm the anorectal control mechanisms.

Stress, neurological disorders and psychiatric disturbance can each inhibit normal colon transit mechanisms. Paraplegia can be complicated by massive colo-rectal dysfunction. Some drugs used in the treatment of mania, depression or anxiety (e.g. diazepam, lithium carbonate) can produce severe colonic faecal retention by either inhibiting peristaltic activity or by promoting excessive segmental contraction. If the rectum becomes overloaded, incontinence can result. Subnormal mental states are commonly associated with both constipa-

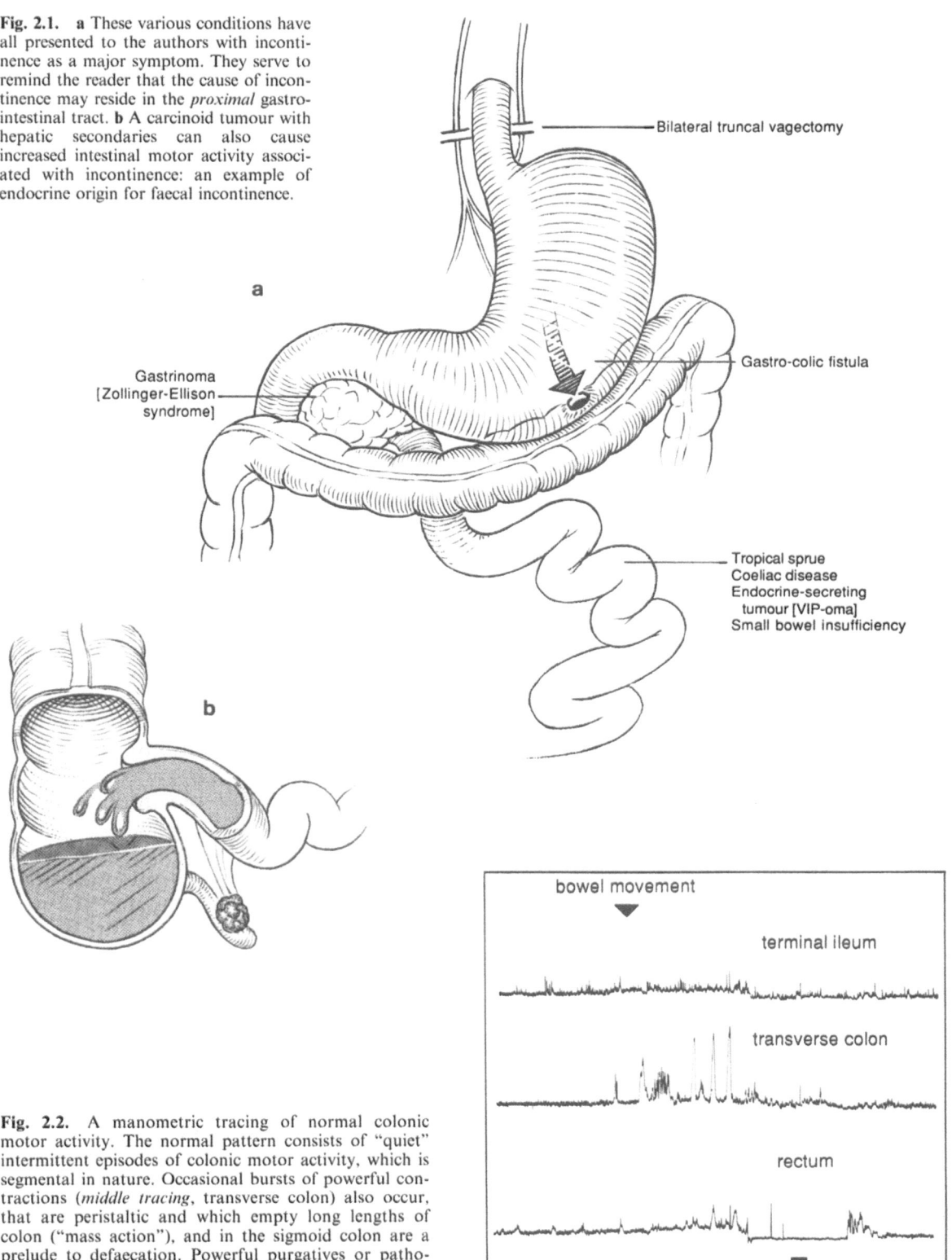

Fig. 2.1. a These various conditions have all presented to the authors with incontinence as a major symptom. They serve to remind the reader that the cause of incontinence may reside in the *proximal* gastrointestinal tract. **b** A carcinoid tumour with hepatic secondaries can also cause increased intestinal motor activity associated with incontinence: an example of endocrine origin for faecal incontinence.

Bilateral truncal vagectomy

Gastro-colic fistula

Gastrinoma [Zollinger-Ellison syndrome]

Tropical sprue
Coeliac disease
Endocrine-secreting tumour [VIP-oma]
Small bowel insufficiency

Fig. 2.2. A manometric tracing of normal colonic motor activity. The normal pattern consists of "quiet" intermittent episodes of colonic motor activity, which is segmental in nature. Occasional bursts of powerful contractions (*middle tracing*, transverse colon) also occur, that are peristaltic and which empty long lengths of colon ("mass action"), and in the sigmoid colon are a prelude to defaecation. Powerful purgatives or pathogenic bacteria precipitate incontinence by producing a combination of fluid stools and violent colonic activity.

bowel movement

terminal ileum

transverse colon

rectum

1 min

tion and incontinence which may be primarily colonic in origin.

Certain generalised medical disorders can be associated with either increased or decreased colonic activity due to the effects of endogenously produced hormones or chemicals. The thyroid gland must be remembered in patients who have diarrhoea (hyperthyroidism) or constipation (myxoedema), and other endocrine hormones can also enhance or diminish colonic motility (e.g. acromegalic constipation). High blood levels of calcium can be associated with both diarrhoea or constipation depending on the degree to which colonic muscle contractility is affected, and a low sodium level (e.g. Addison's disease) can paralyse the colon. Renal failure associated with uraemia can be associated with diarrhoea by direct action of the urate salts on the nerves and muscles of the colon wall.

It is essential to remember in the selection of patients for surgical correction of incontinence that such procedures depend for their best results on a normally functioning colon. *Unless the ano-rectal organ is presented with stools of normal shape, size and consistency, and in a properly regulated way,* incontinence may persist despite a good ano-rectal operation. If the patient has a problem of constipation as well as incontinence, this may be aggravated after surgery. If the patient is obsessed, demented or severely neurotic, the results of any surgical intervention can be catastrophic due to post-operative, centrally mediated colonic dysfunction. If the surgeon mistakenly operates in good faith on a secondary local cause for incontinence, and over-looks the primary severe hormonal or metabolic disorder underlying the patient's condition, both the patient and the surgeon's reputation can be irreparably harmed. *The ano-rectal organ, which is the material out of which a surgical procedure for incontinence is constructed, is but the end-organ of the entire gastro-intestinal tract: failure to recall this essential fact can lead to disappointment, failure and litigation.*

Ano-rectum [3,4,5,8,10]

The rectum is not normally full of faeces because the rectum responds to faecal filling by triggering the defaecatory response. However, if the defaecatory response is suppressed by cortical inhibition reinforced by voluntary contraction of the external sphincter muscle, the rectum is able to act as a reservoir for the faeces until such time as defaecation can be performed more conveniently.

Normally the rectum lies supported in the pelvis by the muscles of the pelvic floor and while it is empty the rectal walls exhibit minimal tonic activity. The neuromuscular responses of the ano-rectum are parasympathetic. When the rectum is stretched by the distending effects of faeces entering it rapidly through the recto-sigmoid junction, the rectal walls contract at the same time as the pelvic floor is raised by contraction of the levator ani muscle in response to stretch receptors in the pub-orectalis muscle. Simultaneously the pub-orectalis muscle together with the deep part of the external sphincter, after an initial contraction, relax and allow the entrance of the anal canal to open. As faeces enter the anal canal, reflex inhibition of the anal sphincters, both internal and external, takes place. As a result of the inhibition of the anal sphincter muscles, rectal wall contraction (reinforced by voluntary breath-holding and abdominal straining) promotes rapid emptying of the rectum. At the conclusion of the process, an abrupt return of sphincter tone occurs, the anal canal closes and the pelvic floor returns to its normal level.

The defaecatory response occurs through a reflex arc, the afferent stimuli of which reside probably both in the rectal wall *and the pararectal tissues* (esp. muscles): we deduce this from the fact that reflex sphincter relaxation can be triggered by stretching the pararectal tissues, *even when the rectum has been entirely removed* [7]. It is thought the stretch receptors are modified end-organs within the muscles of the pelvic floor, especially puborectalis. The spinal segments of the arc are L4–S3, and the efferent impulses are transmitted through roots S3 and S4. Puborectalis and the deep external sphincter muscle have more Type 1 muscle fibres (75%–80%) than the rest of the muscles of the pelvic floor [3,4,14,15], which makes them capable of sustained tonic contraction, and they only relax during defaecation; as has already been pointed out they can be conveniently regarded as one functional unit [13,14]. Consistent with this unity, both these muscles receive their innervation from the peritoneal surface via S3, while the rest of the external sphincter is innervated by perineal branches of the pudic nerve – the inferior haemorrhoidal nerves proper.

There is no convincing evidence that sympathetic nerves have any significant effect on the tone or activity of the anal sphincter muscles, although sympathetic fibres accompany the arterial blood supply.

The normal tone of the anal canal can support pressures of 25–85 cm water, which can be raised for a few minutes to 120 cm water (or more) by voluntary contraction of the external sphincter muscle. The normal rectum can tolerate distention by a balloon of up to 150 ml volume but at this point the anal sphincter is inhibited and expulsion should occur.

The integrity of the nerves supplying the muscles of the pelvic floor and sphincter complex can be tested electromyographically. Responses to electrical stimulation can be carried out (1) indirectly on the spinal cord at various levels; (2) by pudendal nerve stimulation; and (3) by direct resting and stimulated responses from the muscular components of the pelvic floor and sphincter muscles. The electrically stimulated responses can reveal where any abnormalities of neuromuscular function reside. By analysing recordings obtained by both single-fibre and concentric needle electrodes, good information can be obtained of the contributions being made by each of the components of the muscular complex controlling continence (puborectalis, external sphincter and internal sphincter) [4,5]. Neural deficit is shown up by delayed

transmission of impulses by the pudendal nerve ("pudendal nerve latency")

Applied Physiology

The causes of faecal incontinence are shown in Table 2.1

Although a surgeon may feel that physiological laboratory methods [12] are essential to investigate a patient with incontinence for whom surgical correction is being considered, this is not true for most cases [2]. An adequately detailed history and examination will reveal any general medical causes which contraindicate surgical intervention (for example, disease or disorder of the central nervous system; endocrine and metabolic disorder; psychosis and psychoneurosis). Simple but thorough clinical testing will eliminate diabetes, uraemia and collagen-vascular diseases such as scleroderma. An alert physician should pick up the possibility of a specific lesion of the proximal gastro-intestinal tract [for example a gastro-colic fistula (Fig. 2.1a) or an endocrine secreting tumour (Fig. 2.1b)] which can then be confirmed by the appropriate biochemical and radiological techniques. Once the clinician has narrowed the cause of the incontinence to a local defect within the pelvis, readily available out-patient observations can be employed to assist in further analysis of the nature of the problem (Table 2.1). The sensibility of the perianal skin should be tested by touch, temperature and pin-prick: these will pick up the occasional spinal lesion or cauda equina tumour which is the hidden cause of the anal sphincter weakness. Pin-prick testing and coughing can be used to observe the reflex contraction of the anal sphincter which should occur in response to such stimuli; absence of this reflex contraction, especially if it is associated with a lax sphincter, will implicate central or peripheral neuropathic origins for the incontinence [1,8,9,10].

Table 2.1 Important or common causes of faecal incontinence

A *Congenital*
  (i)   Spina bifida

  (ii) Ano-rectal anomaly 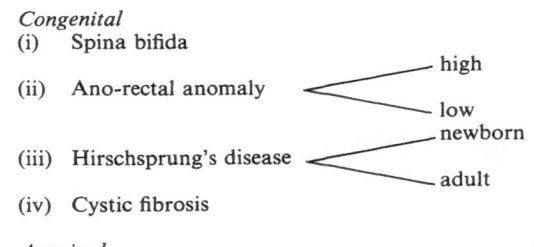 high
                                                low

  (iii) Hirschsprung's disease   newborn
                                                adult

  (iv) Cystic fibrosis

B. *Acquired*
  (1) *Colonic origin* (or higher in the G.I. tract)
       (i)   Chronic diarrhoea due to parasites, inflammatory bowel diseases or drugs
       (ii)   Gastro-colic fistula
       (iii) Malabsorption, including shortgut syndrome
       (iv)   Food allergy, including coeliac disease
       (v)   Laxative abuse
       (vi)   Endocrine tumours, including gastrinoma, VIP-oma and carcinoid
  (2) *Rectum*
       (i)   Diminished rectal sensation (diabetes, old age)
       (ii)   Diminished reservoir capacity (fibrosis; irradiation; trauma)
       (iii) Resection (low anterior resection)
       (iv)   Rectal inflammations (non-specific proctitis; Crohn's disease; tropical diseases)
       (v)   Rectal tumours (villous adenoma; carcinoma)
  (3) *Anus*
       (i)   Poor anal tone (old age; prolapse)
       (ii)   Neurological deficit (pudendal neuropathy; diabetic neuropathy; multiple sclerosis; dementia)
       (iii) Trauma (injuries; fistula surgery; obstetric trauma; anal stretch procedures)

Digital assessment of anal sphincter tone is quite accurate, and it is possible to assess the strength of voluntary anal squeeze (external anal sphincter), and the contractions of the ano-rectal junction on coughing (puborectalis and the deep part of the external sphincter). With the finger in place, the patient can be asked to strain down as if defaecating. This may elicit:

1. Enhanced contraction of the puborectalis ("paradoxical pelvic floor contraction")
2. An abnormal degree of sphincteric inhibition and gaping of the anal orifice (common with rectal prolapse or anal abuse)
3. Obvious descent of the perineal floor often accompanied by ballooning out ("perineal descent syndrome")
4. Evidence of mucosal or rectal wall prolapse

With the finger it is also possible to confirm areas of weakness of the sphincter ring, especially related to the scars of previous trauma, and to measure the length of the anal canal. The finger can also be used to assess the strength of the recto-vaginal septum and to confirm the presence of a rectocele, while in a few patients an internal rectal wall intussusception can be felt and/or the presence of loops of bowel in the low anterior peritoneal pouch that characteristically accompanies a complete rectal prolapse. Finger pressure can be used to assess rectal sensibility, and detect the loaded rectum that is commonly associated with loss of afferent sensibility. Digital examination is not complete without palpation of the anterior surfaces of the lower sacral vertebral bodies: bone deformity or distortion (e.g. from chordoma, meningocele) or an obvious deficiency (congenital, neoplastic) may draw attention to the spinal origin for the patient's symptoms. Vaginal examination provides extra access for the assessment of the pelvic floor and its associated organs, and in females pelvic floor muscular weakness commonly causes associated problems of procidentia and cystocele for patients with functional rectal problems or a prolapse.

Table 2.2 Flow chart for the assessment of suspected functional disorder of the ano-rectum

1. *COMPLETE MEDICAL HISTORY*
Detect neurological causes of incontinence e.g. *central* (due to psychiatric disturbance, senility or stroke) or *peripheral* (diabetic neuropathy, spinal tumours or multiple sclerosis)

Proceed to:

2. *THOROUGH GENERAL MEDICAL EXAMINATION WITH CAREFUL ABDOMINAL ASSESSMENT*
Detect general medical, drug-dependent, endocrine and metabolic diseases or proximal disease of the gastro-intestinal tract e.g. gastro-colic fistula, gastrinoma, coeliac disease

Proceed to:

3. *ASSESSMENT OF ANO-RECTUM AND PELVIS IN THE CLINIC BY:*

A. *Visual observation of:*
(i)   State of closure of anal orifice e.g. gaping or closed: dirty or clean: moist or dry.
(ii) Abnormalities on and around the anal orifice e.g. faeces, inflammatory skin changes, scars.
(iii) Reaction to voluntary straining e.g. anal gaping, perineal descent, rectal prolapse.
(iv) Absence of reflex anal contraction to cough and pin-prick e.g. indicating centre or peripheral nerve damage.

B. *Neurological testing of perineal and perianal skin sensation by:*
(i)   Tactile appreciation.
(ii) Temperature sensibility.
(iii) Anal sensibility and reflex contraction to pin-prick.

C. *Digital assessment of*
(i)   Length, tone and anatomical integrity of anal canal.
(ii)   Reaction of puborectalis to straining and coughing.
(iii) Sensibility of anal wall to pressure.
(iv)   Presence of faecal loading.
(v)   Evidence of intussusception or prolapse of rectal wall.
(vi)   Status of recto-vaginal septum and perineal body in women.
(vii) Integrity of sacrum and pelvic organs.

D. *Per-vaginal examination of:*
(i)   Pelvic organs.
(ii) Vaginal vault for evidence of procidentia or cystocele.
(iii) Posterior vaginal wall for rectocele.

E. *Proctoscopy for:*
(i)   Presence of anal diseases e.g. haemorrhoids, mucosal prolapse.
(ii) Presence of diseases of lower rectum, e.g. anterior mucosal prolapse, solitary ulcer syndrome.

F. *Rectoscopy for:*
(i)   Presence of rectal disease e.g. proctitis, solitary ulcer syndrome, carcinoma.
(ii) Abnormal contents e.g. faecal loading, blood, excess mucus.
(iii) Exaggerated complaints of pain e.g. neurotic personality.
(iv) Empty rectum, but loaded sigmoid colon.

Proceed to (in selected cases):

4. *COLONOSCOPY*
(i)   To assess status of whole colon in appropriate cases e.g. cathartic colon.

5. *RADIOLOGY*
(i)   Contrast studies to exclude colorectal disease e.g. cathartic colon or large villous adenoma.
(ii) Proctography to show rectal defects (e.g. rectocele) or rectal wall intusussception.
(iii) Ultrasound of ano-rectum to demonstrate defects of anal sphincters e.g. due to trauma (*"anal endosonography"*)

6. *PHYSIOLOGICAL LABORATORY TESTS* (Table 2.3)
(i)   *To eliminate those cases unsuitable for surgical help, and to confirm the exact nature of a functional deficiency not able to be assessed by simpler methods.*
(a)   Manometric tests
(b)   EMG
(c)   Rectal distention tests
(d)   Defaecography (video)
(e)   Continence provocation tests.

Clinical assessment is not complete without proctoscopy (to inspect the anal canal and lower rectum), rectoscopy (to inspect the rectum, recto-sigmoid junction and lower sigmoid colon) and possibly colonoscopy and radiology (to investigate the colon).

Proctoscopy will give additional information on the presence of prolapsing anal tissues (haemorrhoids, rectal mucosal prolapse, anterior rectal wall prolapse) and other rarer abnormalities commonly associated with abnormal pelvic floor function (e.g. "solitary ulcer syndrome").

Rectoscopy can be used to assess the rectal wall for changes associated with prolapse (proctitis, "solitary ulcer syndrome", internal intussusception) as well as to give a measure of rectal function. For example, excessive faecal loading will lead to suspicion of psychiatric disorder or disease of the central nervous system. Complaints of pain during the examination may be out of proportion and indicate an anxious or obsessive personality disorder. An empty rectum in association with symptoms of "something always pressing there" will warn the physician that he may be dealing with a patient who has subjective rather than objective problems. An empty rectum but a loaded sigmoid colon will give good grounds for suspecting that colonic inertia is contributing to the defects of ano-rectal control.

It can be seen from this account that the vast majority of cases of ano-rectal functional disorder can be adequately investigated by a combination of an alert physician using standard office procedures. However, the occasional patient presents who has a strong history that is unsupported by convincing physical signs. Some of these patients have a history of previous surgical procedures. In these cases, scientific testing in an ano-rectal physiological laboratory (Table 2.3) will provide objective data that are independent of the patient's psyche of the tone and integrity of the anal sphincter complex and its responses to stimulation. Such information may provide the surgeon with good reasons for further surgical efforts. *It may also give the strongest possible grounds for avoiding operative procedures which are likely to end in disappointment or a legal settlement.*

Provided the clinician is aware of the complex disorders that may underlie a "simple" complaint of incontinence, and

Table 2.3 Physiological laboratory tests

1. *Anal manometry*
    - this is tested by perfusion of an indwelling multiple unit of open-tipped pressure recording tubes.
    - the length and resting pressure of the anal sphincters can be demonstrated.
    - the strength of a voluntary anal "squeeze" and a maximal anal contraction can be ascertained.
    - the absence of a normal ano-rectal inhibitory response to straining can be demonstrated.
2. *Electromyography*
    - the presence and bulk of the two separate anal sphincter muscles can be ascertained.
    - the presence of a deficit (e.g. caused by trauma) can be demonstrated and its severity explored
      (= "anal sphincter mapping").
    - pudendal nerve latency can be shown in patients with nerve damage.
3. *Rectal distention tests*
    - this is tested by "distention" of a balloon placed in the rectum.
    - the volume of fluid that first elicits rectal sensation is established.
    - the maximal volume of fluid that can be tolerated is established (normal = 150 ml).
    - a neuropathic rectum demonstrates delay in recognising distention and tolerates extreme balloon distention.
4. *Defaecography*
    - demonstrates the ano-rectal angle and the process of defaecation.
    - is able to demonstrate internal procidentia and rectal wall intussusception.
    - is also able to demonstrate the extent of perineal descent (> 35 mm is abnormal) by measuring the descent of the ano-rectal junction on straining against the bi-ischiatic and pubo-coccygeal lines.
5. *Continence tests*
    - anal sphincter continence can be tested by infusion of liquid into the rectum (the first leak in normal subjects does not happen before 1–5 litres have been instilled) or by resistance to traction on a solid intrarectal sphere (a normal sphincter can resist traction forces of up to 1000 grammes).

follows the orderly progressive method of assessment outlined in Table 2.2 an accurate diagnosis can be made in almost all cases. Once the cause of the incontinence has been established, it may prove to be one that is amenable to surgical correction. Before giving patients the benefit of an operation, they should be aware of the difficulty of achieving success. Overoptimism may be the prelude to litigation if the patient is led to expect a "guaranteed" good result. Nevertheless, it is the authors' experience that cures can be achieved in many cases, and that, provided patients are correctly motivated and accurately assessed, most of them benefit from increasing use of the surgical measures described in the ensuing chapters.

References and Further Reading

1. Bartolo DCC, Read NW (1983) The role of partial denervation of the pubo-rectalis in idiopathic faecal incontinence. Br J Surg 70: 664.
2. Hallan RI, Marzouk DEMM, Waldron DJ, Womack NR, Williams NS (1989) Comparison of digital and manometric assessment of anal sphincter function. Br J Surg 76: 973
3. Henry MM (1987) Pathogenesis and management of faecal incontinence in the adult. Gastroenterol Clin North Am 16: 35–45
4. Henry MM, Swash M (1985) Coloproctology and the pelvic floor: physiology and management. Butterworths, London
5. Henry MM, Swash M (1985) Physiology of faecal continence and defaecation in coloproctology and the pelvic floor: physiology and management. Butterworths, London, Chap. 3A, pp 42–47
6. Kumar D, Wingate DL (1985) Colo-rectal motility in coloproctology and the pelvic floor: physiology and management. Butterworths, London, Chap. 3B, pp 47–59
7. Lane RHS, Parks AG (1977) Function of the anal sphincters following colo-anal anastomosis. Br J Surg 64: 596
8. Neill ME, Parks AG, Swash M (1981) Physiological studies of the anal sphincter musculature in faecal incontinence and rectal prolapse. Br J Surg 68: 531
9. Nicholls J, Glass R (1985) Coloproctology diagnosis and out-patient management. Springer-Verlag, Heidelberg and New York
10. Parks AG (1975) Anorectal incontinence. Proc R Soc Med 68: 681
11. Parks TD, Spence RAJ (1989) The colon in Scientific foundations of surgery. Ed. Kyle and Carey. Heinemann, Oxford, pp 424–426
12. Read NW, Bannister JJ (1985) Ano-rectal manometry: techniques in health and ano-rectal disease in Coloproctology and the pelvic floor: physiology and management. Ed. Henry and Swash. Butterworths, London, pp 65–87
13. Scharli AF, Kiesewetter WB (1970) Defaecation and continence: some new concepts. Dis Colon Rectum 13: 81
14. Thomas PA, Mann CV (1981) Alimentary sphincters and their disorders. Macmillan, London, p 17
15. Thompson P, quoted by Smith WC (1923) The levator ani muscle: its structure in man and its comparative relationships. Anat Rec 26: 175

CHAPTER 3

Abdominal Techniques

General Introduction

One of the commonest causes of incontinence is complete rectal prolapse. Although complete rectal prolapse is predominantly a disease of old people, it can occur in other age groups throughout adult life. In females the incidence is maximal in the fifth and subsequent decades but in males it is evenly distributed through the age range. Although in western countries approximately 80% of patients are women, the condition occurs more frequently in those who are childless. Uterine and rectal prolapse may occur together and it is not uncommon for the patient to have undergone hysterectomy before the condition presents. In eastern countries rectal prolapse is seen less rarely than in western societies in younger males – possibly as a result of the squatting position for defaecation practised by Moslems. The aetiology of complete rectal prolapse is unclear but there are a number of anatomical abnormalities which are common to all patients [18]. These are:

1. Lack of normal fixation of the rectum to its bed within the sacral curvature
2. Intussusception of the upper rectum
3. An abnormally deep anterior peritoneal recto-vaginal (or recto-vesical) pouch
4. Atrophic pelvic floor musculature with weakness of the levator ani and anal sphincter muscles

It has always been a matter for debate as to whether the weak anal sphincter and pelvic floor muscles are the cause of the rectal prolapse or the result of the rectal intussusception with secondary sphincter stretching by the prolapse. Patients with neurological defects, such as cauda equina lesions [1], develop complete rectal prolapse but in most cases there is no apparent neurological abnormality.

Constipation with the habit of straining to defaecate is a symptom found in three-quarters of the patients and this persists after surgery if it is not treated [8,10,15]. In many patients, because of the weakness of the anal sphincter muscles (which often persists even after successful replacement of the prolapse) the constipation is difficult to manage because, if laxatives are given, incontinence ensues. This is a factor that must be taken into account when choosing the rectopexy procedure to employ for the individual patient.

Approximately half of the patients with rectal prolapse will also be incontinent of faeces, or of mucus and flatus, and on testing will be shown to have reduced resting anal sphincter pressures with a poor voluntary squeeze pressure. Studies have shown that such patients have evidence of muscle denervation in both anal sphincter and levator muscles [13], changes exactly similar to those seen in patients with idiopathic faecal incontinence [20]. It may be that both conditions have a common aetiology.

Many patients, however, remain continent despite having complete rectal prolapse and have relatively normal sphincter muscles. Constipation and other functional bowel symptoms are most common and severe in this group of subjects, who frequently complain of incomplete or inadequate evacuation of stool.

After correction of the rectal prolapse the majority of incontinent patients will regain continence [10]. This may not be immediate and can take 6–8 months to occur, presumably by gradual recovery of muscle tone and nerve function. If return of anal tone does not occur spontaneously, the patient may need a late second-stage procedure for incontinence such as a post-anal sphincter repair. A small number of patients who are apparently continent before correction of the rectal prolapse become incontinent after surgery. The aetiology of this paradox is not clear but it is thought that the intussuscepting rectum acts pre-operatively as an obturator compensating for the coexistent pelvic floor and sphincter weakness. Again, recovery may occur in the post-operative period; some of these patients, however, will also require a second-stage sphincter repair. There is evidence to suggest that the Delorme procedure (see Chapter 7) may avoid this paradoxical post-operative incontinence.

Even after full anatomical correction of the rectal prolapse, many patients are disappointed to find that symptoms of constipation, lack of rectal sensation and inadequate evacuation persist. Post-operative management by aperients, dietary manipulation and evacuant suppositories may need to be continued for life [7,10,15].

With improved surgical techniques the majority of patients can have complete anatomical cure of their rectal prolapse. It is clear, however, that functional results remain a common post-operative problem; this reinforces the belief that rectal prolapse is an anatomical abnormality that is secondary to a preceding physiological abnormality in many of these patients [12,13].

In the following chapters, a number of different surgical techniques are described which can all be used to correct complete rectal prolapse in adults. Every technique has its advocates; each its disadvantages and its advantages. Each is described and its relative merits considered, with particular emphasis on the post-operative functional sequelae – especially the relation to incontinence.

Abdominal Rectopexy with Prosthetic Implant (Syn. Wells Technique) [19]

Introduction

The technique of using Ivalon (polyvinyl alcohol sponge) was developed in the 1950s by Wells of Liverpool [19] and has remained one of the standard methods for rectal fixation by the abdominal route [7,10,14]. The principle is to mobilise the rectum fully and to wrap a thin sheet of inert sponge around it to encourage adhesion-fixation of the bowel to the presacral fascia and lateral walls of the pelvis: intense inflammatory reaction occurs around the sponge and later resolves to a dense fibrosis which fixes the rectum to surrounding tissues. With time the sponge disintegrates by fragmentation and is slowly absorbed. In recent years some surgeons have advocated the use of Teflon or polypropylene (Marlex) mesh [7]. The operation is identical using either material but for simplicity the classical technique using Ivalon is described. As with all operations involving the implantation of foreign materials, sepsis is a recognised complication. Sepsis can be of serious consequence requiring the implant to be removed if the patient is to recover.

Indications and Selection of Patients

The operation is suitable for nearly all patients with rectal prolapse. Although an abdominal exploration and a general anaesthetic are required, as a consequence of modern surgical and anaesthetic techniques very few patients will be found unfit to withstand the procedure [10]. The operation may be considered inappropriate for male patients, especially the young, as the low pelvic dissection might lead to sexual impotence. As sepsis is a serious consequence for this operation, the implant procedure should never be performed in combination with other abdominal operations where the lower gastro-intestinal tract is opened. Incidental cholecystectomy or routine appendectomy must not be performed. As with operations for idiopathic faecal incontinence, operations for rectal prolapse may be contraindicated in those subjects who are habitual strainers with psychiatric problems. Severe diverticular changes of the pelvic colon, or severe degrees of colonic constipation and/or cathartic colon, may indicate the need for a left hemi-colectomy [11] or even a sub-total colectomy as part of the operative treatment in a patient with complete prolapse. In such cases, the prosthetic material must be omitted or an alternative technique (e.g. Goldberg 1975) employed [2,3].

Preparation

The majority of patients with complete rectal prolapse are elderly and require pre-operative assessment with particular attention to cardiovascular, respiratory and renal problems. Pre-operative physiotherapy should be commenced at least 1–2 days before operation and the patient encouraged to be ambulant and active in the ward. Both the use of graduated compression stockings and a prophylactic regime of low-dose subcutaneous heparin are advisable to prevent thrombo-embolic complications. Many patients will have stubborn constipation before surgery and whenever possible this needs to be corrected. Although the bowel is not opened during rectopexy it is advisable to empty the lower bowel as completely as possible before operation as this makes the operation easier and the post-operative management more straightforward. An empty bowel can be achieved in most cases by the use of Picolax sachets and a pre-operative rectal wash-out. In addition to mechanical bowel preparation it is advisable to give the patient two separate doses of systemic antibiotics to cover the operation. Cephradine 250 mg or cefuroxime 250 mg plus metronidazole 500 mg are used by the authors, of which the first doses are given i.v. at the time of surgery and the second after 12 hours. An indwelling catheter is necessary during and immediately after surgery.

The operation described is designed to correct anatomical defects present in patients with complete rectal prolapse. The operation aims to:

1. Elevate, straighten and refasten the prolapsed rectum in the pelvis
2. Prevent intussusception of the rectal wall
3. Promote adhesions between the back of the rectum and front of the sacrum
4. Tether the back of the upper and middle parts of the rectum to the front of the sacral promontory
5. Remove the excessively deep anterior peritoneal pouch

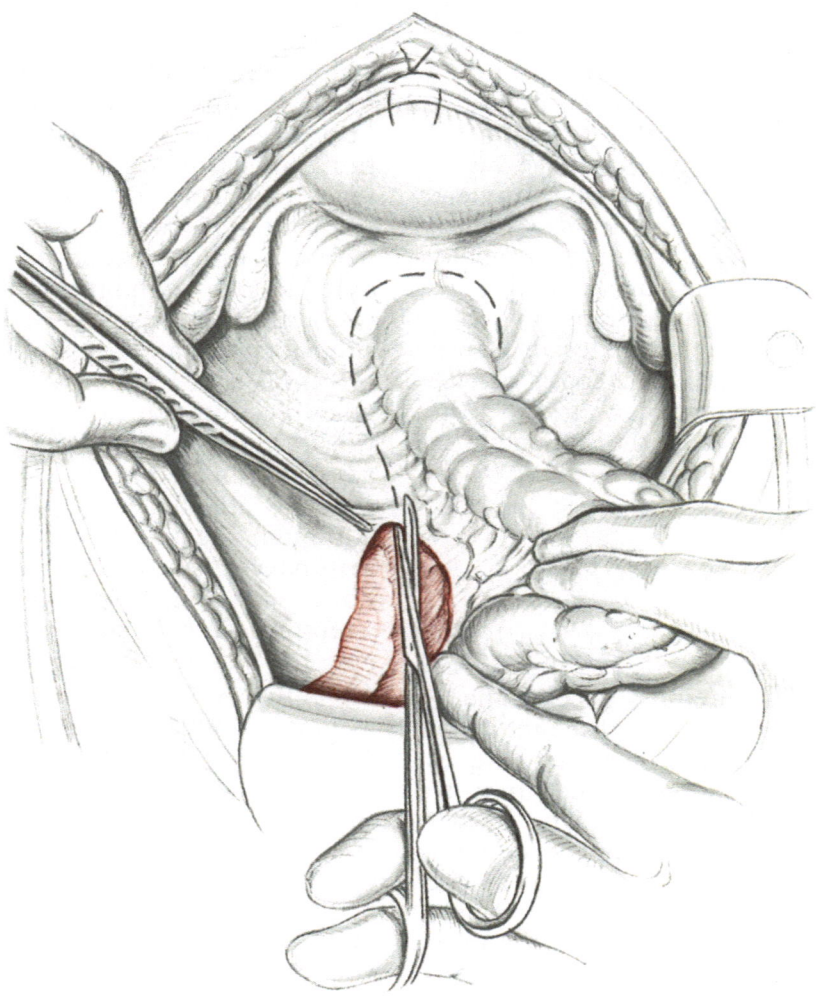

Fig. 3.1. Drawing to show the exposure necessary for the procedure. Note the "hitch stitch" to the lower rectum holding the uterus forwards. The mobilisation of the long sigmoid loop is commenced by dividing the congenital adhesions on the left side of the sigmoid mesentery, and by opening the peritoneum as shown on each side and across the base of the deep anterior peritoneal pouch.

6. Strengthen the recto-vaginal septum and obliterate the deep recto-vaginal peritoneal pouch
7. Ventrosuspend the uterus (if present)
8. Restore the peritoneal floor at the level of the pelvic brim

This operation will therefore correct nearly every pelvic and rectal defect that is present in the patient with the exception of:

1. The weak levator ani muscle with its lax puborectalis sling

2. The atonic anal sphincter muscle

Because of these continuing muscular weaknesses, some patients are not cured of their incontinence and require additional help by secondary anal procedures later.

Operative Technique

The abdomen should be opened by a lower midline or left paramedian incision. The incision should be extended well down to

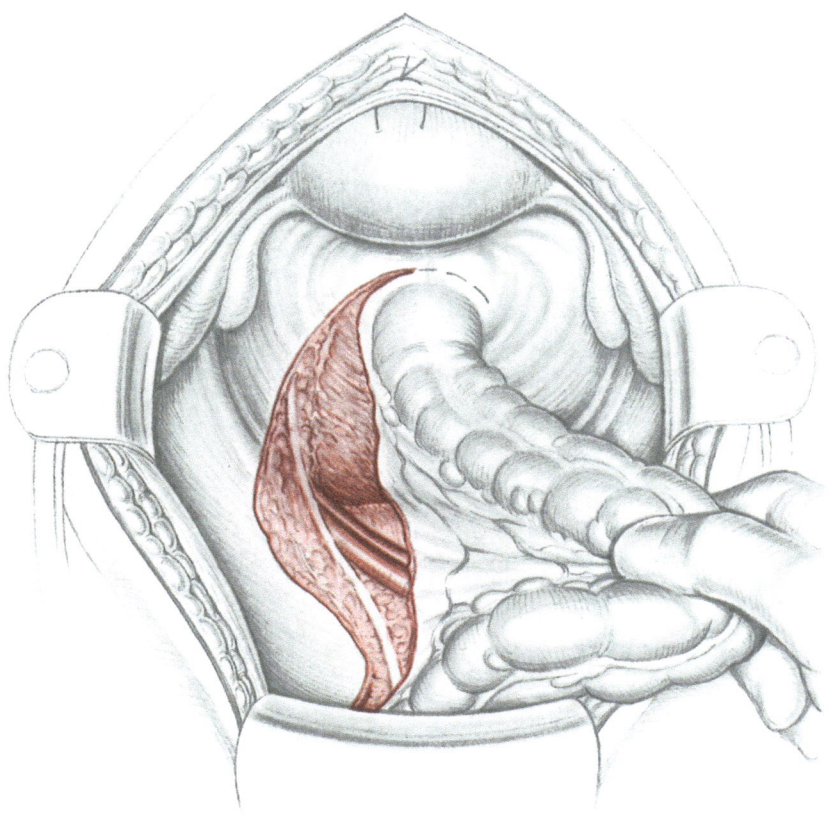

Fig. 3.2. The sigmoid colon and recto-sigmoid junction being mobilised, and the colon elevated on its mesentery.

the pubis but may not need to extend above the umbilicus. As soon as the abdominal cavity is opened the wound edges are separated with a self-retained retractor and after a full inspection the small bowel held back by abdominal packs. The patient is then placed in a moderately steep Trendelenburg tilt position. The excessively deep anterior peritoneal pouch will be clearly seen. The sigmoid colon is often suspended by an elongated excessively mobile mesentery. At this stage of the procedure it is best to hitch up the uterus to the anterior abdominal wall with a stout non-absorbable stitch, such as No. 1 nylon (Fig. 3.1). This will improve exposure as well as access to the deep pelvis and will assist in elevating the anterior rectal wall at the completion of the operation. The sigmoid colon is now held firmly towards the right side of the patient and the congenital adhesions binding it and the meso-colon to the posterior parietal peritoneum are divided with scissors (Fig. 3.1). This frees the entire sigmoid loop and allows it to be lifted up on its elongated mesocolon as far as the midline. The mobilisation of the rectum proper now begins by dividing the peritoneum at the base of the sigmoid mesentery (Fig. 3.2), just lateral to the inferior mesenteric vessels approximately at the level of the bifurcation of the abdominal aorta. The mobilisation of the rectum for complete rectal prolapse differs from that used for abdomino-perineal excision in that particular care is taken to prevent damage to the autonomic nervous system by preserving the pre-sacral nerves and their

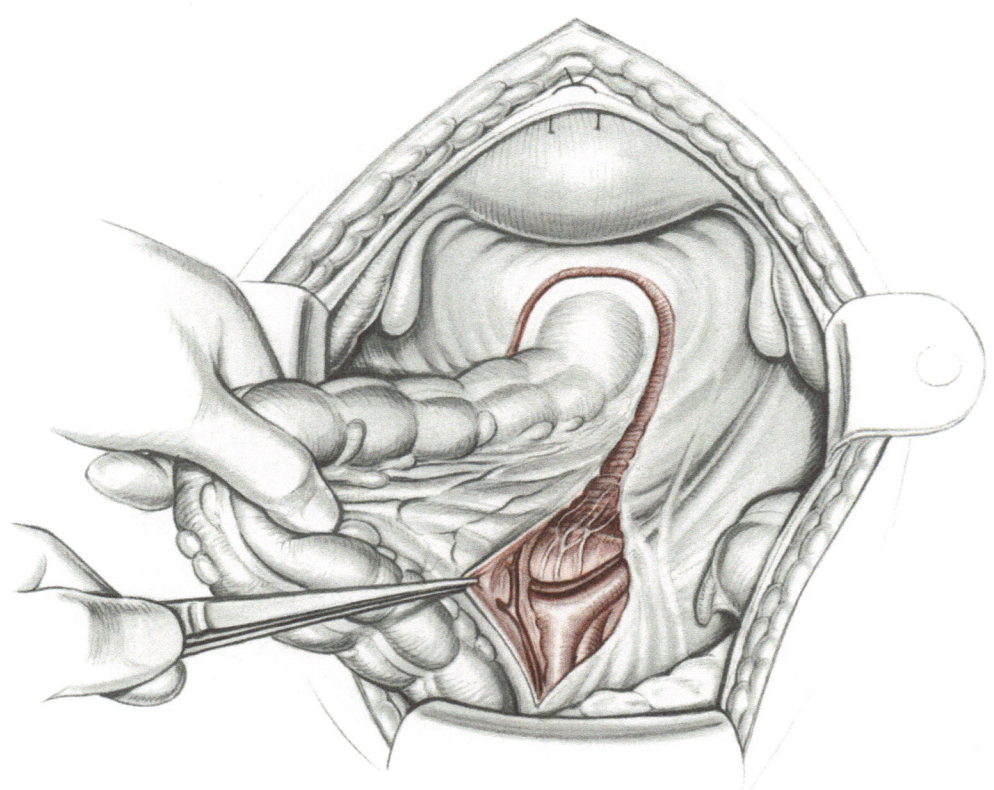

Fig. 3.3. The preservation of the pre-sacral nerves during posterior rectal mobilisation by dissecting in the plane between the inferior mesenteric artery in front and the nerves behind.

branches by dissecting anterior to the nerves at the pelvic brim and keeping close to the rectum on the back and side walls of the pelvis. The blood vessels to the rectum are also preserved. The incision of the peritoneum is carried on near to the side of the rectum and is continued adjacent to the bowel as far as the bottom of the recto-vesical or recto-uterine pouch. The incision is then taken across to the other side and joined by another similar incision descending from the opposite side of the mesocolon. The posterior dissection is developed at the sacral promontory between the inferior mesenteric vessels anteriorly and the pre-sacral nerves posteriorly (Fig. 3.3). The plane of separation is usually well marked in patients with rectal prolapse and the pelvic parasympathetic nerves must be seen and preserved. It is important at this stage of the dissection to identify both ureters so they cannot be inadvertently injured. The

post-rectal space is now entered and with mainly sharp dissection the rectum is raised (Fig. 3.4a) thus opening up the pre-sacral connective tissue sufficiently for the hand of the operator to be passed downwards behind the bowel as far as the tip of the coccyx (Fig. 3.4b). Attention is next turned to the anterior aspect. The divided edge of the peritoneum, just behind the cervix uteri in the female and just above the prostate in the male patient, is lifted forwards and, again employing sharp dissection, anterior mobilisation commences keeping close to the bowel (Fig. 3.5a). A lipped anterior Lloyd-Davies retractor held by an assistant is useful to press the cervix and upper vaginal wall forward at this stage. The dissection is continued approximately halfway down the posterior vaginal wall in females and to the level of the prostate in male patients (Fig. 3.5b). This anterior dissection taken with the completed posterior dissec-

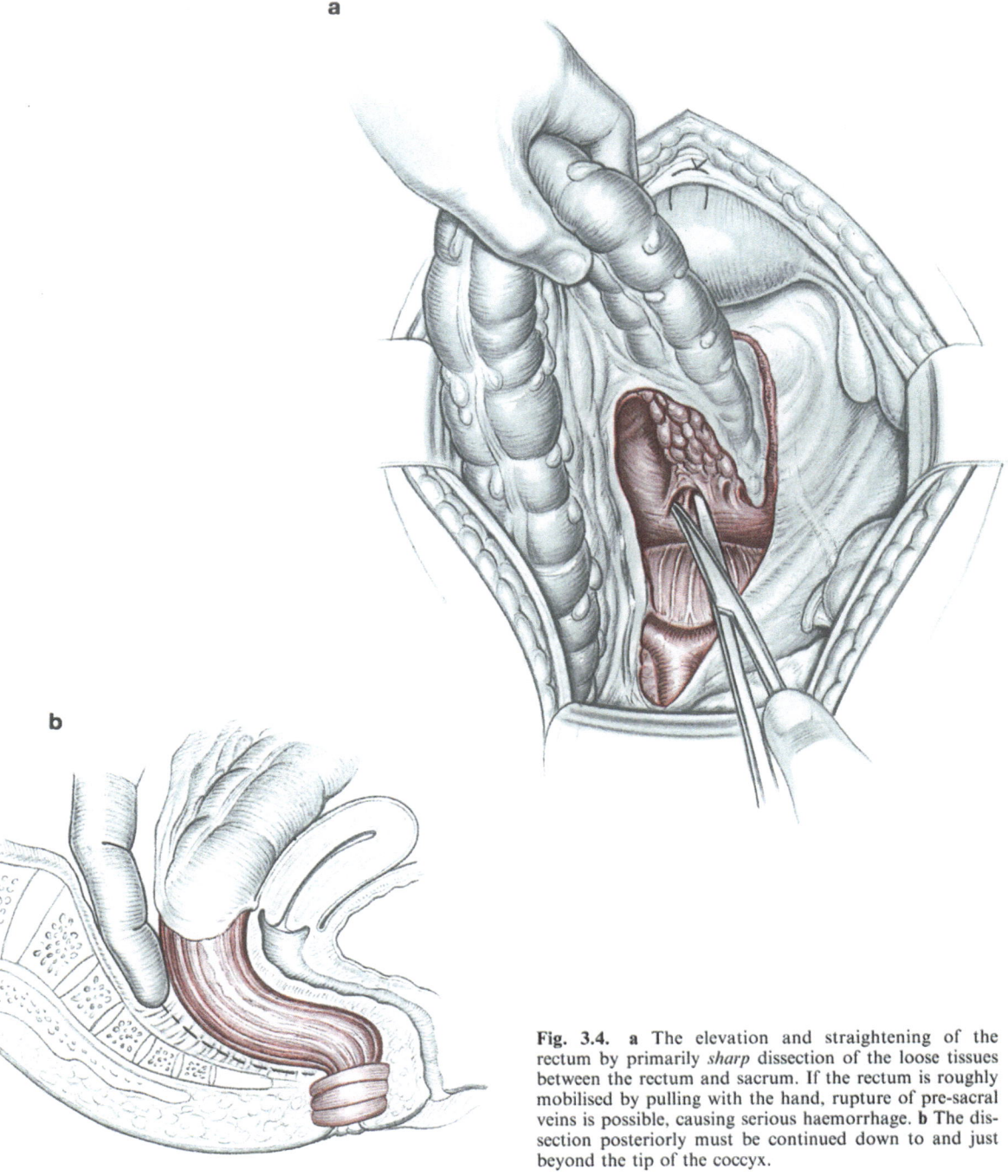

Fig. 3.4. a The elevation and straightening of the rectum by primarily *sharp* dissection of the loose tissues between the rectum and sacrum. If the rectum is roughly mobilised by pulling with the hand, rupture of pre-sacral veins is possible, causing serious haemorrhage. **b** The dissection posteriorly must be continued down to and just beyond the tip of the coccyx.

tion isolates the lateral rectal ligaments, which are often attenuated and flimsy in patients with complete rectal prolapse. Each ligament is now divided quite close to the bowel (Fig. 3.6). Blood vessels may need to be coagulated by diathermy but in the majority of cases the ligaments can be divided between clamps without requiring formal haemostasis. Mobilisation of the rectum is now complete.

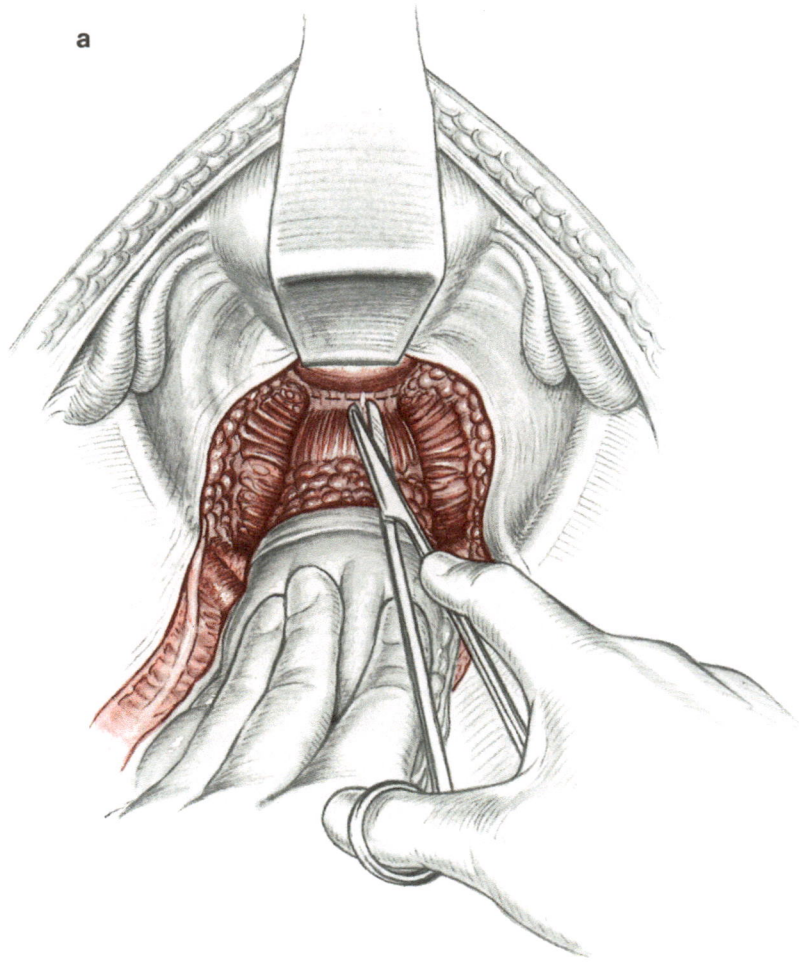

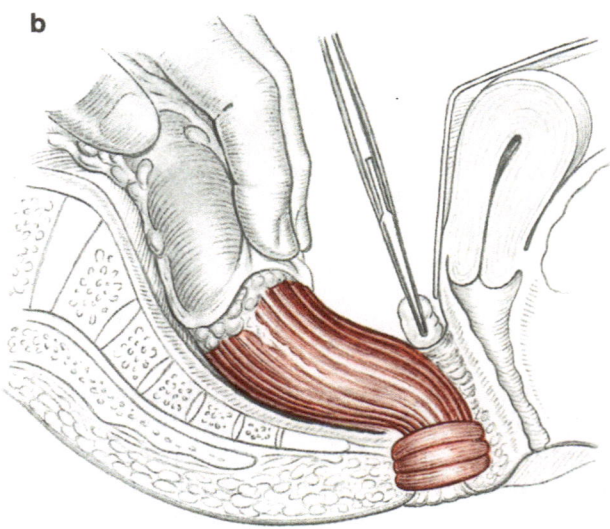

Fig. 3.5. **a** The division of the tissues anterior to the rectum and behind the cervix and posterior fornix of vagina. **b** The extent of the anterior dissection.

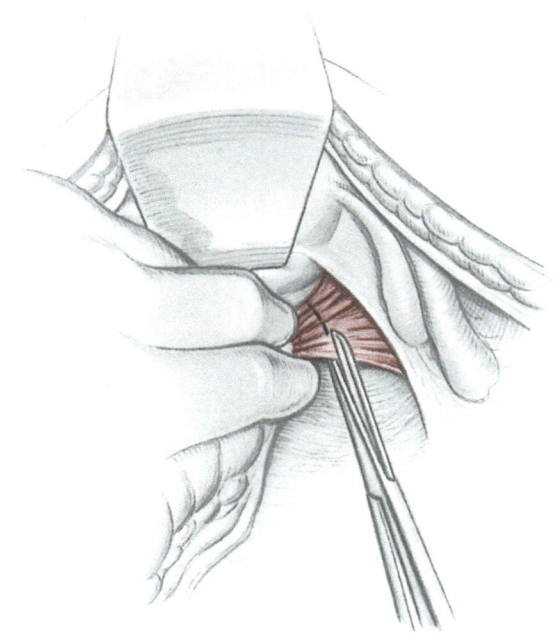

Fig. 3.6. The final manoeuvre of rectal mobilisation by isolation and division of the lateral ligaments on each side.

A hot pack may be placed in the pelvic cavity to aid haemostasis and can be left while the Ivalon sponge is being prepared. A suitable sheet of Ivalon sponge is soaked in saline, then squeezed dry and spread out while it is trimmed to fit the pelvis and the rectum of the patient. The authors prefer to attach the Ivalon sponge to the lateral and posterior aspects of the rectum rather than to formally fix the sponge to the pre-sacral tissues, as it is felt that formal fixation to the sacrum is unnecessary and at times can lead to troublesome bleeding from torn pre-sacral veins. The Ivalon is trimmed to the shape of a modified "T" with a "tongue" that sits at the apex of the posterior dissection at the level of the coccyx. The distal end of the "T" is now stitched to the front of the coccyx (Fig. 3.7). The lateral limbs of the Ivalon are fixed with 00 chromic catgut stitches to the bowel, taking care not to pierce the mucosa (Fig. 3.8). The lateral ligaments of the rectum are now fastened to the sacral promontory, above their original attach-

ment, with interrupted 00 stitches. At this stage of the procedure haemostasis should be minimal. It is permissible to leave a small suction (Redivac) drain (which must be removed after 24 hours) if oozing from the post-rectal space is excessive, but it is advisable to avoid putting in a corrugated drain because of the risk of introducing organisms.

The recto-vaginal septum (or recto-vesical septum in the male) is now repaired and buttressed with interrupted chromic catgut stitches. If the recto-vaginal space is voluminous a further small piece of Ivalon sponge may be placed anteriorly between the rectum and the posterior vaginal wall (Fig. 3.9a). It is important, however, that the rectum should not be completely encircled by Ivalon or stenosis and obstruction will develop (Fig. 3.9b). Retractors are removed and the rectum allowed to fall back into the sacral hollow, although it will remain tethered at the sacral promontory by its lateral ligaments. Finally the pelvic peritoneum is reconstituted to cover the rectum completely and most importantly to exclude the Ivalon sponge from the abdominal cavity (Fig. 3.10). (If sponge is exposed, the intra-abdominal contents, particularly small bowel, can become adherent and produce a possible dense post-operative obstruction.) The abdomen is closed in the usual fashion.

Post-operative Management

Post-operative management is important and involves the general care of an elderly patient who has undergone an abdominal procedure. Bleeding should be minimal at closure and the Redivac drain (if one has been required) must be removed at 24 hours. Oral fluids may be commenced as soon as the patient shows any sign of intestinal activity. The majority of patients, as mentioned previously, have a sluggish bowel and aperients such as magnesium sulphate mixture or Milpar (Cremaffin, Boots) in a dose of 15–20 ml three times a day, should be started as soon as the patient can toler-

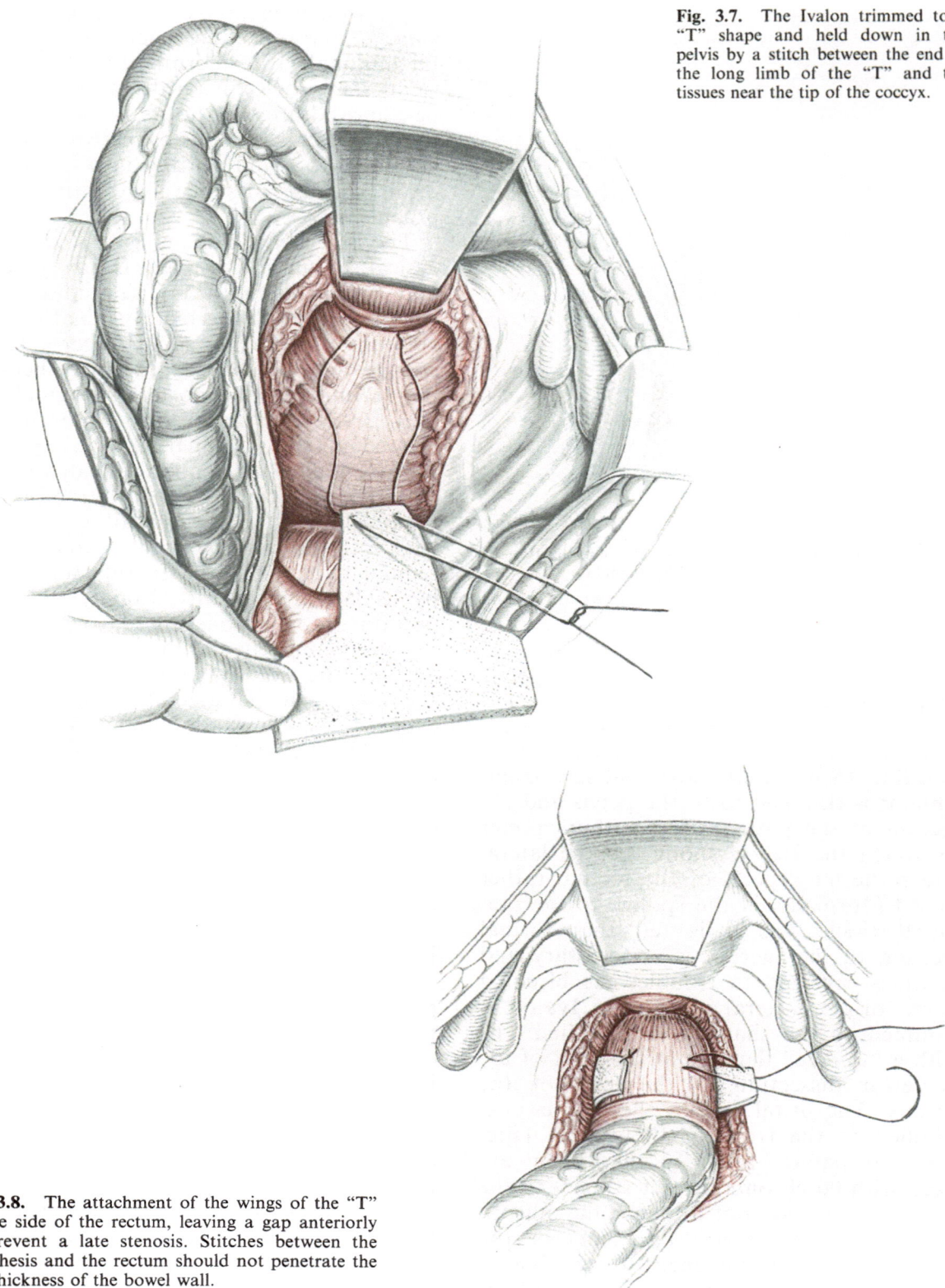

Fig. 3.7. The Ivalon trimmed to a "T" shape and held down in the pelvis by a stitch between the end of the long limb of the "T" and the tissues near the tip of the coccyx.

Fig. 3.8. The attachment of the wings of the "T" to the side of the rectum, leaving a gap anteriorly to prevent a late stenosis. Stitches between the prosthesis and the rectum should not penetrate the full thickness of the bowel wall.

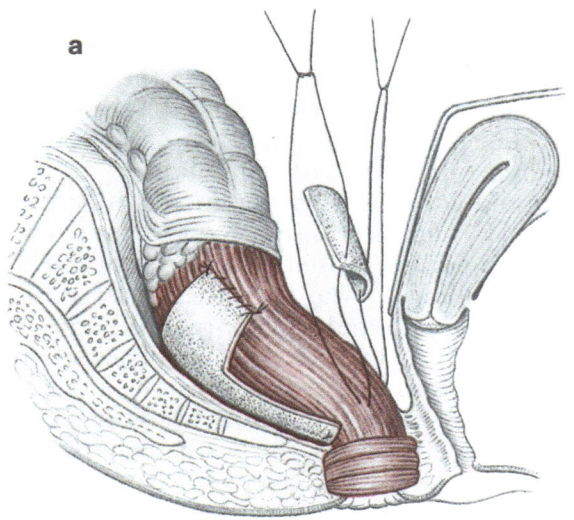

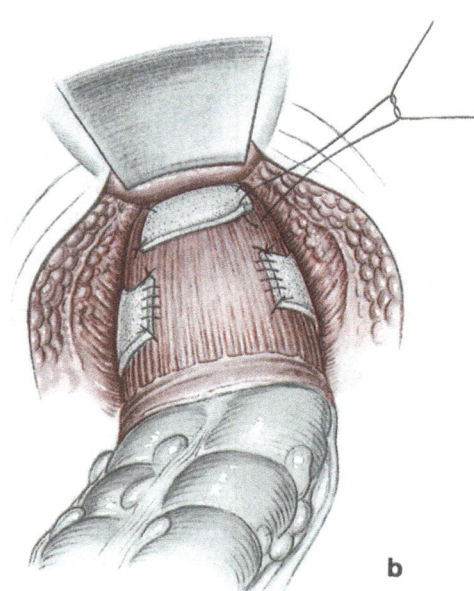

Fig. 3.9. **a** A small additional piece of prosthetic material railroaded down anteriorly to promote fibrous thickening of the upper part of the recto-vaginal septum. The stitch holds the material in the depths of the anterior dissection. **b** The gaps carefully left between the prosthetic edges to prevent strictures developing post-operatively.

Fig. 3.10. The final closure of the peritoneum across the floor of the pelvic brim. All prosthetic material is excluded from the abdominal cavity to prevent adhesions to the small bowel.

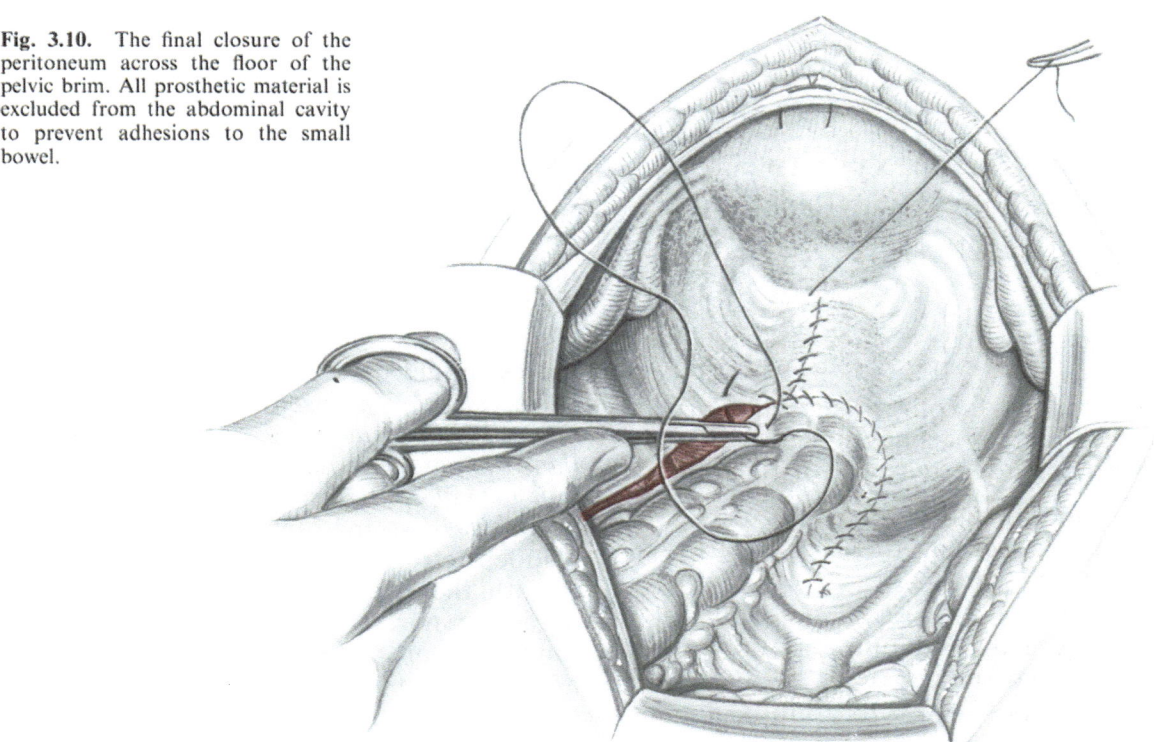

ate oral fluids. The Ivalon sponge induces a marked inflammatory reaction which can be felt easily on rectal examination. This, coupled with the long redundant sigmoid colon, can produce a partial obstruction with immediate severe post-operative constipation. This is prevented by the laxatives which can easily be reinforced by evacuant suppositories or, if persistent, by early and repeated use of disposable phosphate enemas. Careful management and control of bowel function is required if a proper bowel habit is to be restored post-operatively. Long-term aperients are often necessary and in some cases enemas or evacuant suppositories.

After correction of the prolapse it is hoped that the patient will, if previously incontinent, be restored to continence. This may not occur immediately in all cases, and the patient must be reassured and observed closely for signs of functional recovery over the post-operative months. If at 6 months the patient remains incontinent and has clinical evidence of persistent anal sphincter dysfunction with a weak pelvic floor [20], a secondary post-anal repair can be considered.

Abdominal Rectopexy with Prosthetic Sling (Syn. Ripstein Technique) [6,9,16,17]

Introduction

Many surgeons favour this as the procedure of choice for a patient with complete rectal prolapse. The reasons for this are:

1. It is quicker and involves less extensive pelvic dissection than a Wells-type operation
2. The risks of sepsis are reduced by keeping to a minimum the amount of prosthetic tissue inserted
3. It is easy to perform to a uniform standard of excellence

Experience has shown that the safety of the operation is no better than for the Wells procedure [5], except that the risk of implant-related sepsis is reduced. Obstruction at the pelvi-rectal junction as a consequence of forward angulation of the sigmoid colon is a particular post-operative hazard, and is caused by the long loop resulting from mobilisation of the sigmoid colon falling forward on the "fixed point" of the tethered pelvi-rectal junction (Fig. 3.17). To reduce the incidence of this complication, extra care must be taken to prevent the sigmoid colon becoming overloaded (with faeces) or distended (by gas) in the post-operative recovery period. Some surgeons prefer not to have a complete sling across the recto-sigmoid junction to prevent this particular hazard of angulation/obstruction (Fig. 3.17 (insert)).

Indications and Selection of Patients

These are the same as for the Wells procedure, with one exception. Because the dissection is confined to the gap between the posterior wall of the rectum and the front of the sacrum, and does not involve the lateral and anterior aspects of the pelvic cavity, the risk of damage to the pelvic autonomic nerves is very small: great care must still be exercised not to damage the autonomic nerves where they cross the pelvic brim but, providing the surgeon is careful to stay close to the posterior walls of the rectum from the moment the pelvic dissection is commenced, the autonomic nerves should be completely protected from harm. *The advantageous consequence of this reduced risk to the pelvic autonomic nerves is that it is possible to apply the Ripstein operation to male patients without risks of sexual impotence post-operatively*, or of permanent bladder detrusor weakness in either sex.

Both the Ripstein and the Wells procedures are noteworthy for their safety, and can be applied to almost every patient, however old or enfeebled. Selection is mainly one of exclusion of those patients who are absolutely unfit for any major surgical intervention, for whom a perineal operation (e.g. Delorme procedure) remains an option.

Preparation

As for the Wells procedure, abnormal bowel habits (if present) should be corrected pre-operatively. Other colo-rectal diseases must be discovered, and evaluated in relation to the rectal prolapse and its surgical cure. Severe diverticular changes of the pelvic colon may contraindicate surgical treatment limited to the prolapse, as any impedance to emptying of the pelvic colon may precipitate inflammatory complications; and as discussed previously (pp. 23–24) the pre-operative investigations may reveal such a serious loss of normal colonic motility that large bowel obstruction may occur if the recto-sigmoid junction is constrained by a prosthesis (cf. pp. 34 and 39 and Figs. 3.16, 3.17). Such contraindications to an abdominal rectopexy of the Ripstein type only account for 1%–2% of the total number of cases presenting with complete rectal prolapse.

The patient's general condition is assessed in the usual ways, and pre-operative physiotherapy to encourage respiratory function and ambulation is essential. The patient's lower intestine is emptied mechanically before surgery by a combined purgation and mechanical cleansing. The authors favour purgation by Picolax sachets–the first given on the morning of the day prior to surgery and the second 6–8 hours later: these are followed by a light rectal wash-out 2–4 hours pre-operatively. While mechanical preparation is in progress, the patient is kept on a fluids-only oral intake. The operation itself is covered by antibiotics active against aerobic and anaerobic organisms: at present the authors use cephradine (250 mg) plus metronidazole (500 mg) given i.v. at the induction of anaesthesia, followed by one further similar dose of each drug 12 hours post-operatively. It is usual for the patient to be fitted with anti-thrombotic pressure-graded stockings when sent to the operating theatre,

and for these to be kept on until the patient is fully ambulant after the operation. The use of per-operative low-dose subcutaneous heparin is advocated to prevent post-operative thrombo-embolic complications. An indwelling catheter is required during and after surgery until the patient is able to use a commode.

Operative Technique

The patient is positioned on the table in Lloyd-Davies stirrups and opened either through a lower midline or left paramedian incision. The abdomen is inspected and the intestines packed back in the usual way. The pelvic cavity is exposed and the presence of the characteristic deep peritoneal pouch in front of the rectum is confirmed.

The peritoneum is incised through short transverse incisions on each side of the recto-sigmoid junction at the level of the peritoneal reflection from the front of the brim of the pelvis opposite the lumbo-sacral promontory (Fig. 3.11). The incisions can be joined, if the surgeon chooses, across the front of the rectum. Although in some cases it is not necessary to unite the dissected area by joining the peritoneal incisions made on each side of the rectum, in most patients there are definite advantages to be gained by joining the peritoneal incisions anteriorly across the front of the rectum at the lowest point of the recto-uterine (or vesical) pouch because this allows the peritoneum to be raised off the front of the upper rectum, which in turn facilitates the subsequent placement of the prosthetic sling (Marlex, Teflon) across the front of the upper rectum. The peritoneum is replaced over the mesh at the conclusion of the technique, excluding the mesh from contact with the general abdominal cavity.

Care is taken to keep the dissection immediately posterior to the inferior mesenteric and superior rectal vessels (see p. 27) so as to preserve the autonomic nerves where they cross the brim of the pelvis (Fig. 3.12). By a gentle combination of sharp and blunt dissection, and the use of

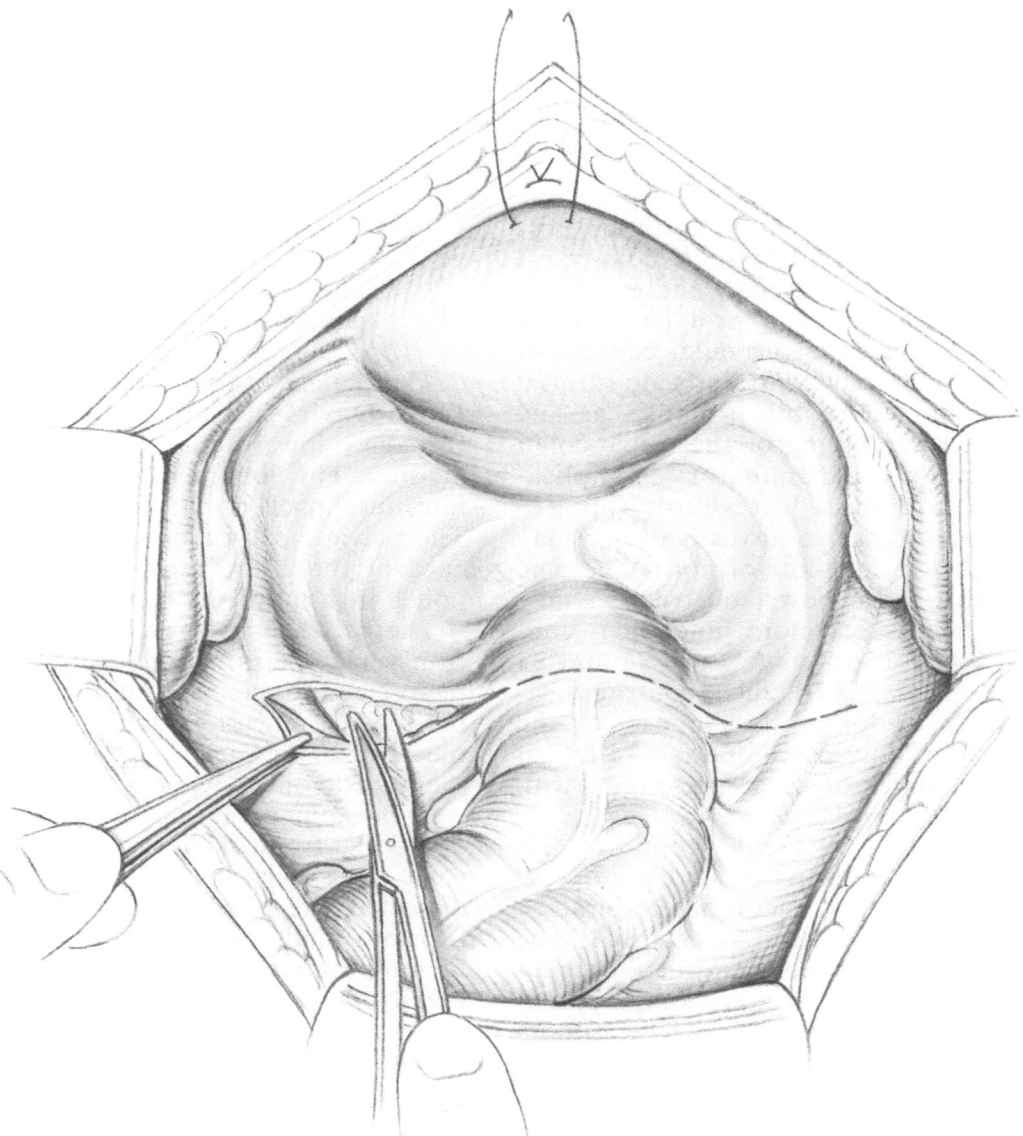

Fig. 3.11. Transverse incisions on either side of the rectum to permit dissection posterior to the rectum. These incisions can be joined across the front of the recto-sigmoid junction if the surgeon chooses.

deep pelvic retractors, the posterior aspect of the rectum is freed to a low level from the front of the sacrum. A long deep Lloyd-Davies retractor with a lip to press the rectum forward is invaluable during this mobilisation of the posterior aspect of the rectum. When the dissection has been carried down as far as the coccyx the rectum can be elevated and straightened by gentle traction (Fig. 3.13).

At this point the sacral promontory is identified and, at a point just below the common iliac vein, a loop of Marlex mesh is attached just below the maximum convexity of the sacral promontory (Fig. 3.14). The mesh encloses the rectum at the level

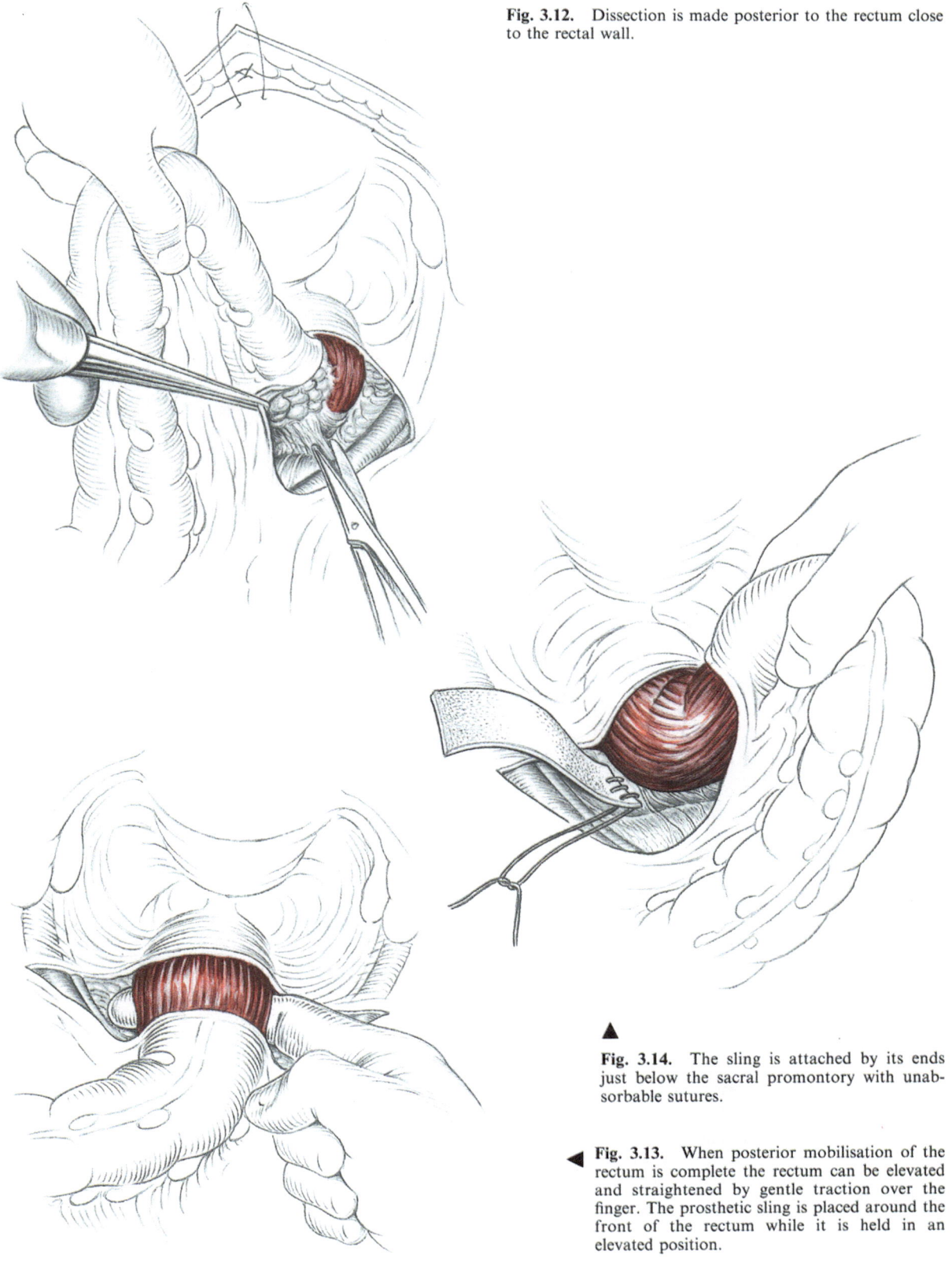

Fig. 3.12. Dissection is made posterior to the rectum close to the rectal wall.

▲

Fig. 3.14. The sling is attached by its ends just below the sacral promontory with unabsorbable sutures.

◄ **Fig. 3.13.** When posterior mobilisation of the rectum is complete the rectum can be elevated and straightened by gentle traction over the finger. The prosthetic sling is placed around the front of the rectum while it is held in an elevated position.

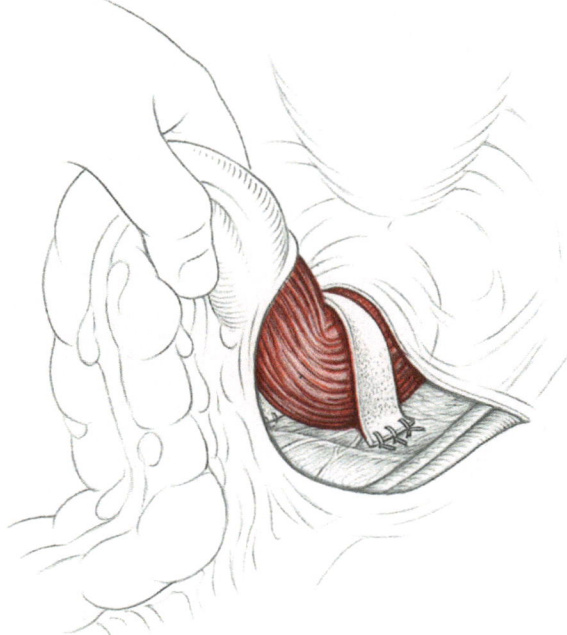

Fig. 3.15. The sling in position.

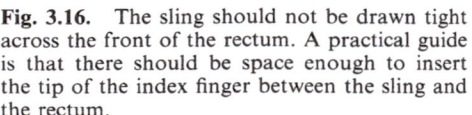

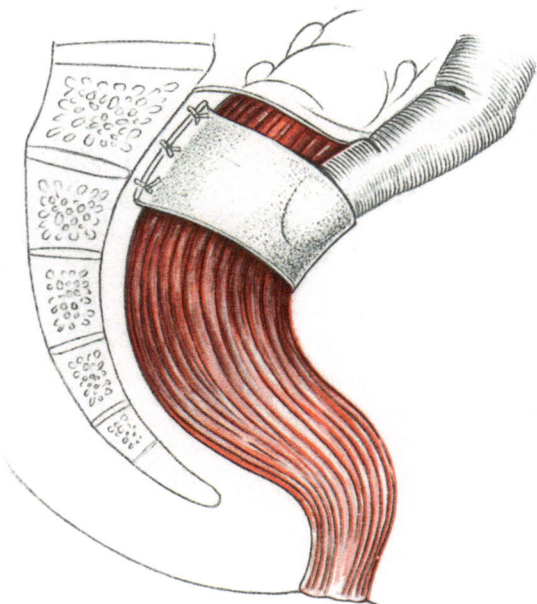

Fig. 3.16. The sling should not be drawn tight across the front of the rectum. A practical guide is that there should be space enough to insert the tip of the index finger between the sling and the rectum.

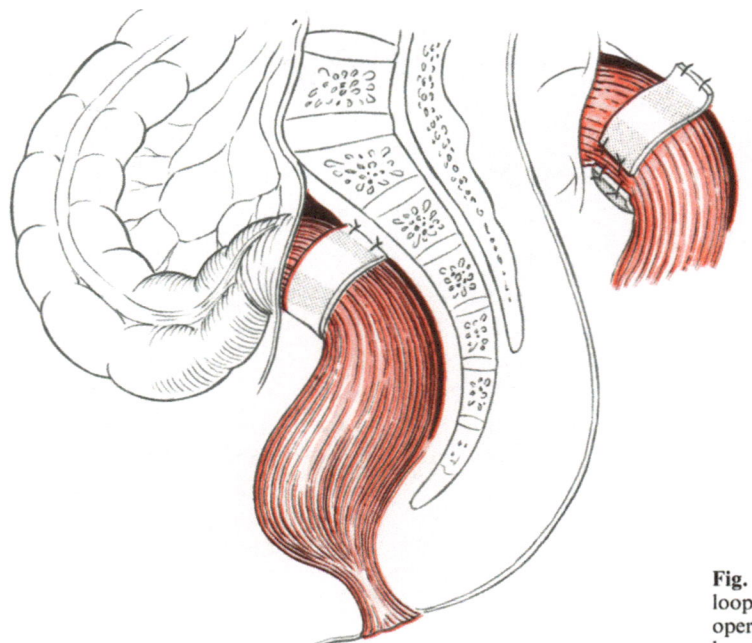

Fig. 3.17. Forward angulation of the sigmoid loop on the sling may occur. This particular postoperative hazard of the Ripstein procedure may be minimised by an "incomplete" sling (see insert).

necessary to hold the rectum in its elevated position (Fig. 3.15). The mesh should be not less than 5.0 cm in width, and should be attached to the fascia of the sacral promontory by unabsorbable sutures: the mesh loop should not be too tight, and should permit the easy insertion of the tip of the index finger between it and the rectal wall (Fig. 3.16). The edges of the loop are tacked to the side of the rectum by interrupted fine unabsorbable sutures that do not penetrate the rectal wall too deeply. At the finish of the suspension of the upper rectum by the mesh, the recto-sigmoid junction should be held without undue tension opposite the brim of the pelvis.

The peritoneal incisions are closed anteriorly and on each side of the rectum to exclude the pelvic dissection (and mesh) from the abdominal cavity in order to minimise post-operative adhesion formation. If the endo-pelvic dissection has been carried out with due care there should be no bleeding from the large pre-sacral space which was opened up during rectal mobilisation, and a drain is not needed.

The abdomen is closed by a standard conventional method, but it is wise to ensure that the loop of the pelvic colon is laid across the posterior abdominal wall in the best position to prevent forward angulation during the post-operative period (see Introduction and Fig. 3.17).

Post-operative Management

This is the same as for the Wells procedure (see pp. 20–30).

Abdominal Rectopexy plus Colon Resection (Syn. Goldberg Technique) [2,3,4]

Introduction

This type of operation is best suited to a patient with a resistant constipated bowel habit and generally should be avoided if the patient is incontinent. However, this statement needs qualification. Many patients with complete prolapse and constipation cannot tolerate the use of laxatives because they are unable to control a soft or semi-liquid stool. A few patients have poisoned the neural tissue of their large bowel and rectum by long-standing laxative abuse ("cathartic colon") and will continue to both strain and purge themselves after rectopexy, with continuing incontinence. Recurrent faecal impaction with faecal leakage and loss of control can sometimes be predicted after rectopexy, especially in elderly patients with diminished rectal sensibility and ingrained habits of straining defaecation. Therefore, while in most cases of complete rectal prolapse correction of the prolapse will cure any problems that the patient has with incontinence, in some patients this will not be enough, and in others the rectopexy can aggravate pre-existing disease, e.g. diverticulitis. It is permissible, therefore, for special reasons, to recommend that an incontinent patient with prolapse should have a colectomy and the clinician must learn to identify those patients where it is indicated: for example the patient with obstipation who is unable to tolerate laxatives, or with a history of diverticulitis. Appropriate testing (see Chap. 2) by radiological or electro-myographic techniques may be necessary in some patients before deciding to employ colectomy as part of the surgical correction for prolapse.

Indications and Selection of Patients

Some patients with prolapse and incontinence are confirmed pre-operatively to have serious pathological disease of the left colon–usually diverticular changes (with or without complications) but also neoplasms e.g. polyps or carcinomas. In such patients, the prolapse repair must be accompanied by an appropriate colectomy.

Other patients combine prolapse with pronounced functional inertia of the colon and/or rectum sufficient to precipitate problems with incontinence either spontaneously or if medications are used. Patients who are unable to tolerate laxatives to relieve straining defaecation prior to rectopexy for complete rectal prolapse should have a left-sided colectomy synchronous with the rectopexy, especially if combined constipation and incontinence are present.

It is important to stress that some patients with complete prolapse have almost total loss of anal sphincter tone. Some elderly enfeebled subjects have shortened anal canals with disappearance of anal muscle mass: others are not able to appreciate rectal distention, and have lost all normal recto-anal responses when tested in the clinic laboratory. All such patients will be unable to control frequent liquid or semi-solid stools, and should not have a resection as part of their prolapse repair.

Preparation

The pre-operative assessment and preparation of these patients is the same as for any major abdominal operation. All cardiovascular, respiratory and urological problems are treated actively and corrected as far as possible. The bowel is emptied by vigorous pre-operative treatment: this is usually accomplished by Picolax sachets — the first given 24 hours before surgery and the second 6–8 hours later. For patients with faecal retention (disclosed by either a history of severe constipation or as a result of radiological investigation) it may be necessary to give the patient laxatives (e.g. magnesium sulphate) to soften or liquify the stools prior to purgation. A high rectal wash-out 2–4 hours before surgery completes the mechanical preparation. In order to reduce faecal residues the patient should be restricted to fluids for several days prior to surgery. Antibiotics are given to cover the operation: both the aerobic and anaerobic bacteria should be treated by "combination" regimes, or by a single agent active against both types. At present the authors favour a combination of cephradine (250 mg) plus metronidazole (500 mg)

given intravenously at the time of surgery, and one further dose of each 12 hours after the operation. The previously mentioned precautions against thrombo-embolism (p. 21) should be used.

Because resection of a length of large bowel inevitably increases the risks of the operation, it is advisable to give extra time to obtain informed consent to the operation, and the patient warned that some complications (e.g. anastomotic leakage) may require a colostomy: *it is wise to obtain colostomy permission in all cases where a colectomy is planned.*

Operative Technique

The patient is positioned on the table in Lloyd-Davies stirrups with an indwelling catheter in the bladder. The abdomen is opened through a lower midline or left paramedian incision and the usual full laparotomy carried out. At this stage, the extent of the colectomy is decided. If a carcinoma or diverticular changes have indicated the need for a colectomy the extent of the resection is determined by the requirement to provide adequate treatment for the pathological process involved. For patients with colo-rectal inertia, a sigmoid resection is insufficient and the authors recommend a formal left hemi-colectomy for such patients. For patients whose main cause of incontinence is the prolapse itself, or who have problems with anal sphincter competence, a sigmoid colectomy combined with rectal fixation is all that is required [3,11].

Mobilisation of the rectum posteriorly (down to the coccyx and pelvic floor) and laterally is carried out in the usual way. The lateral ligaments of the rectum are defined and divided near to the rectal wall: the point of division is decided by the need to re-attach their shortened stumps to the top of the sacrum just below the sacral promontory (Figs. 3.18, 3.19). Once the rectum has been mobilised sufficiently to straighten it and to bring the recto-sigmoid junction opposite the

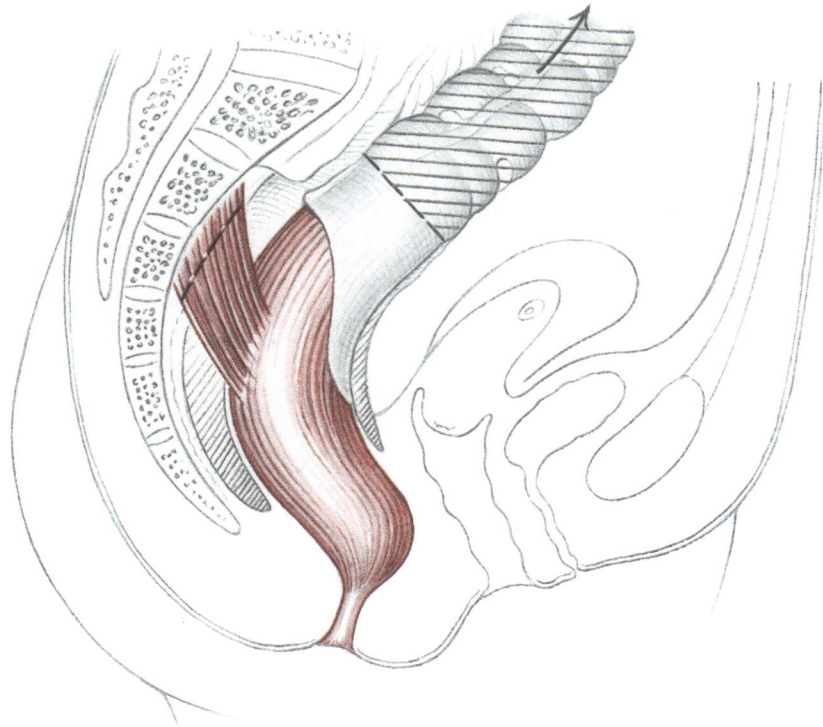

Fig. 3.18. The mandatory thorough mobilisation of the rectum down to the pelvic floor to enable the rectum to be elevated and straightened. The lateral ligaments need to be divided in most cases. The figure shows the usual point of division of the colon just below the recto-sigmoid junction.

level of the pelvic brim, the bowel resection is carried out. The anterior peritoneal coat must not be removed as the colo-rectal anastomosis will be more secure if the peritoneal coat on the anterior wall of the rectum is preserved (Fig. 3.19) and the lower point of bowel division is usually just below the recto-sigmoid junction. Once the bowel resection is completed, a direct colo-rectal anastomosis is performed either manually or by means of a stapling device. The lumen should be as widely patent as possible.

The rectum is re-attached by the stumps of the lateral ligaments to the upper sacrum, using unabsorbable stitches (00 monofilament nylon) (Fig. 3.19). *No prosthetic material is inserted.*

Providing haemostasis is meticulous, no drains are needed.

The peritoneal floor of the pelvis is reconstituted and the abdomen is closed in the usual way.

Post-operative Management

No special precautions are required, other than the routine care of a patient who has undergone a major colonic operation. Once the bowels have acted, a light diet is started, with added stool softeners to ensure that the right faecal consistency is achieved for easy evacuation: a suitable preparation is lactulose (10–15 ml twice daily).

Any tendency to retention of faeces in the rectum is prevented by regular use of two glycerine suppositories to stimulate defaecation. The catheter is removed as soon as the patient is able to drink enough to

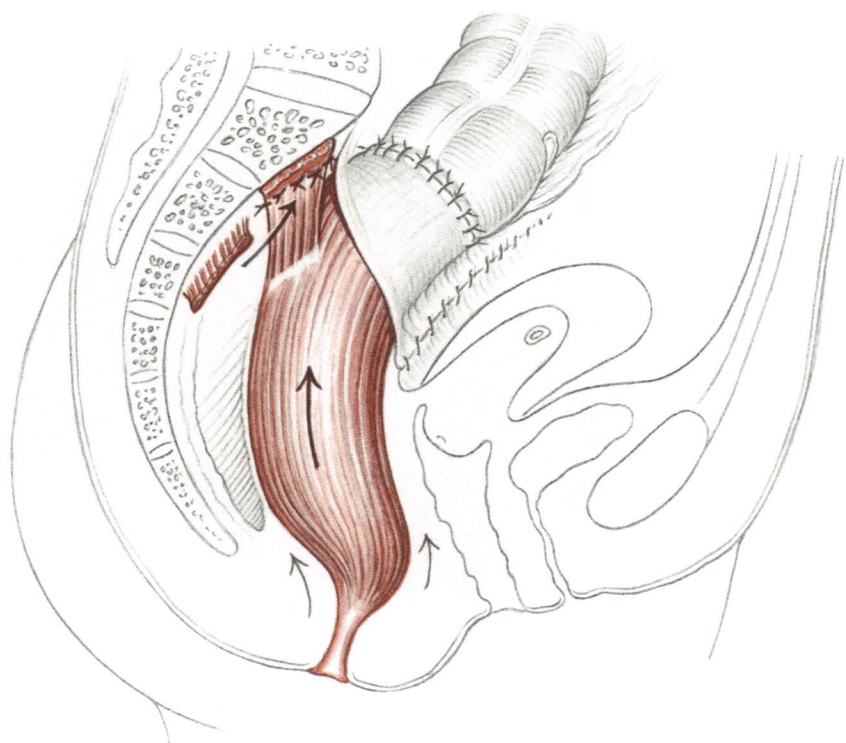

Fig. 3.19. The lateral ligaments attached to the undersurface of the sacral promontory. The anastomosis is shown completed opposite the level of the pelvic brim.

discontinue i.v. fluids. The patient is mobilised at an early stage to discourage venous thrombosis and respiratory problems, and a high roughage/high fluid intake is established before the patient leaves hospital.

Results

As far as the rectal prolapse is concerned, the results are excellent, with less than 10% recurrence rate. The constipation/incontinence problem is always alleviated providing proper selection of cases has been achieved: however, if anal sphincter weakness persists post-operatively, a second stage perineal repair (see Chapters 4, 5, 7) is indicated, and can be confidently expected to produce a good result in these cases. The Delorme procedure gives good results in such cases.

Laparoscopic Rectopexy for Rectal Prolapse

Introduction

Video-assisted colorectal surgery is one of the latest additions to the range of operations being performed laparoscopically. Laparoscopic surgery for rectal prolapse is now firmly established and offers many advantages to the patient. The technique is entirely similar to that of open abdominal rectopexy, but requires an experienced laparoscopic surgeon and up-to-date video and laparoscopic equipment of the highest standard. The recent introduction of commercially available stapling instruments for hernia repairs, and experience in intra-

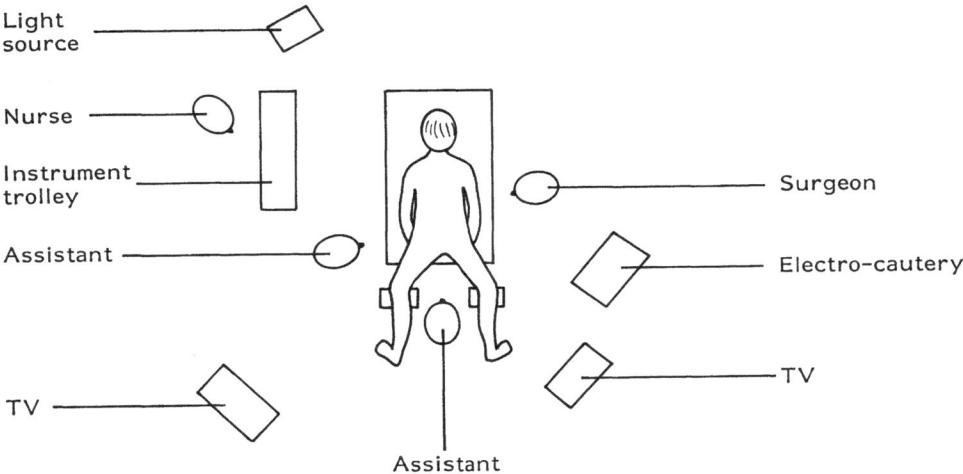

Fig. 3.20. Theatre set-up for laparoscopic rectopexy.

corporal suturing techniques, have provided the necessary techniques for laparoscopic abdominal rectopexy. Experience so far with laparoscopic rectopexy has been more than encouraging, with early mobilization and early discharge from hospital a marked feature. Control of rectal prolapse seems excellent, but as open techniques appear safe for the majority of patients and perineal techniques are available for those patients judged unsuitable for open abdominal rectopexy, the place for laparoscopic rectopexy is not established and long term results are not available yet.

Operative Technique

The pre-operative preparation of the patient for laparoscopic rectopexy is identical to that for open abdominal surgery. The patient is placed in the Lloyd Davies position (Fig. 3.20) and a catheter passed into the bladder. The Lloyd Davies position allows an assistant to stand between the patients legs, and in female patients allows access to elevate the cervix (Fig. 3.20). Pneumoperitoneum is established and a 12 mm port placed in the sub-umbilical position. A 10 mm 0° telescope is inserted through the port and initial laparoscopy

performed. Some surgeons find a 30° laparoscope advantageous for rectopexy and the pelvic dissection. Further 12 mm ports are placed as shown in Fig. 3.21, and a suprapubic 10 mm port placed under direct vision to avoid bladder injury.

The camera is now inserted into the right iliac fossa port and an endoscopic Babcock forceps passed through the left iliac fossa port to hold the rectosigmoid anteriorly and to the left. A second Babcock is passed through the suprapubic port to elevate the middle third of the rectum, which puts tension on the peritoneal reflection on the right side of the recto-sigmoid junction. The peritoneal reflection is now divided

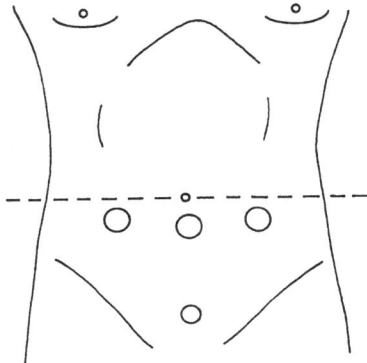

Fig. 3.21. Position of ports for camera and instruments.

using endoscopic scissors, and by careful dissection, the avascular plane between the rectum and the fascia of Waldeyer is developed. Diathermy is restricted until each ureter is identified and moved away from the plane of dissection. As the dissection is carried behind the rectum, the nervi erigentes should be identified and preserved. In female patients it may be advantageous to elevate the uterus by ventrosuspension (which can be performed as with the open technique using calipers). On occasion it may be advantageous for an assistant to elevate the cervix using cervical forceps, thus shallowing the Pouch of Douglas. Having mobilized the rectum down to the pelvic floor, and behind to the lowermost portion of the sacrum, a strip of Marlex mesh is introduced into the abdomen through the subumbilical port. After elevation of the rectum by the assistant and surgeon, the mesh is placed in the presacral space, and when the correct position is established, it is secured to the front of the sacrum with an endoscopic stapler (Fig. 3.22). Approximately three to four staples are used to fix the mesh in the midline.

After fixation, the rectum is moved first to the left and the right hand limb of the mesh secured to the serosa of the rectum

with either staples or a 2/0 vicryl suture on a curved needle using an intracorporeal suturing technique. The rectum is then moved to the right and the left hand limb secured in similar fashion. After the mesh has been secured, the peritoneal edges are approximated using the endoscopic stapler.

Post-operative Management

The post-operative management of the patient is entirely similar to that of a patient undergoing an open abdominal rectopexy. However oral fluids may be commenced the following day with aperients as prescribed for an open procedure. After laparoscopic rectopexy early mobilization is easier and the patient will be expected to be discharged as soon as the bowel habit is controlled and established. As with open abdominal rectopexy the correct management of the patient's bowel post-operatively is more important than an inappropriately early discharge from hospital.

References and Further Reading

1. Butler ECB (1954) Complete rectal prolapse following removal of tumours of the cauda equina; 2 cases. Proc R Soc Med 47: 521
2. Frykman HM, Goldberg SM (1969) The surgical treatment of rectal procidentia. Surgery 129: 1225
3. Goldberg SM, Gordon PH (1975) Treatment of rectal prolapse. Postgrad Med J 35: 97
4. Goldberg SM, Gordon PH, Nivatvongs S (1980) Essentials of ano-rectal surgery. Lippincott, Philadelphia, pp 257–259
5. Gordon PH, Hoexter B (1978) Complications of the Ripstein procedure. Dis Colon Rectum 21: 277
6. Jurgeleit HC, Corman ML, Coller JA, Veidenheimer MC (1975) Procidentia of the rectum: Teflon sling repair of rectal prolapse, Lahey Clinic experience. Dis Colon Rectum 18: 464
7. Keighley MRB, Fielding JL, Alexander-Williams J (1983) Results of abdominal rectopexy using polypropylene (Marlex) mesh in 100 consecutive patients. Br J Surg 70: 229
8. Keighley MR, Shouler PR (1984) Colonic function in patients with rectal prolapse and faecal incontinence. Br J Surg 71: 892
9. Launer DP, Fazio VW, Wheatley FL, Turnbull RB, Jagelman DG, Lavery IC (1982) The Ripstein procedure: a 16 year experience. Dis Colon Rectum 25: 41

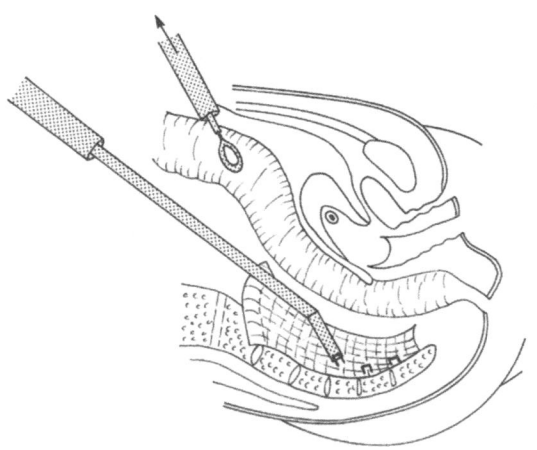

Fig. 3.22. Anterior retraction of the rectum with an endoscopic Babcock forceps allows dissection within the pre-sacral space. The Marlex mesh is secured to the fascia overlying the sacrum with and endoscopic stapling instrument.

10. Mann CV, Hoffman C (1988) Complete rectal prolapse: the anatomical and functional results of treatment by an extended abdominal rectopexy. Br J Surg 75: 34
11. Muir EG (1962) Treatment of complete rectal prolapse in the adult. Proc R Soc Med 55: 1086
12. Neil ME, Parks AG, Swash M (1981) Physiological studies of the anal sphincter musculature in faecal incontinence and rectal prolapse. Br J Surg 68: 531
13. Parks AG, Swash M, Urich H (1977) Sphincter denervation in ano-rectal incontinence and rectal prolapse. Gut 18: 656
14. Penfold JCB, Hawley PR (1972) Experiences of Ivalon-sponge implant for complete rectal prolapse. St Mark's Hospital. Br J Surg 59: 846
15. Porter N (1980) Results of Ivalon-sponge repair for rectal prolapse in surgery of the colon and rectum. Ed. Pichlmaier, Grundmann. Stuttgart, pp 45–49
16. Ripstein CB (1965) Surgical care of massive rectal prolapse. Dis Colon Rectum 8: 34
17. Ripstein CB (1972) Procidentia – definitive corrective surgery. Dis Colon Rectum 15: 334
18. Todd IP (1959) Aetiological factors in the production of complete rectal prolapse. Postgrad Med J 35: 97
19. Wells C (1959) New operation for rectal prolapse. Proc R Soc Med 52: 602
20. Womack NR, Morrison JFB, Williams NS (1986) The role of pelvic floor denervation in the aetiology of idiopathic faecal incontinence. Br J Surg 73: 404

CHAPTER 4

Anterior Perineal Techniques [2]

General Introduction

Anterior approaches to the pelvic floor and anal sphincters have been developed, but remains less well-known than posterior techniques. This is surprising when one considers that it is the anterior wall of the rectum that is exposed when the pelvic floor gives way. Rectal prolapse manifests itself by an initial *anterior* invagination and descent of the rectal wall; mucosal prolapse is most often apparent on the *anterior* aspect of the lower rectum: childbirth trauma to the recto-vaginal septum and perineal body occurs in the *anterior* quadrant; solitary rectal ulcer and the mucosal lesions of anal abuse (sexual or otherwise) preferentially occur on the *anterior* aspects of the rectal lumen. The mechanical effects of stretching, tearing and compression are found most often (and to their greatest extents) on the tissues *in front of* the rectum and anal canal, and the anal sphincter muscles are shorter and less well-defined anteriorly than they are laterally and posteriorly (especially in female subjects). Logic would seem to dictate that we should give

at least equal prominence to the development of anterior techniques for the surgical correction of ano-rectal incontinence which arises as a result of anterior rather than posterior causes. When one also considers that the nerve supply to the pelvic floor and anal muscles enters from the posterior and lateral aspects, one becomes even more surprised by the current surgical emphasis on *posterior* approaches for the perineal correction of ano-rectal incontinence, which must frequently sever or damage these important nerves.

If the surgeon can be satisfied by clinical assessment and investigation that the cause of incontinence resides in anterior weakness or distortion of the muscular framework of the pubo-rectalis and sphincter muscles, an anterior repair should always be considered. Common causes that fall into this category include:

1. A floppy recto-vaginal septum, often associated with an absent perineal body (clinical examples of this origin are

anterior mucosal prolapse; rectocele; and possibly solitary ulcer syndrome)

2. Weakening of the normal anatomical buttresses of the anterior rectal wall by stretching (childbirth) or organ removal (hysterectomy) (clinical examples of this aetiology include patients with complete rectal prolapse and solitary ulcer syndrome)

3. Trauma [clinical examples of this are episiotomy, surgical operations (especially for a high recto-vaginal fistula), wounding and forcible anal dilation]

Although surgical trauma is a common cause of damage to the anterior quadrant of the ano-rectum in western societies, particularly after treatment of fistulas or tumours of the vagina and lower ano-rectum, in areas of endemic tribal conflict or during more extensive international wars, explosions and bullets are the most frequent causes of perineal wounds of the ano-rectum.

Because of the nature of the causes of anterior weakness of the ano-rectum, many of these patients are young. A perineal approach to their incontinence problem spares such patients the problems of the prolonged hospital stay and subsequent convalescence which is associated with extensive abdominal operations. A perineal approach also avoids additional damage to the pelvic autonomic nerves.

All patients should have their bowels emptied prior to operation using the appropriate method. To achieve this the authors favour the use of Picolax Sachets or Clean-Prep, plus a subsequent disposable phosphate enema administered 4 hours before surgery. An elemental diet is advised over the operative period, with a small dose of Milpar (one or two tablespoons daily) given by mouth to prevent faecal bolus formation. Prophylactic antibiotics are advisable (see p. 25) to cover the operation and an indwelling self-retaining catheter is used for at least 48 hours. All perineal wounds heal best by preventing activity until the stitches are removed, and after those operations where wound closure is achieved "under tension", skin stitches should be left in situ for at least 10 days, and the patient confined to bed until sound healing is obtained. If primary healing of the wound edges does not take place, it may be many weeks before healing by granulation is finalised. All these wounds are likely to become infected, and infection is inevitable if a closed haematoma forms in the depths of the wound; for this reason the authors advocate routine use of a small suction catheter (Redivac) which is left in the wound for 24 hours having been introduced at surgery by a separate stab incision. Patients should not leave hospital before they can defaecate normally, and should have proper counselling on medications for bowel regulation and diet prior to discharge. A high roughage diet with a bran supplement, plenty of clear fluid, the regular use of a hydrophilic colloid such as Normacol or Fybogel, and in some cases planned resort to glycerin suppositories, are all invaluable aids (separately or in combination) for preventing constipation and straining after a weak ano-rectal organ has been successfully reinforced by surgery. In a few patients, aperients may be required to promote adequate rectal emptying, especially in the early weeks or months after the operation when the anal canal may appear a little "too narrow". *It is a rule that with time all perineal repairs by any route tend to become looser, and that a tight repair becomes adequate with time, but a loose repair will only become laxer and will be a failure from the beginning.*

The techniques described are those selected by the authors as representing the best methods currently available for the correction of the different causes of incontinence by an anterior approach. A covering defunctioning stoma (colostomy or ileostomy) is not used for any of these techniques.

Anterior Plication of Pubo-rectalis and Anal Sphincter (Syn. Anterior Buttress Technique, Anterior Levatorplasty)

Indications and Selection of Patients

This technique is very suitable for patients in whom a floppy recto-vaginal septum is causing a rectocele or anterior mucosal prolapse associated with incontinence. It is also the best approach to employ in those cases who have suffered direct anterior trauma to the anal sphincter muscles that has *not* resulted in complete division of the sphincters, which is best repaired by an overlap technique to rejoin the divided ends (p. 121). Some patients with complete rectal prolapse or solitary rectal ulcer, in whom anterior intussusception of the rectal wall appears to be a predominant factor, can be submitted to this operation before other approaches are considered. If a recto-vaginal fistula is repaired through an anterior approach within the layers of the recto-vaginal septum, the fistula repair can be reinforced by utilising some parts of the technique to turn in and bury the suture line as an additional precaution against breakdown. In those patients with rectal prolapse who are so frail or unhealthy that an abdominal rectopexy is out of the question, a perineal approach may be the only possibility for surgical correction: in some of these cases an anterior repair may be chosen, especially if there is a good indication that anterior weakness of the pelvic floor has been the precipitating cause of the prolapse e.g. after extensive gynaecological surgery. Patients with either a central neurological deficit (senile dementia, psychopathic diseases and multiple sclerosis amongst others) or a peripheral neuropathy, may not be suitable for a major abdominal operation; in these patients a perineal repair of the prolapse is indicated when incontinence is the major disability caused to the patient. In such cases an

anterior approach can be employed either on its own or in combination with a simultaneous posterior approach (="total perineal pelvic floor repair"). In many cases of idiopathic incontinence, a rectocele is present and when these patients are selected for a perineal repair it is always advisable to incorporate an anterior levatorplasty as part of the procedure; when it is remembered that post-anal repair only achieves modest success in such cases, a combined (total) approach should be preferred.

As well as the preparations for all such cases described in the general introduction to this chapter it is wise to counsel the patient for possible disappointment with the result, especially if the operation has been done as a last resort. *Patients who make pain rather than the associated incontinence the reason that has brought them to seek surgical help are probably unsuitable for any procedure as their pain is unlikely to be cured.* Patients who are clearly obsessed by anal hygiene or are otherwise demanding of a "complete cure" of their incontinence should be told firmly that they cannot have such an assurance and this should be recorded: operations for functional disorders in and around the anal canal have become a prime source of income for lawyers, who are only too happy to encourage patients who are overtly psychoneurotic concerning their ano-rectal organ and the functions of their lower intestine.

Since sepsis is the main cause whereby a technically satisfactory operation can be destroyed, every precaution should be taken to minimise bacterial contamination of the wound by:

1. Pre-operative bowel preparation
2. Perfect haemostasis
3. An indwelling suction drain
4. Per-operative antibiotic cover by cephradine and metronidazole
5. Meticulous surgical technique

The repair should be protected post-operatively against faecal disruption, and if necessary the bowels should be confined and a low (or nil) residue diet given until sound healing has taken place. An indwelling catheter facilitates keeping the patient inactive post-operatively while the wound heals. It is best to carry out these operations in those hospitals where medical and nursing attendants are familiar with this type of surgery, and to insist on frequent and accurate bed-side assessment of healing and bowel function after the operation. The drain should be removed after 24 hours.

Provided proper selection and counselling of the operated patients has been carried out, good results will follow in direct proportion to the skill and experience of the surgeon.

Operative Technique

The patient is positioned in the lithotomy position and a catheter is put in. The anus is closed with a circumferential 00 chromic catgut stitch. The vagina and the interior of the ano-rectum are cleaned with a mild antiseptic solution (aqueous chlorhexidine 1:200) before draping. If there is more than minimal faecal contamination in the rectum, an immediate on-table rectal lavage, also with 1/200 aqueous chlorhexidine, should be carried out. Skin preparation of the perineum is again with aqueous chlorhexidine solution. Drapes are positioned to give good exposure of the perineum between the tip of the coccyx behind, the ischial tuberosities laterally and the pubic arch anteriorly. Perfect lighting is essential and a head-lamp an advantage. The perineal tissues of the recto-vaginal septum (with special emphasis on the submucosal plane of the vaginal epithelium) are infiltrated with up to 100 ml of a 1:300 000 solution of ephedrine (adrenalin) in normal saline: the infiltration should extend laterally for several centimetres, and should be carried upwards into the retroperitoneal tissues behind the cervix. The anaesthetist must be informed while the infiltration is in progress (Fig. 4.1).

Two incisions can be employed depending on the local assessment: if a large recto-

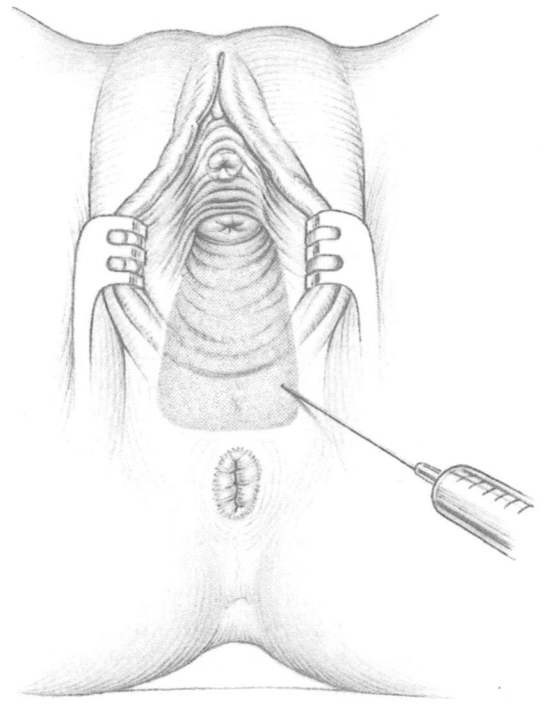

Fig. 4.1. The extent of the infiltration with 1:300 000 ephedrine (adrenaline) in physiological saline. In order to achieve the proper degree of haemostasis, the infiltration should be generous, and given time to work.

cele is present, some of the redundant vaginal epithelium may need trimming: in such cases a vertical incision through the posterior vaginal wall is ideal (Fig. 4.2a). In patients who only need the puborectalis apposed across the front of the rectum, or who need the anal sphincter muscle tightened or repaired, a transverse incision midway between the anus and the vaginal orifice is sufficient (Fig. 4.2b). This will allow separation of the intact posterior wall of the vagina and the front of the anorectum without exposure of the subsequent repair to the possibility of infection through a vaginal defect. The incision should be at least 10 cm in length and can be increased by curving the lateral ends of the cut forwards alongside the vagina, as shown in Fig. 4.2b. Once the correct plane has been entered between the vaginal wall in front and the rectum behind, cautious use of blunt and sharp dissection will allow the

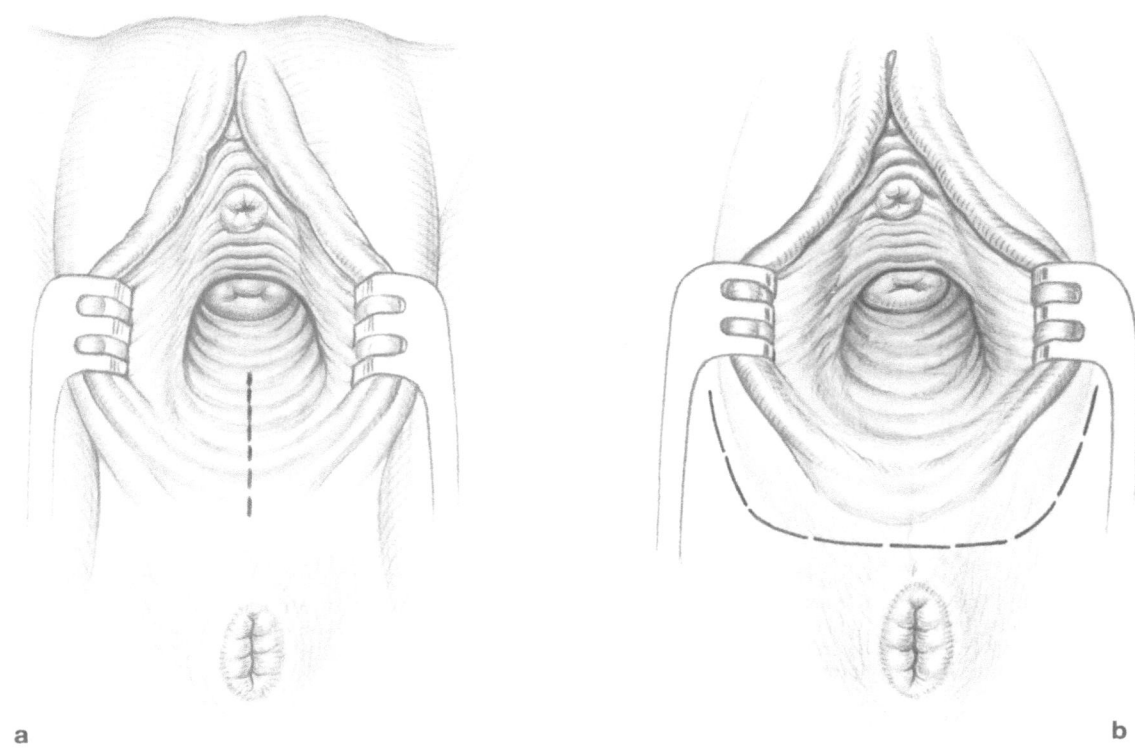

a

b

Fig. 4.2. **a** A vertical incision through the posterior vaginal wall is ideal if redundant vaginal epithelium needs trimming back. **b** The standard approach, which is sufficient for most cases.

tissues to be separated: if the correct plane has been opened up, bleeding should not be profuse. If bleeding is severe, the plane is almost certainly too anterior and the vaginal venous plexus is being encountered.

Separation of the tissues is continued upwards behind the level of the posterior fornix, at which point there is sudden easy entry into the loose extraperitoneal tissues. Blunt sweeping motions with a mounted swab will now allow good retraction of the tissues in the depths of the wound and permit adequate exposure for purposes of the repair.

After insertion of thumb and index finger laterally in the retroperitoneal tissues, the anterior limbs of puborectalis can be identified on each side as they pass forwards to the pubic bone (Fig. 4.3). A large (0) monofilament Vicryl or Prolene (polypropylene) stitch can now be passed through each limb as far forward as poss-

ible, and then securely tied; this brings together the limbs of puborectalis and ischio-coccygeus muscles under tension across the front of the rectum at mid-rectal level. The apposition of the puborectalis muscle is continued vertically downwards by a series of Vicryl sutures, which then brings the operator onto the anterior surface of the deep portion of the external anal sphincter (Fig. 4.4) which can also be narrowed down by similar stitches (see later). A second layer of stitches can be inserted over the first in many cases, which augments the strength of the repair.

Once the decision is made to tighten the external anal sphincter as well as the puborectalis muscle, it is easy to continue the plication process across the front of the external sphincter down to the anal verge. If the anal sphincter has been divided, a formal sphincter repair (see Chap. 8) should be carried out before any final deci-

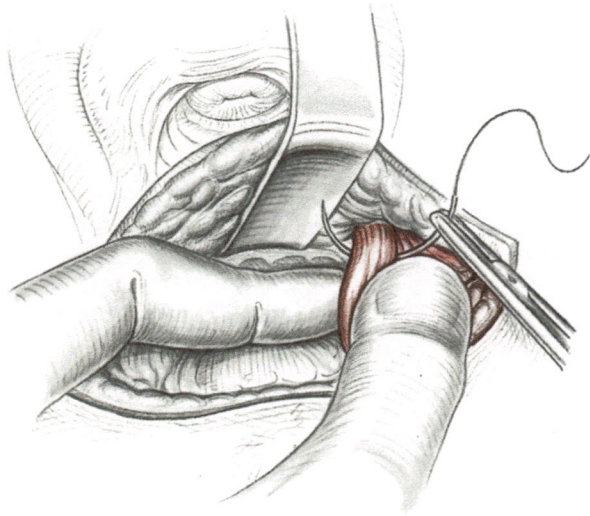

Fig. 4.3. The commencement of the anterior muscle "buttress" by placement of stout stitches of unabsorbable material far forwards into the anterior limbs of the puborectalis muscle.

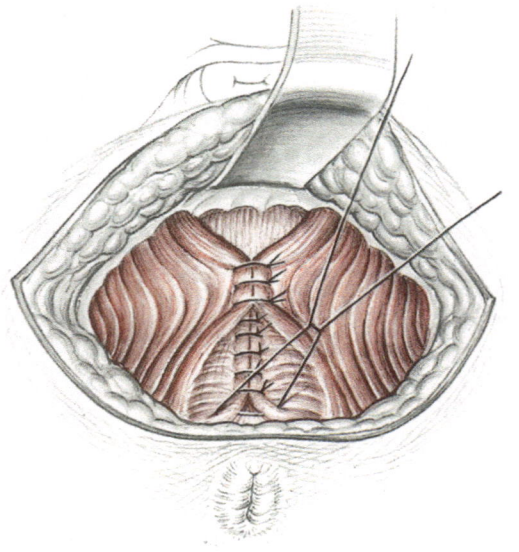

Fig. 4.5. Continuation of the repair of the muscles by plication of the external sphincter ring.

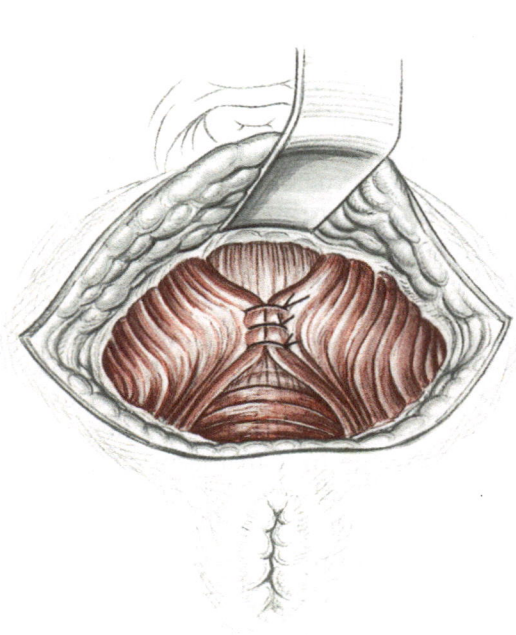

Fig. 4.4. The drawing together of the puborectalis muscle leads the operator "seriatim" as the closure proceeds downwards onto the anterior surface of the external sphincter muscle.

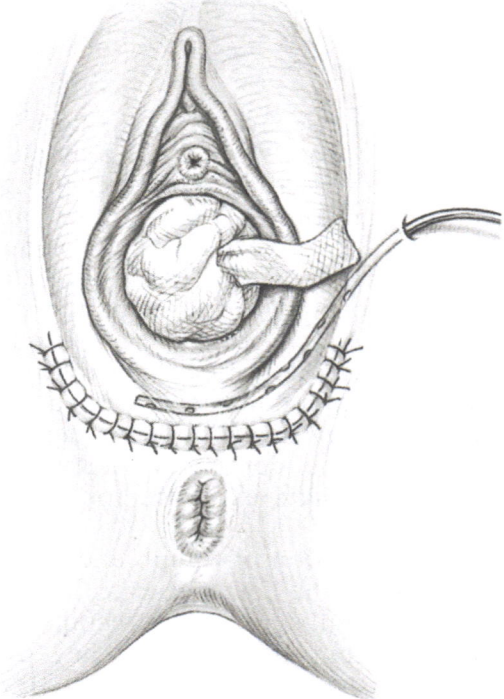

Fig. 4.6. The importance of prevention of a wound collection by combined suction drainage and per-vaginal packing.

sion is made about plicating the external sphincter. The lower stitches in the external sphincter which are close to the anal verge should be of absorbable materials in case superficial infection occurs at skin level. The final position at completion of the muscle repair is shown in Fig. 4.5.

Immaculate haemostasis is essential before the wound edges are closed. If a vertical vaginal incision has been used, redundant vaginal epithelium should be trimmed back. A Redivac suction drain should be placed through a separate lateral perineal stab wound. Vaginal wounds should be closed by a continuous fine (000) Dexon suture. The perineal wound should be closed by fine (000) sutures or clips. A vaginal tampon of gauze soaked in Proflavine Gel is useful to exert light pressure on the posterior vaginal wall during the early postoperative period, but should be removed after 48 hours: this tampon is an extra precaution against a post-operative wound collection (Fig. 4.6), which is not always prevented by the suction drain alone.

This description has focussed on the female: however, the anterior approach is also feasible in males and can be used in both sexes to reinforce suture lines after repair of recto-urethral or recto-prostatic fistulas.

It is important to remember to remove the anal closure stitch before the patient leaves the operating table.

Post-operative Management

The indwelling catheter should remain for at least 5 days and preferably in many instances until the wound has healed by the 7th or 8th post-operative day. Antibiotic cover should be continued by a second i.v. injection of cephradine and metronidazole at 12 hours post-operatively: at this point, the surgeon decides whether the risks of infection justify continuing the antibiotic cover. A low residue or elemental diet ensures that faeces do not accumulate in the rectum, and Milpar (25 ml b.d.) can be given to liquefy any faeces that form. The

extremes of diarrhoea or constipation should be avoided by suitable adjustment of medication, as either can be destructive to the operation (diarrhoea by promoting infection, and constipation by causing suture line disruption). Providing precautions are taken against venous thrombosis by graduated compression stockings and physiotherapy, recumbency in bed ensures that these vulnerable perineal wounds are given the best chance to heal. In patients who are judged at special risk of thrombosis/embolism complications, subcutaneous heparin should be used.

Anterior Sling Procedure (Syn. Notaras Technique) [6]

Indications and Selection of Patients

Rectal prolapse is the commonest indication for this operation. Many surgeons report repairs of complete rectal prolapse incorporating anterior strengthening of the pelvic floor structures, especially the puborectalis muscle. The original descriptions of operations devised by Moschcowitz (1912) [5], Roscoe Graham (1942) [1,3] and Hughes (1980) [4] laid emphasis on the importance of elevation and buttressing of the pelvic floor in front of the rectum as an essential safeguard against recurrence of prolapse.

Many surgeons find anterior repair of the limbs of puborectalis and lower fibres of the pubococcygeus muscles by an abdominal approach difficult to achieve, or at least more difficult than a posterior repair: and in elderly patients it is essential to remember that a speedy and effective technique should always be preferred especially if a general anaesthetic can be avoided or shortened. Also complete mobilisation of the rectum can only be obtained if the rectum is first elevated by thorough posterior dissection down to the pelvic floor. Once a posterior dissection has been carried out, most surgeons find that posterior rectopexies become the obvious and simplest methods by which to obtain fixation.

However, if the only aim of the surgeon is to buttress the anterior wall of the rectum and to provide support to the gap in the pelvic floor in front of the rectum, it is possible to achieve this from below. A perineal approach has much to recommend it for its simplicity and safety. Although many cases are suitable for a direct repair of the puborectalis muscle by the procedure already described (pp. 49–53), in some patients even this may be considered as too risky for their parlous general state of health. For these cases an anterior supralevator buttress operation can be used. The Thiersch operation (pp. 79–82) has been long favoured as the last resort operation for the surgical treatment of patients with rectal prolapse who are unsuitable for techniques that are better devised but more severe. Unfortunately the Thiersch procedure is usually unsuccessful. Notaras (1973) [6] developed a technique that incorporates the advantages of a minor procedure through the perineal route with specific anterior support of the pelvic floor. The technique can be used to treat unfit cases of complete rectal prolapse in whom anal sphincter weakness is a major feature. In cases of mucus leakage associated with weakness of the recto-vaginal septum and/or overt anterior rectal wall descent (mucosal or complete) the procedure may be used in preference to other larger operations. In patients where there is doubt whether a complete prolapse is present, or whether "interior" anterior rectal wall intussusception is the only feature that can be discovered in a patient with incontinence, the Notaras approach is a useful technique to employ as a first choice because it offers a good chance of improvement with minimal demands on the patient's constitution: the risks are low, convalescence is brief, and if it does not succeed the patient can be expected to be forgiving. Finally, the operation does not make a subsequent abdominal rectopexy more difficult if a

further operation becomes necessary. The authors present a modified version of Notaras' original description (in which the sling lay below the levator muscle).

Preparation

The patient's poor general condition is usually the prime indication for using the technique, and will need to be treated vigorously before the operation. The anaesthetist should have the opportunity for pre-admission consultation when a general anaesthetic, however light and short it may be, will carry obvious risks. Nerve-blocking techniques by intrathecal, epidural, caudal or local infiltration routes (used singly or in combination) may be preferred to a general anaesthetic for patients with dangerous cardio-respiratory conditions.

The operation can be ruined by postoperative faecal impaction or by infection. For this reason, the patient's rectum should

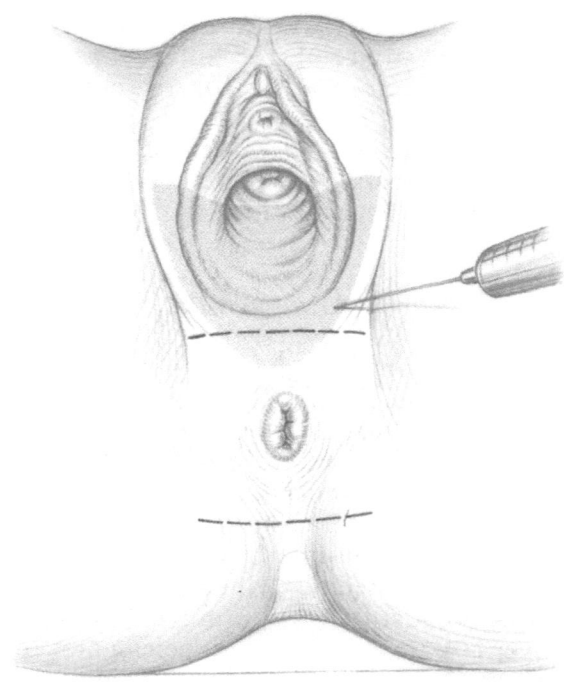

Fig. 4.7. The infiltrated area prior to making the surgical incisions, as shown.

be emptied pre-operatively by an effective stimulant (bisacodyl or phosphate enema) given the night before surgery, subsequently reinforced by a rectal washout 2 hours before the operation. The operation should be protected against infection by per-operative antibiotic cover, usually a single intravenous dose of Augmentin (1.2 g) or a combination of cephradine (80 mg) with metronidazole (500 mg). The bladder should be emptied before the operation by a catheter, which should be retained for 24 hours post-operatively. A preliminary digital examination should confirm that the rectum is empty, and, if not, an "on-table" rectal wash-out using 1/200 aqueous chlorhexidine should be administered.

Operative Technique

The technique used by the authors has been modified slightly from Notaras' original description. The authors advocate a litho-tomy, rather than a prone, position for the operation. The prone position exerts con-siderable pressure on the lower abdomen which can distort the anatomy of the pelvis in an undesirable way around the base of the pelvic floor, and it does not make access for this procedure any easier: it can also aggravate anaesthetic difficulties. The vagina should be thoroughly cleaned with Povidone iodine solution, and the legs and perineum draped in the usual way. The anus is closed by a temporary 00 chromic

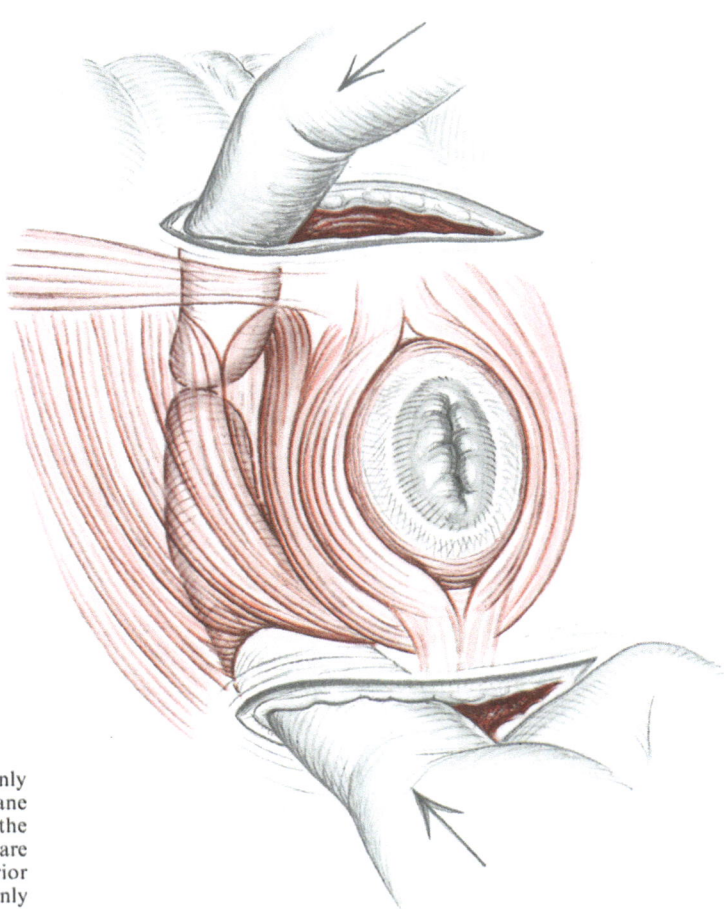

Fig. 4.8. The dissection is carried out mainly by finger pressure which develops the plane close to and on the superior surface of the levator ani muscle. The supra-levator tunnels are completed when the anterior and posterior finger-tips meet on each side of the rectum (only one side shown in figure).

catgut purse-string suture before starting the skin incision.

The recto-vaginal septum is infiltrated with a weak (1:300 000) solution of ephedrine (adrenaline) in physiological saline (Fig. 4.7). In these poor-risk patients the anaesthetist must be extra alert during the infiltration.

After the infiltration has become effective, two transverse incisions 4–5 cm long are made in front of and behind the anus. The *posterior incision* is deepened by blunt and sharp dissection through the tissue behind the anus and rectum and in front of the coccyx until the midline gap between the posterior attachments of the levator muscles is reached and can be entered. Waldeyer's fascia can be incised with the point of a pair of scissors and the index

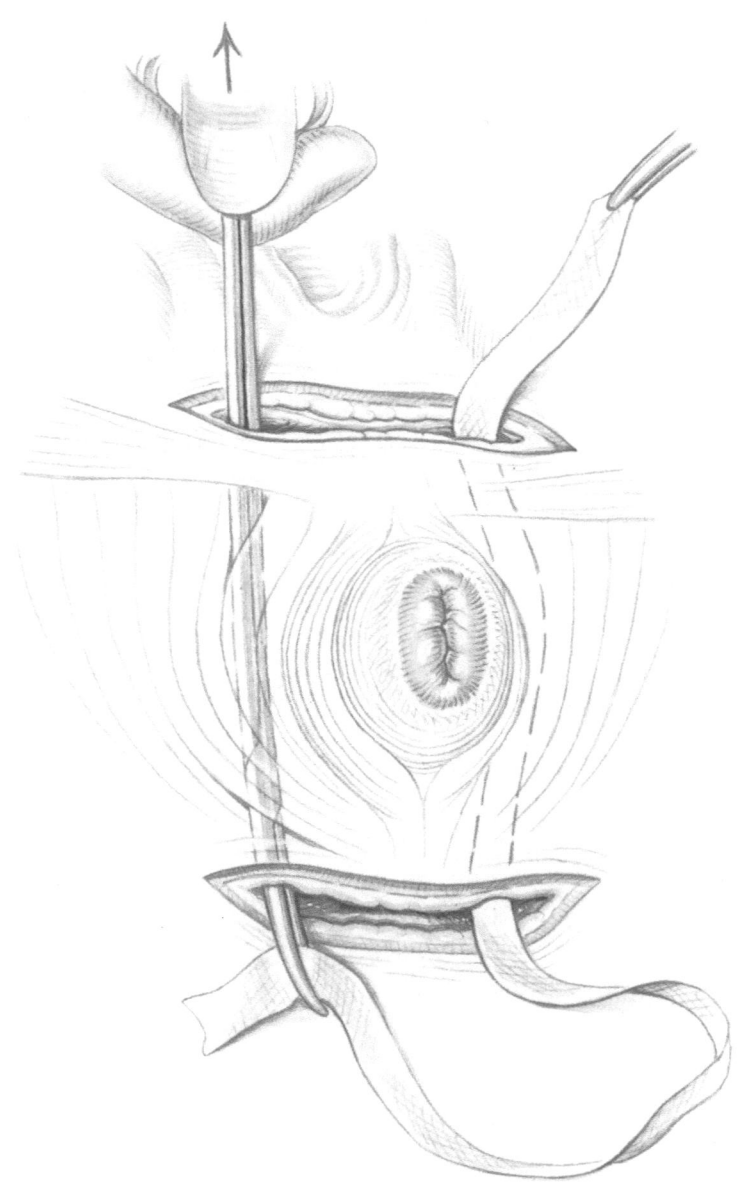

Fig. 4.9. A long, curved instrument (see text) is substituted for the fingers to thread a loop of Teflon ribbon through the supra-levator tunnels on each side of the lower rectum, and drawn snugly against the back of the ano-rectum. Once joined anteriorly and tightened the Teflon loop acts as a sling to support the ano-rectal junction.

finger can be used to free the posterior wall of the rectum upwards from the last two sacral vertebrae. Next the index finger can also be used to develop a plane passing forward on each side of the rectum on the superior surface of the levator ani muscle: during this part of the technique, the finger should be kept as close as possible to the upper surface of the levator ani muscle so that the ureters are not damaged or subsequently entangled by the Teflon sling which is to be used later. Sometimes the tunnels can be formed more easily by breaking through the pelvic muscular floor on each side alongside the puborectalis muscle. *The anterior dissection* is deepened within the layers of the recto-vaginal septum, keeping well away from the anterior walls of the anus and rectum behind: it is safest to keep close to the vagina because inadvertant opening of the vaginal epithelium does not preclude proceeding with the operation: once the level of the upper vagina and posterior fornix are reached, the tissues can be stripped back very easily by finger-tip pressure of the opposed index finger (Fig. 4.8).

At this point, working with the index finger of each hand, the planes on each side of the rectum can be joined up anteriorly and posteriorly (Fig. 4.8) and a suitable long curved instrument passed through anterior-posteriorly: a Moynihan cholecystectomy clamp, a curved Doyens forcep or a Lloyd-Davies artery clamp are used appropriately by the authors for this manoeuvre as indicated by the individual situation (Fig. 4.9).

A Teflon ribbon 2–3 cm wide (other materials such as Marlex or soft Silastic tubing are also suitable) is grasped with the forceps by each end on either side, the ends are drawn forward into the anterior wound and the sling which is thus created around the lowest part of the rectum just above the pelvic floor is drawn firmly against the resistance of the ano-rectal angle (Fig. 4.9).

The two ends of the prosthesis are overlapped and stapled or stitched together with several unabsorbable (00) interrupted sutures across the front of the rectum and the extraneous ends of the ribbon cut away. At this point extra stitches can be conveniently put in to give more strength to the join of the overlapped ends (Fig. 4.10).

Finally, after haemostasis has been secured, and topical antiseptic (povidone iodine) or antibiotic (Tribactrim) spray used to impregnate the surfaces of each wound, wound closure is begun. The deeper tissues can sometimes be drawn together with fine catgut stitches, and the skin is closed with clips or fine (000) sutures (Fig. 4.11). No drains are required. The circumferential anal suture is removed and light dressings are applied.

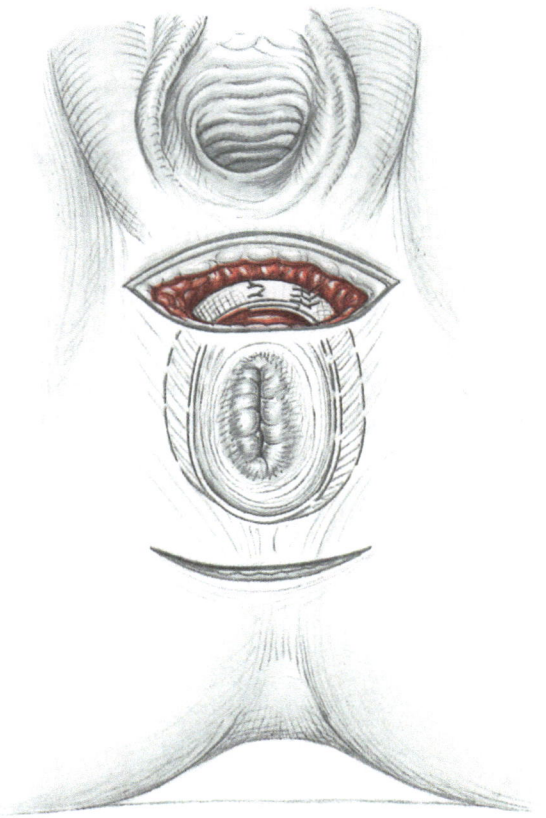

Fig. 4.10. The tightened sling firmly held by "double-overlap" stitching.

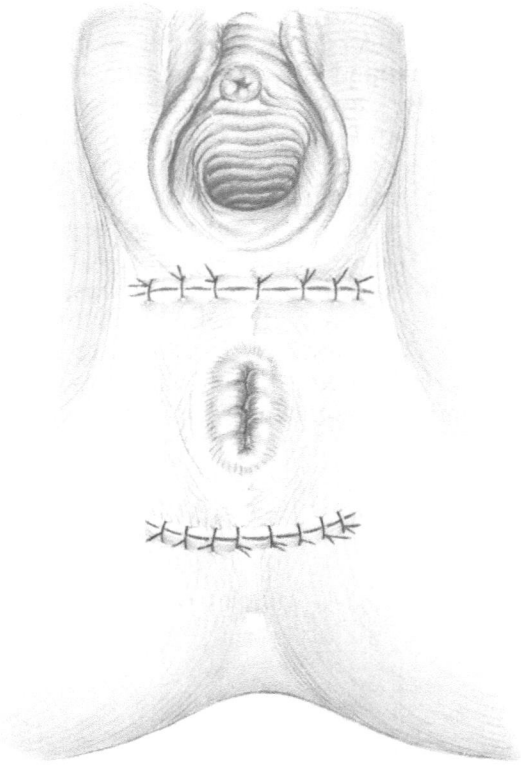

Fig. 4.11. The wounds are closed without drainage.

Post-operative Management

The patient is mobilised the day after operation and the catheter is removed. The bowels are kept open with suitable laxatives and once the patient is ambulant and the bowels controlled he can be discharged home, usually within 3–4 days. The skin stitches can be removed between the 7th and 10th post-operative days.

Results

The long-term results of this operation are not yet known. Unlike the Thiersch operation, cutting out of the circumrectal prosthesis has been uncommon although sepsis does occur. For very unfit patients with incontinence due to a small or "interior-only intussusception" type of complete rectal prolapse in whom long-term control is desirable, the authors prefer it to the simpler (but often useless) Thiersch operation. It is a good alternative to an abdominal rectopexy when anterior wall intussusception or a solitary ulcer syndrome are encountered and the surgeon wishes to avoid a risky abdominal procedure.

References and Further Reading

1. Goligher JC (1957) The treatment of complete prolapse of the rectum by the Roscoe Graham operation. Br J Surg 45: 323
2. Goligher JC (1984) Prolapse of the rectum. In: Surgery of the anus, rectum and colon. Ballière Tindall, London, pp 261–263
3. Graham RR (1942) The operative repair of massive rectal prolapse. Ann Surg 115: 1007
4. Hughes ESR, Johnson WR (1980) Abdomino-perineal levator ani repair for rectal prolapse: technique. Aust NZ J Surg 50: 117
5. Moschcowitz AV (1912) The pathogenesis, anatomy and cure of prolapse of the rectum. Surg Gyn Obstet 15: 17
6. Notaras MJ (1973) The use of mersilene mesh in rectal prolapse repair. Proc R Soc Med 66: 684

CHAPTER 5

Posterior Perineal Techniques

General Introduction

Although the *anterior* rectal wall, recto-vaginal septum and perineal body are prime areas of local weakness of the ano-rectal organ associated with incontinence and prolapse, *posterior* perineal procedures have always been popular when surgical correction has been attempted. From the earliest descriptions of Lange (1887) [8], Tuttle (1903) [13] and Lockhart-Mummery (1910) [9] up to the present day, many surgeons have employed the posterior approach as the method of choice for a perineal fixation of the rectum. One such repair [the post-anal (Parks) operation] [10] demands a high level of familiarity with the sphincteric anatomy. However, most surgeons are familiar with the dissection via the perineum of the tissues in the plane between the lower rectum and the front of the coccyx and sacrum as a part of their training for the abdomino-perineal (Miles) operation for cancers of the lower third of the rectum; this route can also be adapted for fixation of rectal prolapse and repair of the external anal sphincter, as in the Wyatt technique (pp. 70–77).

The post-anal repair (Parks), which is carried out through the intersphincteric plane, is a swift and largely bloodless operation. However, it is painful and can be destroyed if the wound becomes infected. The posterior perineal repair (Wyatt) [14] involves a more formidable dissection in which there are often time-consuming delays caused by the presence of large amounts of fatty tissues and from brisk bleeding by the inferior rectal arteries (and their branches) on each side: however, septic complications of the wound are more likely to settle without destroying the repair. Both types of operation require meticulous attention to prevention of infection. This is achieved by emptying completely the distal bowel pre-operatively by mechanical means and the use of per-operative antibiotic cover.

Because the speed and safety of these perineal operations are usually the determining factors when they are chosen for particular patients, at present most experienced colorectal specialists carry out more intersphincteric than truly post-rectal operations. However, for surgeons outside specialist centres the latter approach may prove more popular, as they will be more at home with the anatomy, and there are fewer risks of injury to the rectum by straying from the correct plane of dissection.

At present, the results of these alternative approaches have not been compared by a prospective trial with convincing follow-up observations. It can be stated with conviction, however, that the surgeon should not expect more than two-thirds of his incontinent patients to be substantially improved, and only 50% at best to be cured [1,7,10,15]. It is also the authors' experience that strict patient selection and meticulous technique are vital to achieving even such modest success. As with all operations there is a learning curve to be passed, and disappointing initial results should not discourage persistence with these procedures when they are indicated on good grounds of safety and a desire to give the patient at least a reasonable chance of a normal social life. In some of these cases, a permanent colostomy may be the sole practical alternative if the problems of incontinence are severe, and the patients are unfit for major surgery.

Post-anal Intersphincteric Repair (Syn. Parks Technique [1,2,10,15]. Posterior Levatorplasty)

Introduction

The operation of "post-anal repair" was developed by the late Sir Alan Parks [10] in an attempt to help patients with *idiopathic faecal incontinence* [5]. The aetiology of the condition is unclear but electro-physiological tests have suggested that it is the result of denervation of the pelvic floor and external anal sphincter muscles. Most patients are female and it is possible that the denervation is caused by traction neuropathy of the nerves supplying the pelvic floor and may be either the result of excessive straining to defaecate, or a consequence of difficult childbirth, especially in those patients who undergo prolonged labour with forceps delivery [11,12].

As a result the muscles of the pelvic floor degenerate and are stretched. Muscle degeneration is found to the least extent cranially in the ileococcygeus muscle and increases progressively in a caudal direction to affect the external anal sphincter most of all. This muscle is usually so severely affected that rarely can any worthwhile active contraction be obtained. There is, however, nearly always some residual function in the pubo-rectalis and pubococcygeus muscles.

The operation of post-anal repair makes full use of this muscle sparing, and by bringing together the opposite limbs of the ileococcygeus, pubococcygeus and puborectalis muscles, shortens their muscle fibres and improves the efficiency of the atonic muscle. In addition, approximation of these muscles reconstitutes the ano-rectal angle which, in turn, restores the flap valve mechanism at the ano-rectal junction [3].

In normal subjects, resting anal canal pressure is mainly due to maintained tonic contraction of the internal sphincter. Resting pressure in patients with idiopathic faecal incontinence is usually low as a result of repeated stretching of the internal sphincter during abnormal pelvic floor descent. Repair of the pelvic floor and external sphincter muscles does to some extent protect the internal sphincter from further damage and promotes some recovery of function.

At present neuropathic damage to muscle cannot be reversed; all that can be achieved is to make the muscle mass act more efficiently and correct anatomical abnormalities [1]. The anatomical changes seen in

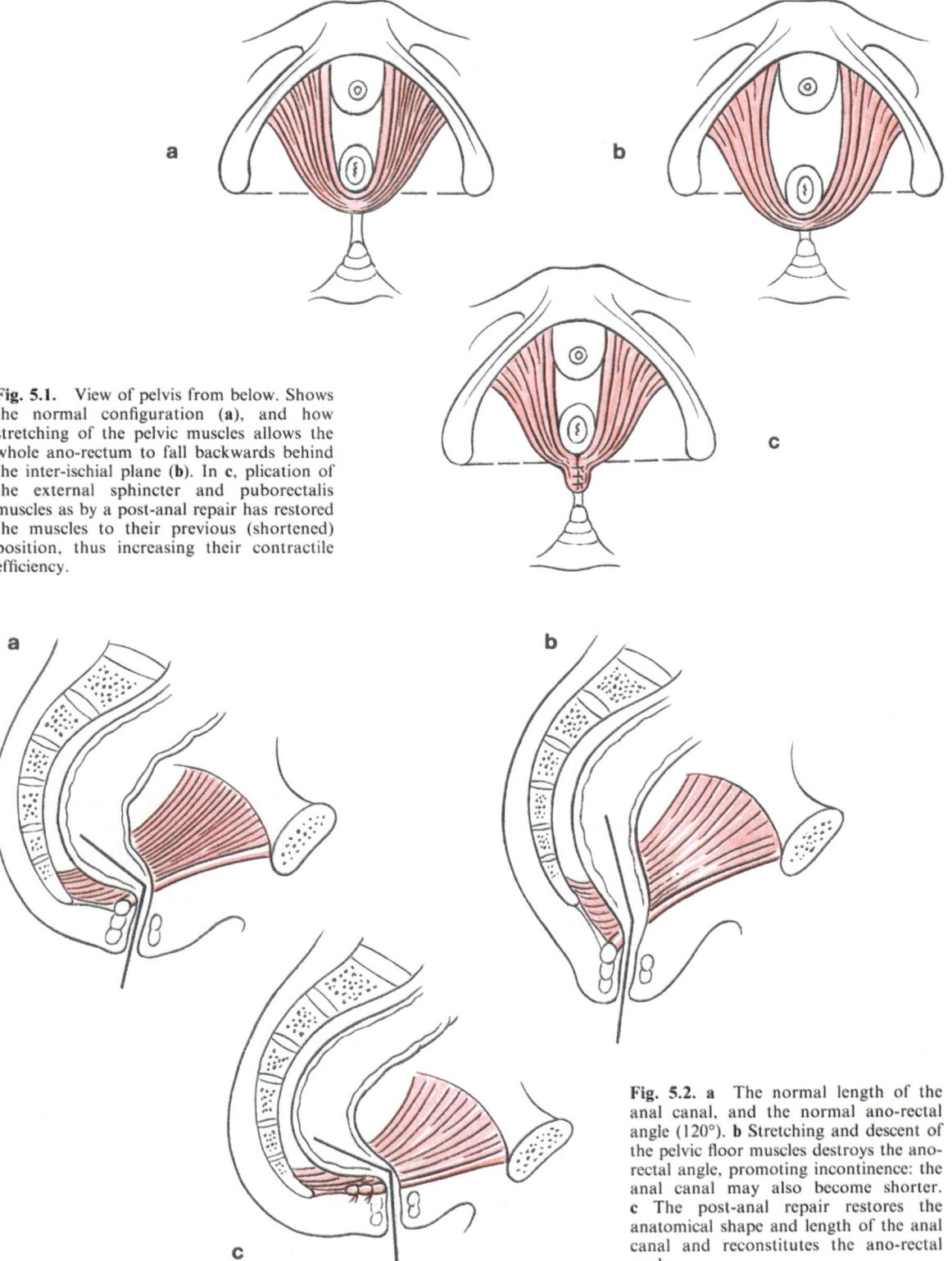

Fig. 5.1. View of pelvis from below. Shows the normal configuration (**a**), and how stretching of the pelvic muscles allows the whole ano-rectum to fall backwards behind the inter-ischial plane (**b**). In **c**, plication of the external sphincter and puborectalis muscles as by a post-anal repair has restored the muscles to their previous (shortened) position, thus increasing their contractile efficiency.

Fig. 5.2. a The normal length of the anal canal, and the normal ano-rectal angle (120°). **b** Stretching and descent of the pelvic floor muscles destroys the ano-rectal angle, promoting incontinence: the anal canal may also become shorter. **c** The post-anal repair restores the anatomical shape and length of the anal canal and reconstitutes the ano-rectal angle.

patients with idiopathic faecal incontinence and the principles of the post-anal inter-sphincteric repair are summarised in Figs. 5.1 and 5.2.

It is now believed that the operation achieves its effects more by lengthening the anal canal than by restoring the ano-rectal junction.

Indications and Selection of Patients

Before a patient is considered for a post-anal repair it is important to exclude colonic disorders that may be contributing to incontinence (see pp. 12–14). In those patients with a loose or poorly formed stool, bulking agents may be of benefit and suppositories can be prescribed as an initial measure to promote complete rectal evacuation. A careful history and examination must be carried out to exclude neurological problems. A co-existing complete rectal prolapse is not uncommon in these patients and must be corrected before considering further surgery (although in some patients with minimal complete prolapse a post-anal repair may be enough, the Delorme procedure (p. 107) is the authors' preferred option). If conservative measures fail and the patient remains incontinent due to weakness of the pelvic floor and sphincter muscles without any evidence of rectal prolapse a post-anal repair should be considered.

The operation is particularly suited to those patients whose symptoms definitely date from prolonged labour or a traumatic (forceps) delivery [12] or for those patients who remain incontinent after abdominal repair of rectal prolapse. Selection of patients in whom the aetiological factor is thought to be prolonged and repeated straining at stool is more critical. Many such patients are of a nervous and obsessive disposition and cannot resist the habit of prolonged and repeated straining at stool. Bio-feedback (p. 188) has not impressed most surgeons as helpful to reverse the trait. Such repeated straining must be curtailed or minimised if a repair is to be successful. Pre-operative coun-

selling may be necessary to explain the aetiology of pelvic floor weakness and the principles of the operation, and inevitable failure must be emphasised if habitual straining is continued after surgery. Many patients will need to use evacuant suppositories in the immediate post-operative period and some of them for life. Not all patients accept this discipline, and their reluctance must be considered during case selection. It is the authors' experience that the best results are seen in those patients with a positive mental attitude both to their condition and to the necessities of post-operative care of their bowel habits.

Preparation

The patient needs to be counselled before surgery against undue optimism (see previous section). The principles of the repair and its post-operative management must be explained. The patient can be reassured, however, that with careful selection the operation of post-anal repair can restore continence in approximately 30% of affected individuals. Many of the remaining 70% will be improved and it is very unlikely that the operation will make the condition worse.

Many patients are elderly and frail and require pre-operative assessment with particular reference to their fitness to withstand a general anaesthetic. Serious health problems should be identified and corrected as far as possible. All sources of infection should be eradicated especially in the lungs, urinary tract and genital tract. If the perineal skin is excoriated a barrier cream should be used for a few weeks before surgery. Pre-operative physiotherapy and graduated stockings should be given to reduce the risk of thrombo-embolism. Anti-coagulants are not required for most patients and should be avoided for fear of a post-operative wound collection.

The authors emphasise that post-operative management of these patients is eased by mechanical cleansing of the bowel *before* surgery. Picolax, one sachet given

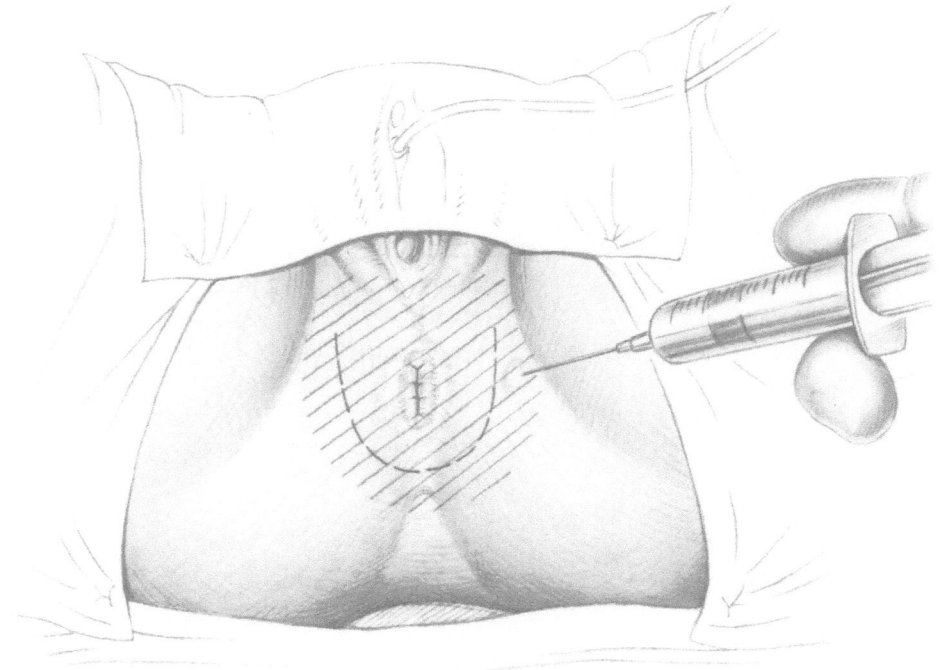

Fig. 5.3. The infiltrated area, and the usual curved incision around the posterior and lateral aspects of the anus. Some surgeons use a transverse incision, especially when the inter-ischial distance is greater than usual.

24 hours before operation followed by a further sachet 6–8 hours later, gives most satisfactory results. A disposable enema or a rectal washout should be given 2–4 hours before surgery. Skin protection is very important during preparation of the incontinent patient, as excoriation can aggravate infection risks. In most patients antibiotic cover of the procedure is not required.

Operative Technique

The patient is positioned in the lithotomy position with the hips well flexed. A urinary catheter is passed into the bladder and the perineum shaved. The patient is draped as shown and at this stage it is often worthwhile to carefully palpate the perineum to identify the inter-sphincteric groove. (In many cases it is best to close the anal orifice with a temporary purse-string suture to prevent faecal contamination.) The opera-tive field is now infiltrated with a weak solution of adrenaline (ephedrine) in saline (1 in 300 000). The area of infiltration of the subcutaneous tissues is shown (Fig. 5.3).

An incision is made between 2 and 3 cm posterior to the anal verge as an opened "U" (Fig. 5.3). If the infiltration has been successful bleeding will be minimal. With fine-toothed dissecting forceps the upper flap is lifted and with scalpel or scissors dissected free towards the anal canal. The upper flap may now be grasped with tissue-holding forceps or skin hooks which should be held by an assistant. The skin flaps should be taken well forward, as shown in Fig. 5.4. Care must be taken not to button-hole the skin when the flap is dissected. Beneath the flap the fibres of the external sphincter (red) will be seen contrasting with those of the internal sphincter (white) and the inter-sphincteric plane is thus identified. The skin flap is now sewn up over the anus with silk stitches (Fig. 5.5). This keeps the

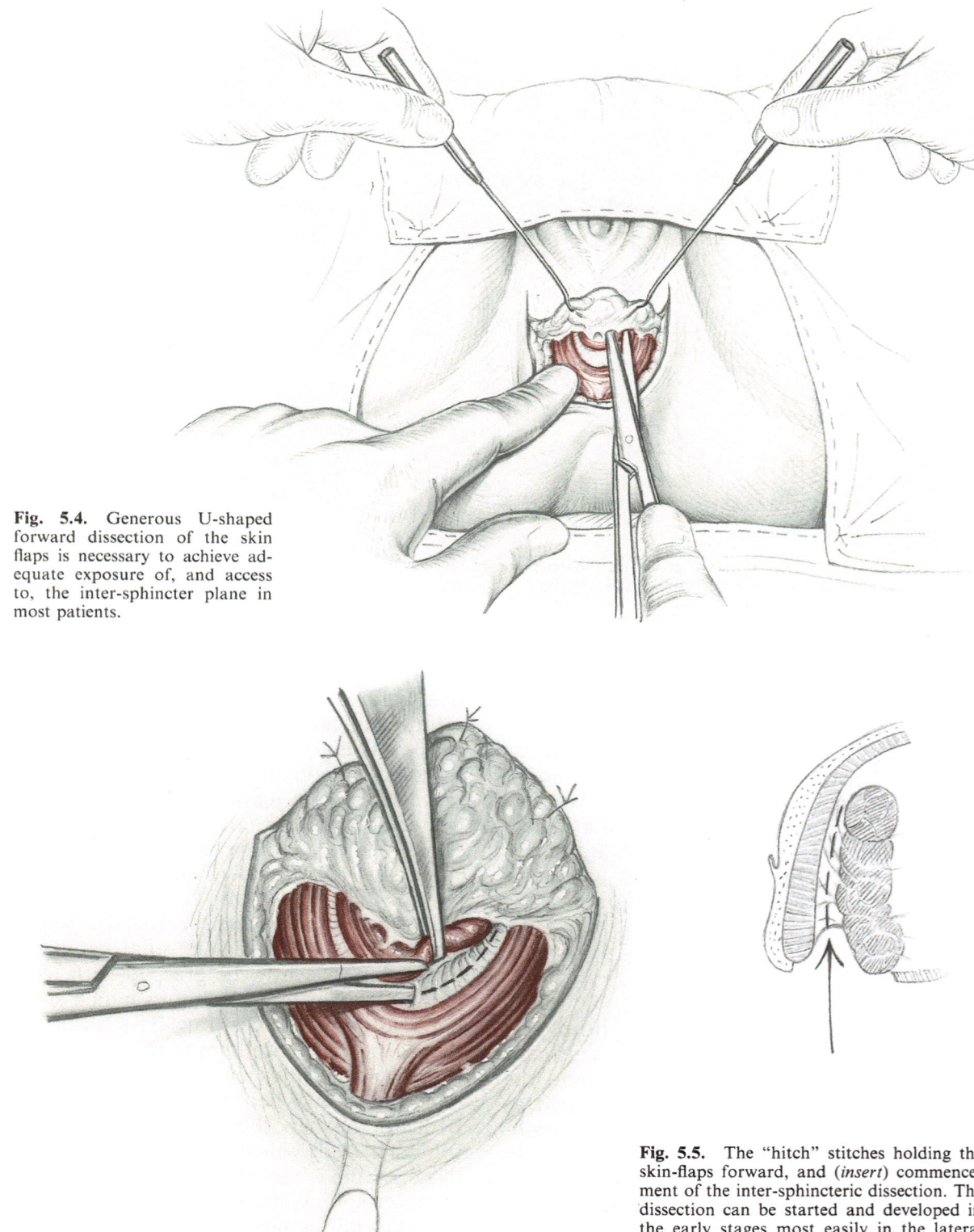

Fig. 5.4. Generous U-shaped forward dissection of the skin flaps is necessary to achieve adequate exposure of, and access to, the inter-sphincter plane in most patients.

Fig. 5.5. The "hitch" stitches holding the skin-flaps forward, and (*insert*) commencement of the inter-sphincteric dissection. The dissection can be started and developed in the early stages most easily in the lateral quadrants (see text).

operative field well exposed and prevents any seepage from the anus contaminating the operative field.

The next stage of the dissection is to identify and deepen the inter-sphincteric plane (Fig. 5.5). The dissection should start laterally as this is the easiest place to develop the inter-sphincteric plane at an early stage: in the midline posteriorly the lowest part of the inter-sphincteric plane is more adhesive and it is easier to open up the inter-sphincteric plane by approaching it from each side until a later stage of the dissection. A muscle stimulator may be of help during this part of the procedure if the anatomy has been obscured (e.g. by previous trauma); contraction of the external sphincter can be seen clearly, in contrast to the internal sphincter which does not react to direct electrical stimulation. As the inter-sphincteric plane deepens, the anal canal is revealed anteriorly covered by the pale circular fibres of the internal sphincter. Langenbeck or Landon straight retractors are needed as the dissection deepens. The entire post-anal circumference of the inter-sphincteric dissection should be joined up and continued as one exposure by this stage. Eventually the puborectalis muscle sling is reached and the rectum can be displaced anteriorly by further posterior mobilisation. It is important to remember that the rectum naturally passes backwards towards the coccyx and sacral concavity (as also does the inter-sphincteric plane) and it is dangerous to continue dissection in a cephalad vertical direction as this may lead to perforation of the rectum. Instead, the surgeon should follow the natural slightly posterior direction of the intersphincteric groove as it nears the level of the pelvic floor. Langenbeck retractors are now conveniently replaced by longer Landon retractors as the dissection proceeds above the

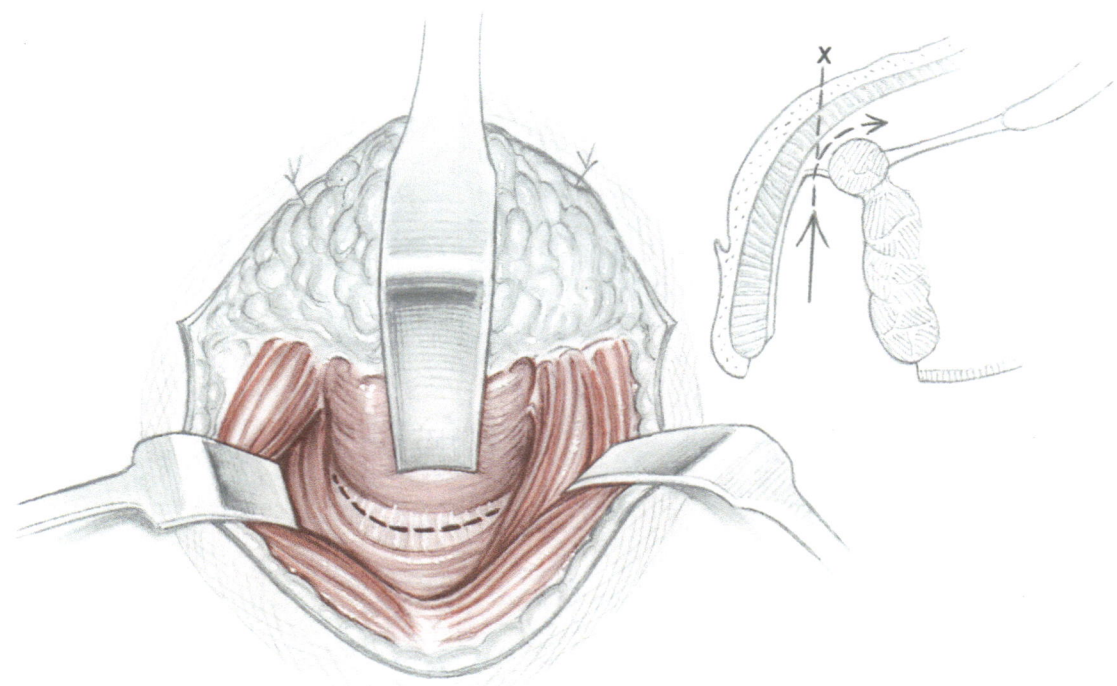

Fig. 5.6. The higher aspects of the dissection. As the surgeon enters the supra-levator plane, the fascia of Waldeyer is seen. This is incised (*insert*) to allow the post-rectal space to be opened up. Note how the angle of dissection must be changed if damage to the posterior wall of the rectum is to be avoided (x).

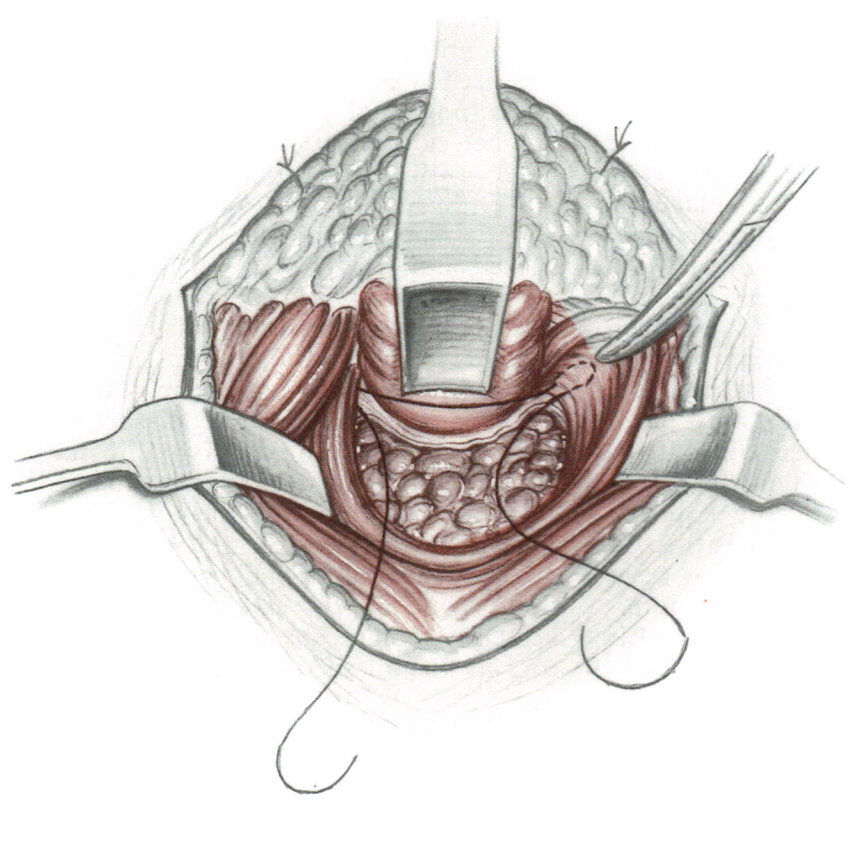

Fig. 5.7. Insertion of the first stitch of the repair, which is placed as high and anteriorly as possible.

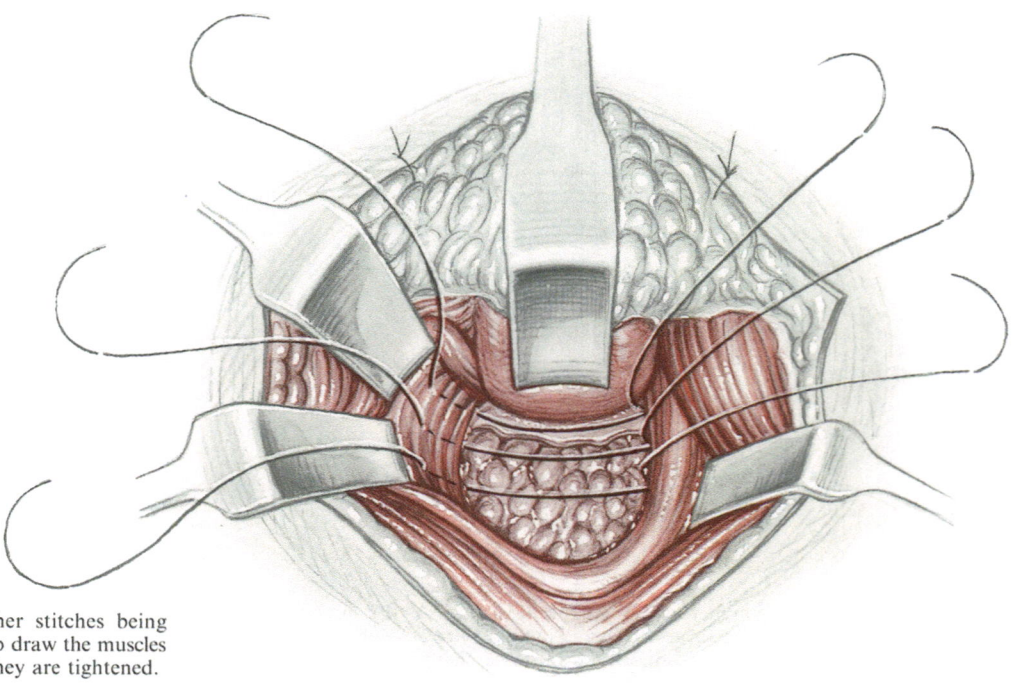

Fig. 5.8. Further stitches being placed serially, to draw the muscles together when they are tightened.

levators to open up the post-rectal space. It is important to make sure that the dissection is also deepened laterally to a high level so that the ischial spines can be easily palpated. As the back of the rectum is displaced forward the fascia of Waldeyer can be identified both visually and by palpation; this should be incised transversely to open up the post-rectal space after which the dissection is nearly complete (Fig. 5.6). The surgeon ensures that he has dissected adequately laterally and anteriorly to the ischial spines and that he has access to the anterior portions of the levator muscle close to the pubic arch. The repair may now proceed. The rectum is mobilised by blunt and sharp dissection posteriorly and freed from the anterior surface of the sacrum up to the 3rd or 4th sacral vertebra. The whole rectum is now held forcibly upwards and forwards by the assistant with a narrow-bladed Deaver retractor.

The authors prefer to make the repair with interrupted polypropylene (Prolene) or Vicryl sutures mounted on a 30-mm round-bodied needle. With the retractor firmly held by an assistant to displace the rectum anteriorly, a deep bite is taken of the levator muscle high up on the left side (see Fig. 5.7). The retractor is now moved to expose the same area on the left side and a similar deep bite of muscle is taken. The Prolene or Vicryl stitch is now clipped, after which the assistant holds this first untied suture anteriorly. Again retractors are placed to the left side of the patient and a further deep bite of musculature is taken. The procedure is again repeated in the right-hand side. Between four and six interrupted sutures are thus placed in the deep part of the levator muscles (Fig. 5.8). These are held by the assistant and with traction the puborectalis muscles from each side can now be made to approximate in the mid line. The sutures are now tied, starting first with the posterior stitch and working towards the anterior stitch. With the most anterior stitch it may not be possible completely to approximate the muscles from each side and a lattice work of stitching results (Fig. 5.9). This does not usually cause problems and it is important not to put too much tension on the muscle that is being sewn together or the repair might cut through in the post-operative period; for this reason many surgeons always prefer a loose darn. After the deep muscle bites have been secured (Fig. 5.10), which re-

Fig. 5.9. The anterior stitches may be impossible to draw together completely, and a lattice results. This is preferred to drawing the muscles together with undue force when the repair will fail because the stitches cut out.

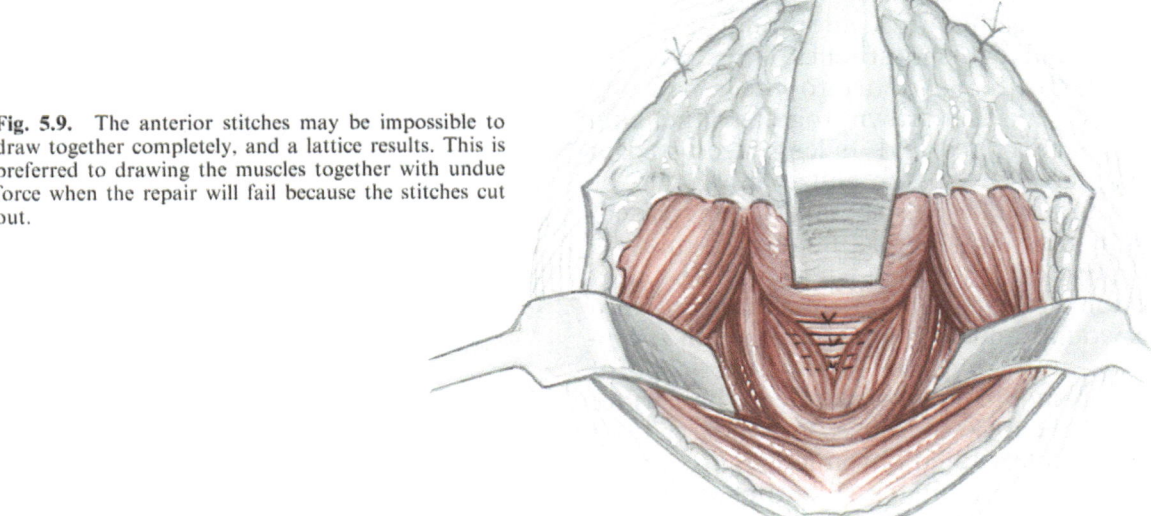

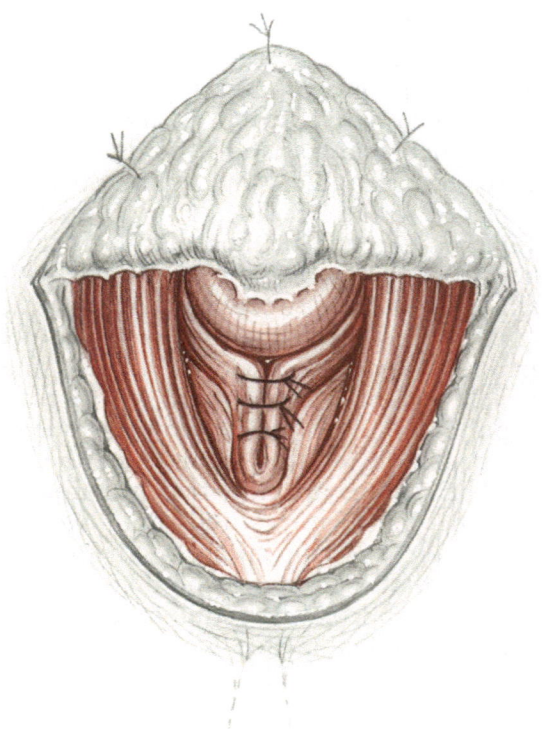

Fig. 5.10. Completion of repair of the inferior levator muscles and puborectalis.

creates a sharp ano-rectal angle, the surgeon now directs his attention to the lower aspects of puborectalis and external anal sphincter muscles. These are now brought together with additional layers of interrupted Prolene stitches (Fig. 5.11) to provide further support to the repair. As these layers are drawn together the anal canal is narrowed and its length restored or even increased. At the end there should be an anal canal of normal (or increased) length meeting the rectum at an angle of 110°. Blood loss should be minimal, but a suction drain (Redivac) can be placed into the wound and brought out through a separate "stab" incision. This final layer of stitches should be covered near the surface (where the risk of sepsis is greatest) by a layer of interrupted chromic catgut sutures. At this stage the black silk stitches holding the anterior skin flap are removed and it will be apparent that the skin edges have

been pulled inwards and backwards as the ano-rectal angle has been elevated and restored and the anal canal lengthened (Fig. 5.12) and that the original "U" shape of the incision has changed to a "Y". It may be impossible to close the incision in it's original "U" shape, and if so, the surgeon has two options. The most common recommended response is to sew up the incision as a "Y" shaped closure. It is the authors' experience that the mid point of the anterior skin flap presents a redundant skin fold and that the top parts of the vertical legs of the "Y" are difficult to approximate without tension. The second (easier)

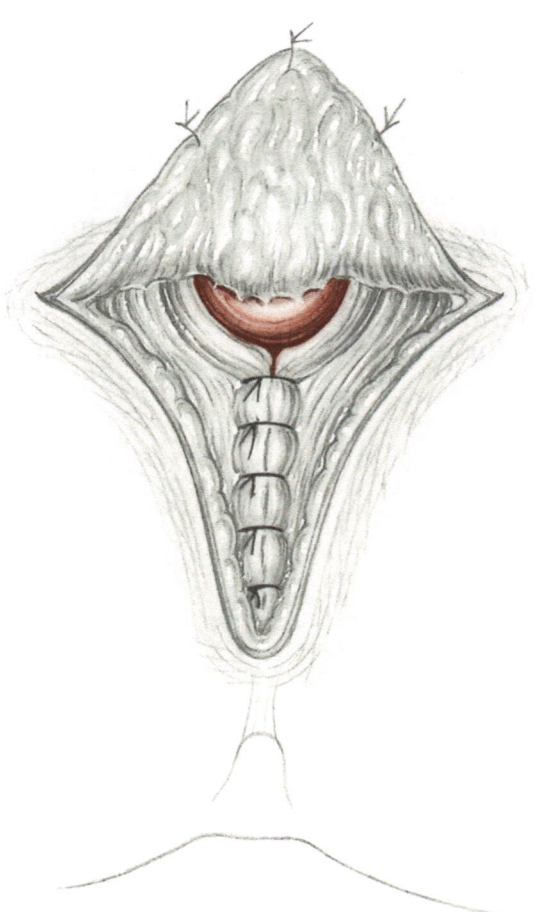

Fig. 5.11. The repair is completed by additional layers of stitches further drawing the puborectalis and external sphincter muscles across: this narrows and lengthens the anal canal.

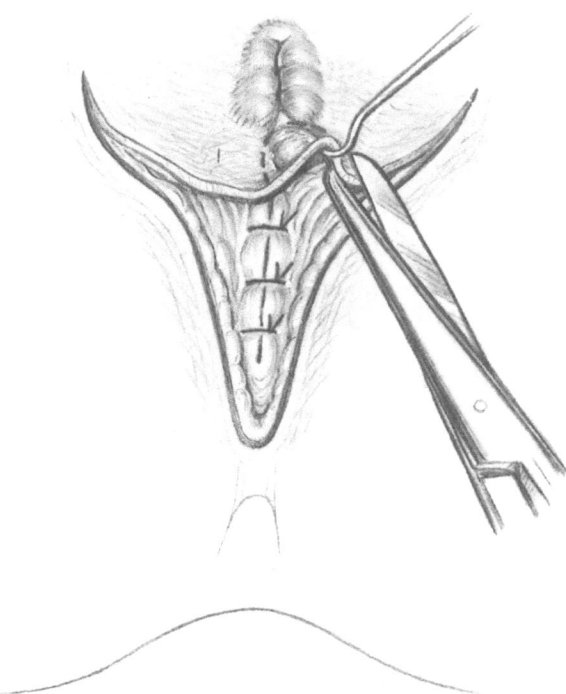

bowels to move until the fourth or fifth day. The patient should remain on complete bed rest for 48 hours. On the second post-operative day the patient should start to take an osmotic laxative such as magnesium sulphate (Epsom salts) or Milpar (Cremaffin, Boots) 25 ml three times daily. This should ensure that the first and subsequent bowel movements will be soft and semi-solid, and pass easily without straining. From the second post-operative day the patient should have the unclosed triangle in the middle of the wound (if present) treated by twice daily saline irrigations to remove debris, and a flat dry dressing applied.

The perineal wound of a post-anal repair is notoriously poorly healing and some separation of the wound edges occurs in a

Fig. 5.12. The skin edges of the "U" shaped incision are distorted by the elevation and anterior displacement of the ano-rectal junction into a "Y" shape.

option is to excise the redundant skin anteriorly leaving a small triangle of skin in the middle (where tension is greatest) which has not been closed (Fig. 5.13). This leaves a wound partially closed without tension. The small open wound causes no post-operative problems and heals rapidly. The operation is now complete, and the wound is covered by a light dressing held in place by a "T" bandage.

Post-operative Management

It is important in post-operative management that the patient should not strain to pass water or to open his bowels, nor move about excessively (which causes disruption of the skin wound). Therefore, the urinary catheter should be kept in place for at least four days and with adequate pre-operative preparation there should be no need for the

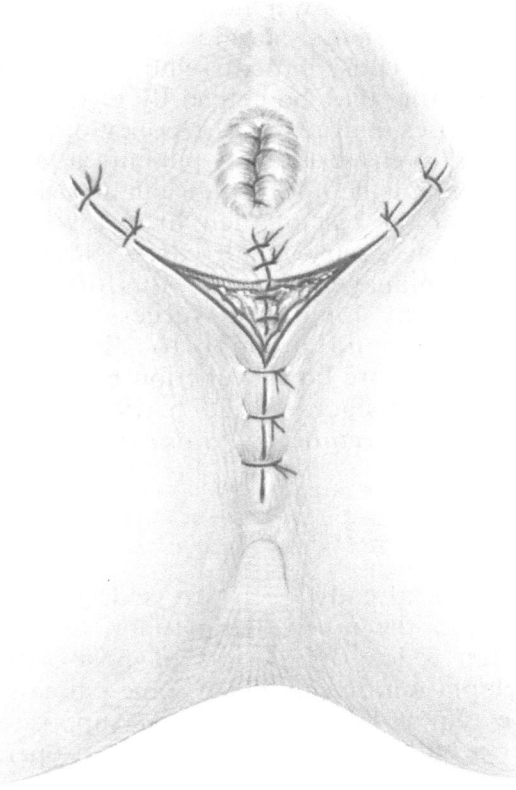

Fig. 5.13. When the wound is closed, it may be desirable to leave a small triangle open as shown at the point of greatest tension.

high proportion. This is of no consequence as long as the separation is confined to the skin and superficial tissues. If there are signs that the wound edges are separating the patient should be advised to continue bed rest and *removal of skin sutures should be delayed until the wound edges are stable.* If the bowels have not moved by the sixth post-operative day it is important that the rectum be examined to ensure that faecal impaction is not threatening. This must be avoided at all costs by using enemas freely. By 7 days post-operatively the patient should have established a satisfactory bowel habit without straining.

The patient may not immediately notice benefit from the operation especially if the stool is liquid from aperients. Moral support for the patient is all-important from the medical and nursing staff during the difficult early days, especially when the wound is healing slowly and is painful. As soon as the bowel habits has been regulated, aperients should be progressively reduced. Those patients who have difficulty evacuating may be helped by glycerine suppositories, and it was the policy of Sir Alan Parks to insist that all patients after post-anal repair should use evacuant suppositories for the rest of their life. However this is not necessary in all cases. Nevertheless bowel management after this operation is crucial to long-term success and there should be no attempt to discharge the patient before bowel function has been seen to be satisfactory. *Early discharge may mean early return with a disrupted repair.*

Results [1,2,7,15]

As has already been stressed, results are best in the motivated patient, as there is often a lengthy period of post-operative adaptation during which some patients may be required to use evacuant suppositories, or a bulk laxative. Frequent post-operative supervision is required to ensure maximum benefit. In patients with anal neuropathy the results are always likely to be partial or poor, with persisting incontinence.

Post-rectal Buttress Repair (Syn. Wyatt Technique) [14]

Introduction

This approach was described by Wyatt (1981) [14] and has been used by the authors on several occasions with good results. However, it is not regarded by them as a substitute for other procedures (such as abdominal rectopexy or direct sphincter repair) when the cause of incontinence can be specifically attributed to a single over-whelming cause (such as rectal prolapse or sphincter damage or a physiologically incompetent puborectalis and external sphincter muscle).

Indications and Selection of Patients

Missiles, trauma (as after falls or high-speed accidents) and the after-effects of operations on the lower spine can produce a patient with severe damage to the muscles of the pelvic floor associated with incontinence. The anal sphincters are commonly included in the destruction, which aggravates the degree of incontinence. Septic complications frequently follow the initial injury and any muscle tissue that remains is hampered by dense scar tissue. Some special tumours (e.g. sacral chordoma, post-anal dermoids) are best removed through a posterior perineal route, and such operations are usually extensive when malignancy is present: these cases may need wide removal of the postero-inferior parts of the levator ani muscle. A large perineal hernia with both constipation and incontinence may then develop, and a similar situation can follow certain specific cancer or inflammatory bowel disease operations that entail sacrifice of the normal muscular supports of the ano-rectal organ (e.g. colo-anal excision of the rectum). Some patients, usually elderly women (but a similar situation can develop at any age after prolonged malnutrition) suffer such extreme thinning of the muscles of the pelvic floor that the clinical features pass beyond simple "perineal descent" to one of "ballooning" of the whole pelvic floor. Many such patients cannot be helped by an intersphincteric procedure as the defect in the weakened posterior parts of the levator muscle and puborectalis needs more substantial buttressing than can be provided by a post-anal repair. The post-rectal perineal approach allows for direct repair of the lower pelvic floor [4] without the need to put a "stretch" stress on incomplete or thinned muscles in order to pull them together: it is also simpler to insert sheets of prosthetic material into large defects through the posterior perineal route. Occasionally in a few patients who have had one or more failed attempts at a post-anal intersphincteric repair, this operation can be offered as it can be carried out through planes free of scar tissue. Not many patients will be willing to accept this offer after previous failures but some patients (and their surgeons) can be surprisingly persistent when the only alternative to continuing incontinence is a permanent colostomy or a life-endangering abdominal operation. Wyatt himself has used the operation for elderly and infirm patients with complete rectal prolapse. The posterior approach offers excellent exposure for an extended repair of the muscles of the pelvic floor ("levatorplasty")

Preparation

Patients need to be counselled not to assume a good result, but they can be reassured that the operation should not make their incontinence worse. If the patient has serious health problems, these should be corrected as usual prior to the operation, at least as far as is possible. If the perineal skin is excoriated, the use of barrier creams to clear up the surface inflammation is indicated: Vasogen and Metanium cream are both useful for this, but the patient may need skilled nursing to enable the skin to heal. All sources of infection should be eradicated, with special attention to the

lungs, urinary tract and the vagina and cervix.

The patient should have thorough pre-operative oral and mechanical bowel cleansing (see p. 25) and per-operative antibiotics are given as usual (see p. 25). Those patients with malnutrition should have their hypo-proteinaemia corrected by either naso-gastric or intravenous hyper-alimentation programmes chosen as most suitable to their requirements.

If spinal nerve damage is present, pre-operative physiological testing should establish whether rectal sensibility remains. No patient should be offered the operation who cannot distinguish the presence of a rectal bolus: such patients will not be able to obtain faecal evacuation post-operatively and will suffer a disastrous combination of incontinence plus rectal impaction of faeces.

Pre-operative physiotherapy and graduated compression stockings should be given to reduce thrombo-embolic risks, but anti-coagulants should be avoided (unless the risks of thrombo-embolism are exceptional) in order to reduce the chances of enhanced operative bleeding and subsequent haematoma formation in the wound.

The bladder should be emptied pre-operatively by an indwelling catheter, which is retained until the patient is ambulant again. Digital examination immediately prior to surgery should confirm that the rectum is empty, and, if it is not, an "on-table" rectal wash-out is administered.

Operative Technique

The operation can be performed in both the prone and the lithotomy positions but the authors favour the prone position, which not only gives excellent access but also reduces bleeding. The anus is closed by a circum-anal stitch and the perineum cleaned in the usual way with aqueous chlorhexidine solution (1:200): inflammable skin preparations must not be used because of the risk of diathermy sparking. The perineum is draped in the usual way to give generous

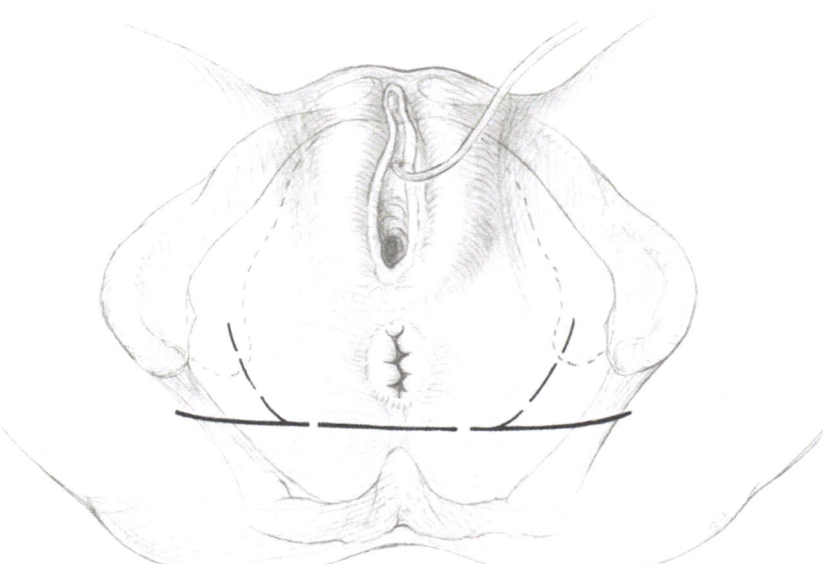

Fig. 5.14. A generous incision is made transversely across the perineum midway between the anus and the tip of the coccyx. In patients with a narrow pelvis, access is facilitated by extending the ends of the incision anteriorly as shown (---).

Fig. 5.15. After the dissection has been deepened into the perineal and ischiorectal fat spaces, a St. Marks pattern perineal retractor is inserted to retract the tissues. After suitable removal of fat, the lower aspect of ileococcygeus can be seen, and Waldeyer's fascia (X) palpated anterior to the coccyx.

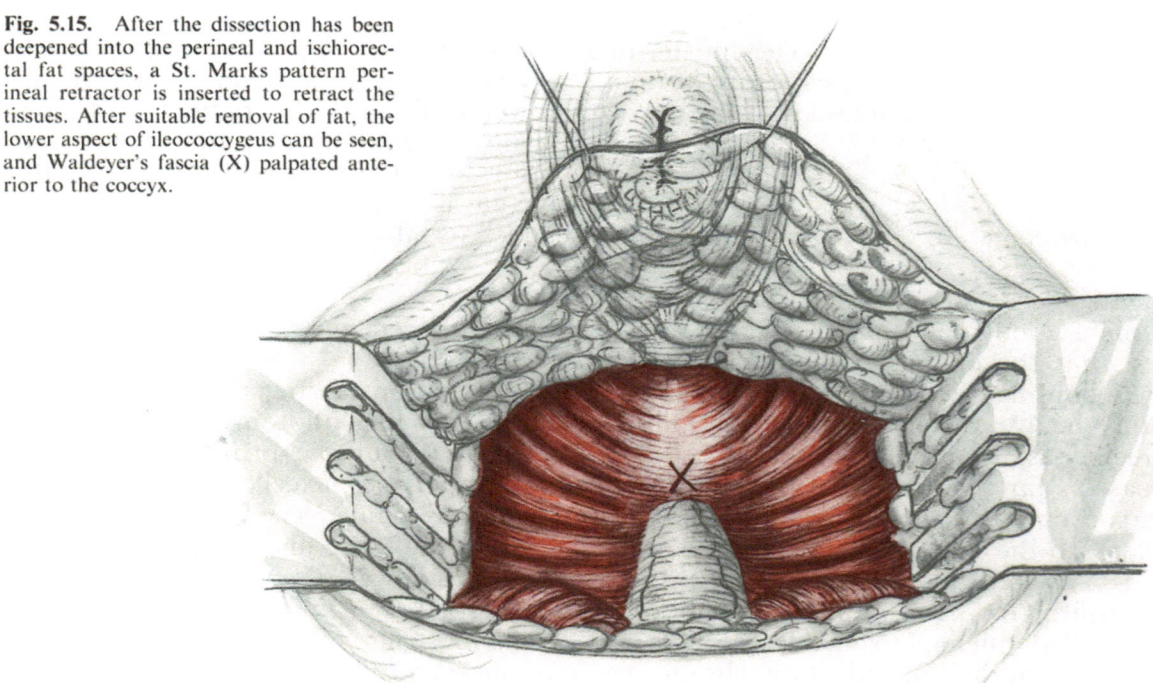

exposure to landmarks: the tip of the coccyx behind, the ischial-tuberosities on each side, and the anal orifice itself, should all be easily identifiable in the operative field. A nerve stimulator should be available so that the pudendal nerves can be identified when necessary and safeguarded. The authors advise free use of a weak solution of ephedrine (adrenaline) in physiological saline (1:300 000) to reduce oozing during the operation, providing the usual precautions are taken by the anaesthetist when the infiltration is given (e.g. to discontinue halothane (or similar) anaesthetic agents). In some patients the desire of the surgeon to reduce operative bleeding from small vessels can be combined with the aim of avoiding certain types of anaesthesia by the use of epidural analgesia techniques.

A large incision, 10–15 cm long, is made transversely midway between the anus in front and the coccyx behind (Fig. 5.14). The incision can be curved forwards at each end alongside the ischial tuberosities to allow maximum retraction of the edges of the incision (Fig. 5.14, interrupted line), and exposure must be planned to anticipate that the operative field narrows as it is deepened. The incision should encircle any previous scar tissue as it is desirable to remove all such tissue in the course of the operation. The retro-anal (and rectal) space is progressively opened up, and the operation plane extends on each side into the fat of the ischio-rectal fosa. It facilitates both exposure (and the subsequent repair) if much of this fat is removed: a sponge holder is useful to do this, in combination with fingers and swabs: brisk bleeding is usual at this point from the divided inferior rectal vessels, which require suture ligation as they do not respond favourably to diathermy coagulation. The amount of fat requiring to be removed is always more than the surgeon anticipated. The ano-coccygeal raphe is divided, and in some patients the coccyx is removed to facilitate exposure.

Eventually, the fascia of Waldeyer, the posterior and inferior aspects of the anal sphincter in the mid line anteriorly, and the ileococcygeus and puborectalis portions of the levator ani muscle will be exposed (Fig. 5.15). The lower surfaces of the muscles should be cleaned, and any defects in the muscle floor of the pelvis should have their edges exposed.

The fascia of Waldeyer is divided transversely, and the back of the rectum covered by its enclosing connective tissue and blood vessels will be seen (Fig. 5.16). The rectum can be separated from the front of the

Fig. 5.16. After transversely incising Waldeyer's fascia, the space between the rectum (in front) and sacrum (behind) can be developed. The space can be opened up as far as the mid-point of the sacral concavity, and the rectum can be pushed upwards and forwards to reduce any prolapse.

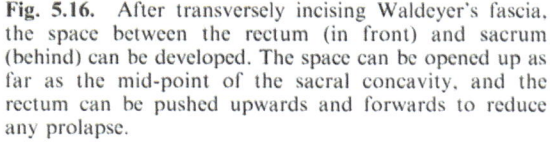
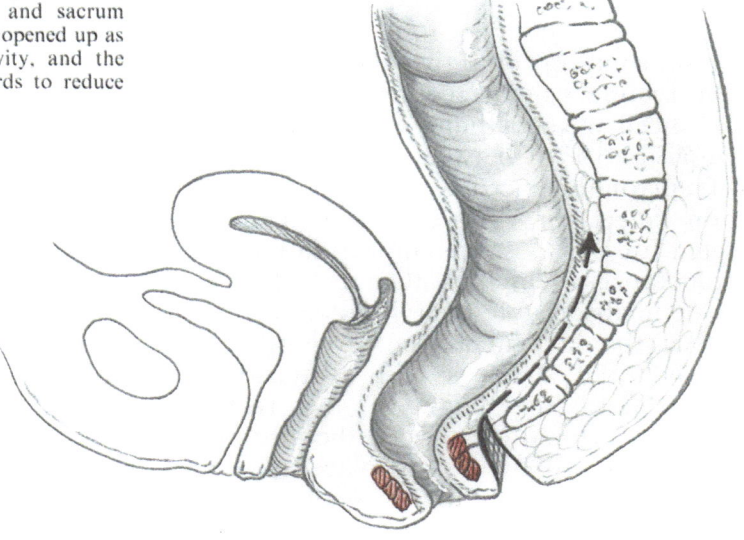

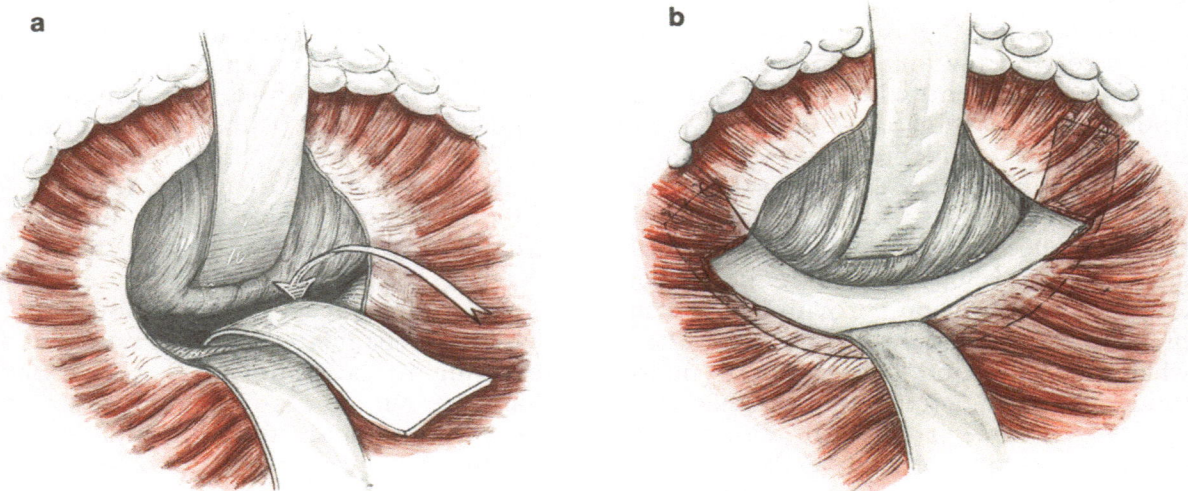

Fig. 5.17. a With a deep retractor holding the back of the rectum in an elevated anterior position, prosthetic material can be inserted and stitched in place as high as S2 to fill the pre-sacral space, or can be used as a supra-levator sling to hold the ano-rectal junction forwards and restore the ano-rectal angle (**b**).

lower three sacral vertebrae by careful blunt and sharp dissection of any loose fibrous strands that are present, until the rectum can be pushed easily forwards in an antero-superior direction (Fig. 5.17a). The upper surface of the levator ani muscle can be separated easily from any loose tissue on each side of the rectum by gentle but firm finger dissection at this point.

The extent of any laxity of the muscles of the pelvic floor, as well as the outline of any defects, can now be fully assessed by the operator, and decisions made on the most appropriate corrective action. Prolapse of the rectum can be rectified by insertion of a sheet of prosthetic material in the space (Fig. 5.17b) between the rectum and the front of the sacrum. Polyvinyl sponge, Teflon sheet or Marlex mesh can be selected for this as seems appropriate to the circumstances, which is then attached by clips or unabsorbable (vicryl) stitches to the front of the sacrum at the level of S2/3. The anchored sheet is then fastened on each side to the back of the rectum (Fig. 5.18a,b). Alternatively the prolapse can be corrected by a sling placed around the posterior and lateral aspects of the ano-rectal junction. The posterior and inferior

aspects of the puborectalis and inferior aspects of the puborectalis and levator ani muscles can be apposed and strengthened by a buttressing darn of unabsorbable (00) stitches (Fig. 5.19a). A wide deficiency of the muscular floor can be rectified by the insertion of a prosthetic sheet (Fig. 5.19b). The external sphincter muscle can be plicated by a latticework of Dexon (no. 1) or other unabsorbable monofilament (00) sutures, or a direct sphincter repair (see pp. 103–106) can be carried out. Occasionally several of these procedures are used together to correct multiple defects as a form of combined repair.

Once the repair is finished, meticulous haemostasis is carried out and a suction drain inserted through a separate stab into the depths of the wound. Topical antisepsis with either a providone iodine or antibiotic (Tribactrim) spray is used to coat the wound surfaces. When possible the fatty tissue is closed with interrupted fine chromic catgut sutures to reduce the wound space and to prevent a large sero-sanguineous fluid collection. The skin is closed with fine (000) stitches. A light gauze wound dressing is applied using a protective adhesive (Op-Site; Nobecutane; Tinct-

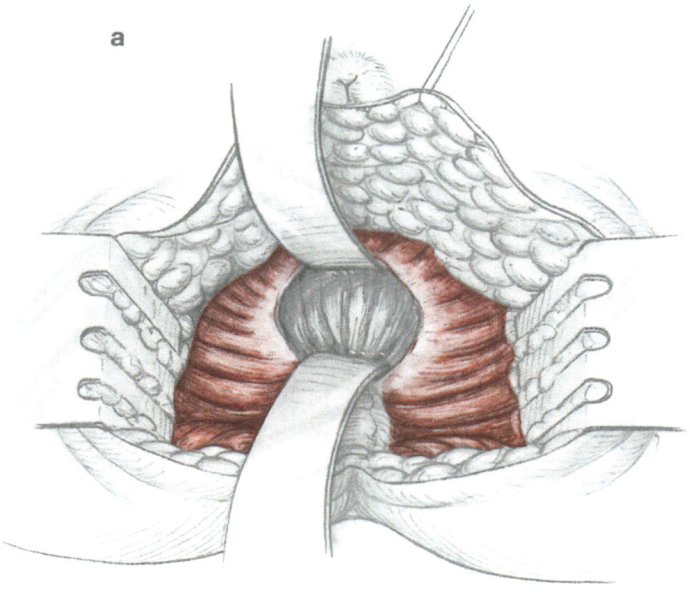

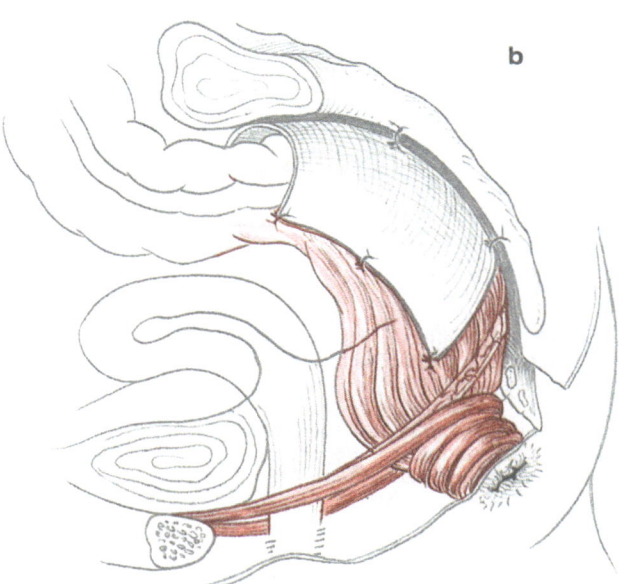

Fig. 5.18. a Through the same approach (shown here in sagittal view) (**b**) a sheet of prosthetic material can also be fastened against the front of the sacrum, as shown, and stitched to the sides of the rectum.

Benz Co, solutions are all suitable). The anal stitch is removed.

Post-operative Management

The patient is confined to bed for 72 hours: movement encourages post-operative oozing in the wound and makes the skin

stitches cut through. The catheter remains until the patient is at least fully ambulant, and preferably until the wound is stable. The suction drain is removed after 24 hours unless it is still draining more than 3 ml hourly. Antibiotic cover is discontinued after 24 hours unless there are special indications for continuing. The I.V. infusion is taken down after 24 hours, by which time

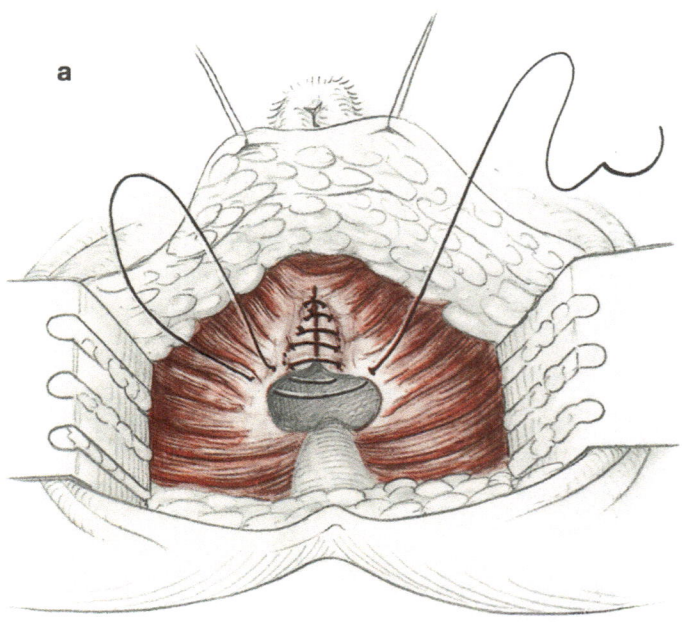

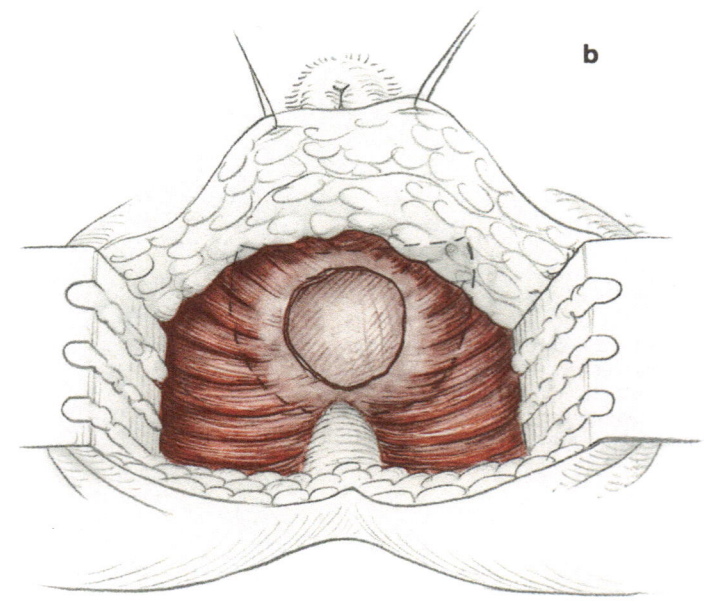

Fig. 5.19. a Whether or not the rectum is supported at a higher level, the muscles of the levator floor can be pulled together by a latticework of stitches, and drawn snugly against the back of the rectum. b Alternatively, wide defects can be repaired or the pelvic floor strengthened by the insertion of a sheet of prosthetic mesh either above or below the levator muscles. This shows a mesh sheet put in as a flat plate on the superior surface of the levator muscles to shut off a large defect causing herniation and distortion of the ano-rectum with resulting incontinence.

the patient should be able to take oral fluids.

The bowels need not be confined after this operation, and a hard bulky stool should be avoided by giving a light aperient (Milpar – 25 ml b.d.) and by daily rectal wash-outs from the third post-operative day onwards until the wound stitches have been taken out. A non-residue or low residue diet is recommended until a regular bowel habit has been established. The patient should not leave hospital until it can be confirmed that the rectum is being satisfactorily emptied by spontaneous defaecation, and once this point has been reached a high roughage diet should be encouraged, with bran or hydrophilic substances added if necessary to ensure that the faeces are of normal bulk and consistency.

Results

Although Wyatt [14] reports good results, there have been no other reported series to enable comparisons to be made with the results of other techniques.

References and Further Reading

1. Browning GGP, Parks AG (1983) Post-anal repair for neuropathic faecal incontinence. Correlation of clinical results and anal canal pressures. Br J Surg 20: 101
2. Browning GGP, Rutter KRP, Motson RW, Neill ME (1984) Post-anal repair for idiopathic faecal incontinence. Ann R Coll Surg Engl Supplement, pp 30–33
3. Duthie HL (1971) Anal continence. Gut 12: 844
4. Espiner HJ (1981) A new operation for repair of complete rectal prolapse in the elderly. Royal Soc Med, Communication to Section of Proctology, Jan 28th
5. Hardcastle JD, Parks AG (1970) A study of anal incontinence and some principles of surgical treatment. Proc R Soc Med 63: 116
6. Keighley MRB (1981) Anal function. In: Jewell D, Lee E (eds) Topics in gastroenterology. Blackwell, Oxford, pp 305–323
7. Keighley MRB, Fielding JWL (1983) Management of faecal incontinence and results of surgical treatment. Br J Surg 70: 463
8. Lange (1887) quoted by Carrasco AB (1934) Contribution à l'étude du prolapsus du rectum. Masson, Paris
9. Lockhart-Mummery JP (1910) A new operation for prolapse of the rectum. Lancet i: 641
10. Parks AG (1975) Ano-rectal incontinence. Proc R Soc Med 68: 681
11. Parks AG, Swash M, Urich H (1977) Sphincter denervation in ano-rectal incontinence and rectal prolapse. Gut 18: 656
12. Snooks SJ, Swash M, Setchell M, Henry M (1984) Injury to innervation of pelvic floor sphincter musculature in childbirth. Lancet ii: 546
13. Tuttle JP (1903) A treatise on the diseases of the anus, rectum and pelvic colon. Appleton, New York and London
14. Wyatt AP (1981) Perineal rectopexy for rectal prolapse. Br J Surg 68: 717
15. Yoshioka K, Keighley MRB (1989) Critical assessment of the quality of continence after post-anal repair for faecal incontinence. Br J Surg 76: 1054

CHAPTER 6

Circum-anal Techniques

General Introduction

As has been stressed before, many patients with incontinence have general problems of old age and ill-health that make them unsuitable for major operative procedures. Some of them have specific health problems (e.g. cardio-respiratory, endocrine or metabolic) that rule out procedures that are better in design but more hazardous in execution. In some countries conditions of life prohibit the luxury of expensive materials or prolonged hospital-related care. Facilities for general anaesthetics may not be available.

For these situations, the relatively minor procedures described in the following pages have a role to play. Performed by a technically adept surgeon they may be the only methods that stand between the patient and social ostracism. No ano-rectal surgeon can be considered a complete expert without knowledge of, and skill at, these time-honoured techniques.

Circum-anal Wire (or Nylon) Encirclement (Syn. Thiersch Procedure) [6,7]

Introduction

Thiersch (1891) [17] attempted the control of complete rectal prolapse (with or without incontinence) by circum-anal narrowing with silver wire. He hoped to control the prolapse mechanically and induce later a permanent fibrous ring to support the weakened anal sphincter muscles and allow the silver wire to be removed. There is little evidence to suggest that silver wire (or any other alternative suture material) can induce such fibrotic reaction and Thiersch procedures only hold back the prolapse within the rectum by the resistance of the material inserted. If the wire or nylon ring is removed or broken, the prolapse immediately recurs. Since Thiersch's original description a number of variations

[10,11,15] have been used, using a variety of different materials, such as silk, fascia, nylon and polypropylene; Corman [3,5] uses a wide band of Silastic/Dacron mesh (Dow Corning, Michigan) and a similar technique has been reported from the Lahey Clinic [8].

To be effective for adequate control the retaining suture (or wire) must be tightened sufficiently to retain the prolapse but must be loose enough to allow passage of faeces: this is a difficult compromise to achieve. The suture must be retained indefinitely. In patients with a large prolapse a Thiersch procedure is rarely successful as the wire (or suture) breaks or cuts through the tissues and becomes exposed, with consequent infection and pain. A Thiersch suture can, however, be introduced under local anaesthetic, and therefore no patient need be considered unfit for the procedure. Consequently it remains a method of treating elderly unfit patients in the United Kingdom, but in the authors' experience it is rarely successful except for patients with small prolapses, and then often for only a few months. In many patients the suture has to be removed; if it is too tight, faecal impaction is precipitated; if it is too loose, it does not cure the incontinence; in too many cases the patient begs for some more effective answer, even if greater risks are involved. In most colo-rectal specialist centres the procedure has been largely abandoned for better alternatives such as an abdominal rectopexy or a perineal type repair. While an abdominal rectopexy is more risky than a Thiersch procedure or a perineal repair, these abdominal techniques are also so safe in modern surgical practice [12] that it is an exceptionally ill patient indeed who must be condemned to treatment by a Thiersch technique.

The Thiersch operation is not suitable for treating patients who have idiopathic incontinence due to patulous sphincters with no accompanying prolapse: the support given by the ring of wire (or nylon) is entirely passive and does not enable any restoration of anal muscle tone to occur.

Indications and Selection of Patients

All patients can be considered fit for a Thiersch procedure providing the surgeon cannot perform a more effective procedure. In patients with severe psychiatric or senility problems the post-operative management of the bowels can be very difficult, often resulting in faecal impaction and overflow incontinent diarrhoea. However, it is even easier to remove the wire (nylon) than it is to put it in, so this makes a Thiersch procedure an acceptable "last-ditch" recourse made in hope rather than expectation, especially for surgeons inexperienced in other perineal type procedures.

Preparation

The procedure can be performed under general or local anaesthesia. Often the perineal skin in these patients is unhealthy and macerated and pre-operative epidermal healing by local hygiene measures supplemented by barrier creams (Vasogen) is essential. Post-operative management is much easier if the rectum is emptied pre-operatively. This can be achieved by the use of Picolax or alternative suitable bowel cleansing agents (Clean Prep). Prophylactic antibiotic cover is not necessary unless a mesh of prosthetic material is used when the authors recommend broad antibiotic cover against both aerobic and anaerobic organisms.

Operative Technique

Although Thiersch originally used a single circle of silver wire and some continue to prefer this material, the authors use a double, triple, or even a greater number of encirclements with No. 2 monofilament nylon. Nylon is easier to use, retains some elasticity, is more comfortable for the patient and, in our experience, is less likely to fragment than wire. The operation may be conducted with the patient either in the

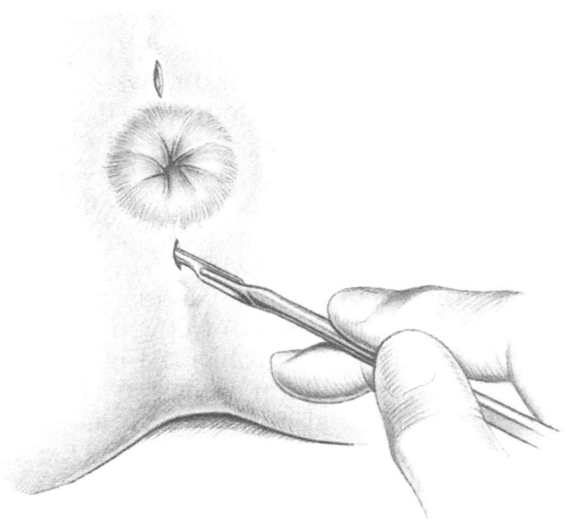

Fig. 6.1. The two small skin incisions (2–5 mm) are made respectively in front of and behind the anal orifice as shown.

lithotomy position or in the left lateral ("Sims") position. This latter position is often easier in patients who must have a local anaesthetic because of cardio-respiratory disease or who have arthritic problems of the hip joints. After cleaning the skin, two small incisions, approximately 2–5 mm long, are made in the midline approximately 2 cm in front and behind the anus (Fig. 6.1). Then a fully curved Doyen needle is passed from the posterior wound through the subcutaneous tissues approximately 1 cm deep to the surface, to appear at the anterior wound (Fig. 6.2). A length of No. 2 nylon is then passed into the eye of the Doyen needle and the instrument drawn back. The needle is unthreaded and then re-passed through the opposite side to reach the anterior wound again (Fig. 6.3). Once more the free end of the nylon is threaded and withdrawn into the posterior

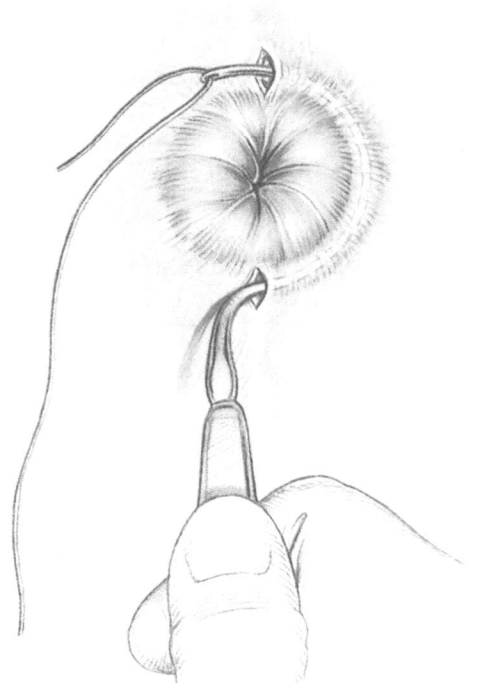

Fig. 6.2. A Doyen (or large aneurysm) needle is passed antero-posteriorly as shown, to appear in the anterior wound. No. 2 nylon is threaded through the eye of the needle which is then drawn back.

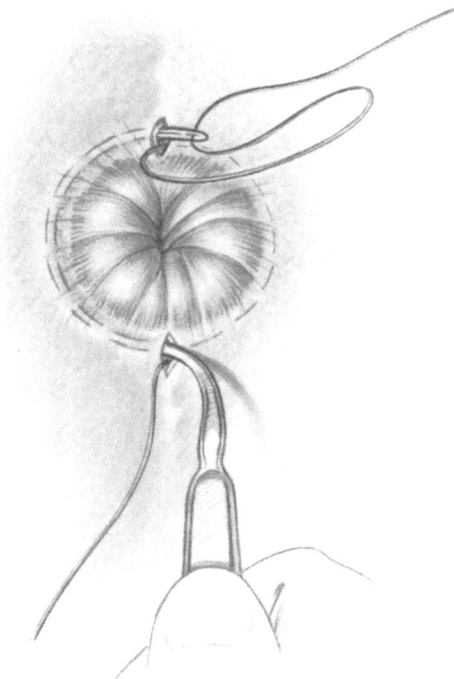

Fig. 6.3. The nylon encirclement of the anal orifice is completed by repeating the manoeuvre on the other side of the anal circumference.

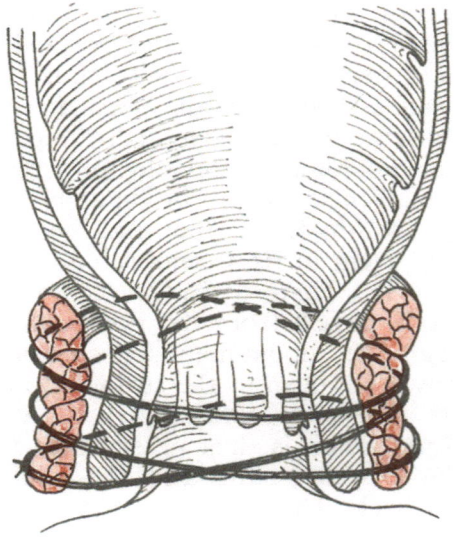

Fig. 6.4. Two (or more) encirclements of nylon are made at different levels to support the length of the anal canal and create a flexible "watch-spring" effect.

wound. This is repeated to allow 2–4 encirclements of nylon to be passed in the subcutaneous and peri-anal tissues. It is an advantage to place the loops at slightly different levels along the length of the anal canal starting as high as is conveniently possible as this produces a "watch-spring" effect that gives flexible support to a longer length of the canal [which may in turn reduce the chances of impaction as well as enhancing the prospects of effective control of the incontinence problem (Fig. 6.4)]. A No. 18 Hegar's dilator is passed (Fig. 6.5) into the anal canal (although an assistant's finger inserted to the second knuckle will act as a suitable alternative) and with the dilator in place the nylon is tied so as to grip the finger (or the dilator) firmly; the dilator (or finger) will prevent overnarrowing of the anal orifice when the suture is tied. The knot requires 4–6 throws to secure it and the knot should be insinuated into the depths of the wound after tying and then buried with a catgut stitch. The cutaneous incision should be closed with interrupted 000 nylon stitches or clips (Fig. 6.6).

Post-operative Management

The stitches (or clips) can be removed early, at latest by the fourth day after surgery. To

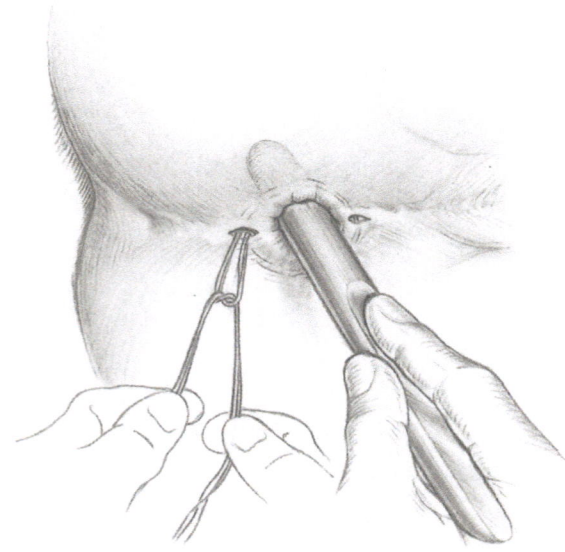

Fig. 6.5. A no. 18 Hegar dilator is inserted as a measure of the extent to which the nylon stitch should be drawn tight. An assistant's index finger (up to the 2nd knuckle) is an alternative to the dilator.

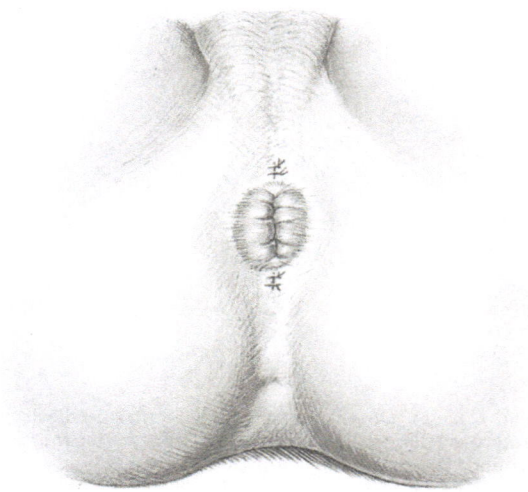

Fig. 6.6. The finish of the Thiersch procedure.

prevent faecal impaction the patient should be given aperients by mouth from the first post-operative day. Osmotic laxatives such as Milpar (Cremaffin, Boots) or a mildly stimulant laxative such as Senokot (Reckitt and Colman) are recommended. Rectal examination should be performed frequently in the post-operative days to confirm proper rectal emptying. Evacuant suppositories or enemas may be necessary. Early mobilisation is essential in these (usually) frail patients and the patient should not be discharged from hospital until a satisfactory bowel habit is established.

Circum-anal Cicatrical Fixation (Syn. Saraffof Technique) [1,16]

Introduction

At present most rectal surgeons are disenchanted with the previously described Thiersch procedure as a method of treating ano-rectal incontinence. This bad opinion of the procedure is maintained *whether the incontinence is associated with a rectal prolapse or not*, and is based upon the poor result of the operation. These are usually because of the notorious tendency of the Thiersch wire (or nylon) to break or cut out in a high proportion of cases, but even if the suture does not fail, too many patients are left with severe residual functional problems: either the ligature is too "tight" and causes faecal impaction, or it is too "loose" and does not control the incontinence (or the prolapse). In some patients septic complications occur, or the patient complains of severe pain (especially at defaecation). For all these reasons, the Thiersch procedure is hardly used at all by most surgeons at present in the treatment of incontinence with or without the presence of a prolapse.

However, if the incontinence is due principally to a lax atonic anal canal, the direct way of providing relief would be by a technique which gives firm all-round support to the weakened anus, but which avoids the complications of the Thiersch ligature. Since fibrous tissue has a well-known tendency to contract, one way of providing a firm "natural" narrowing of the anal canal would be by causing a ring of scar tissue to form around the anal canal.

In 1937 Saraffof [16] devised a method of causing peri-anal fibrosis by a 1.0 cm deep circum-anal incision (with additional removal in subsequent modifications of a circular ring of peri-anal skin 1.0 cm wide). This produces a tight contracture around the external opening of the anus which (theoretically) can be prevented from overnarrowing by subsequent digital anal dilatation if necessary. Most surgeons have found the results of this operation unpredictable but good results have been reported by European surgeons [1]. In patients in whom a Thiersch operation might be indicated if its complications were lower and its results better, the "Saraffof principle" has many advantages because of its freedom from complications, plus the ease and simplicity of the procedure. For these reasons the authors believe that it deserves to be recognised and used more widely than at present. The technique has been modified since originally described by making deeper incisions around the anal canal to provoke peri-anal cicatrisation around the entire length of the anal canal. A patulous anus with mucosal ectropion or a "Whitehead" deformity is the ideal case for a Saraffof operation or one of its variations [1].

Indications and Selection of Patients

Some patients require an operation for incontinence that is minor and is without risk, especially if it can be carried out without the necessity of a general anaesthetic. In other patients, a Thiersch procedure may have been attempted and have failed: a post-anal repair may also have been unsuccessful. Such cases may be considered for treatment by peri-anal cicatrisation. Correction of a "Whitehead deformity"

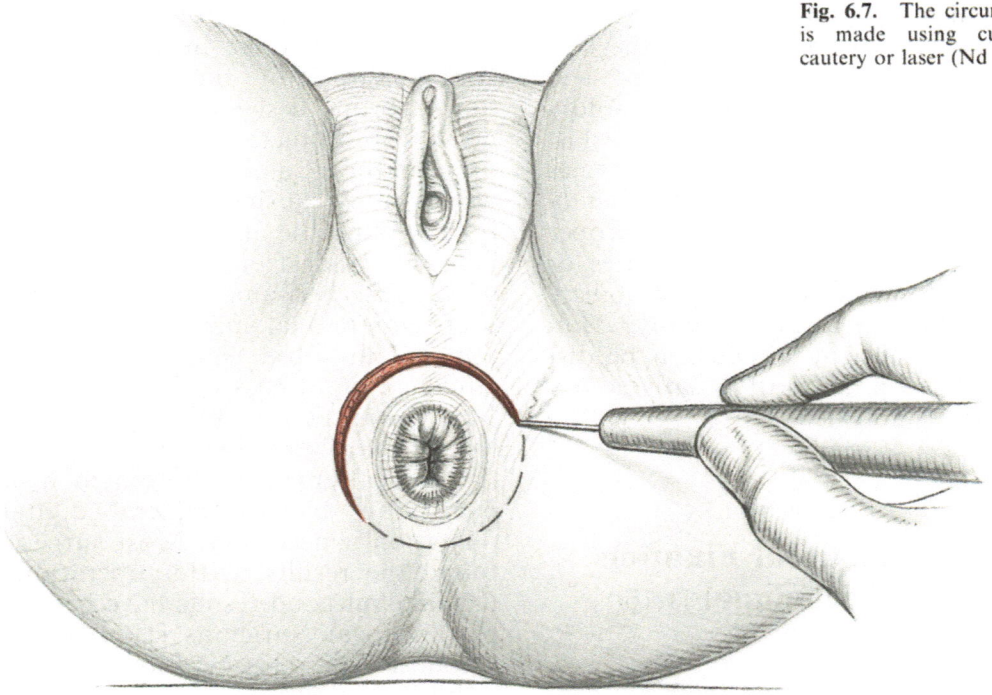

Fig. 6.7. The circum-anal incision is made using cutting electro-cautery or laser (Nd YAG) beam.

with ectropion of rectal mucosa can also be achieved by this technique.

If the patient's incontinence is due to a complete rectal prolapse, whenever possible the prolapse is treated first of all, as successful correction of the rectal descent may render any further operation for incontinence unnecessary. However, in a few patients a second-stage follow-up operation for incontinence may still be required. Usually, a perineal repair (intersphincteric, Delorme) will be the best procedure but occasionally this will not be the case e.g. the patient's circumstances, poor general health or abnormal mental state may indicate the briefest possible time for hospital admission. For such cases, perianal cicatrisation provides an alternative approach.

Because the degree of fibrotic post-operative anal narrowing is difficult to predict, patients must be available for close supervision and follow-up. Otherwise a dense and tight anal stenosis may develop which is impossible to reverse by any subsequent manoeuvre.

Operative Technique

The rectum should be emptied pre-operatively by a rectal washout given 2 hours before surgery.

A general anaesthetic is not a necessity as the operation can be performed under a caudal (or other low spinal or epidural) nerve-blocking technique.

Either the lithotomy or the jack-knife position can be used, and if the patient has difficulty in tolerating either of these, the left lateral ("Sims") position, using strapping to separate the buttocks, can also give the required operative exposure.

Using cutting electro-cautery or a laser, a slow and careful circum-anal incision is made around and outside the anal sphincter muscles (Fig. 6.7). *Behind*, the ano-coccygeal raphe is divided and *in front*, the plane just behind the vagina (but anterior to the perineal body) is opened up (Fig. 6.8). On either side, the fat of the ischiorectal fossa is encountered. An index finger within the anal canal monitors the depth of the

Fig. 6.8. Insertion of the index finger (as shown) aids the estimation of the correct depth of the cut. The depth of the wound should be almost up to the ano-rectal bundle or ring to ensure that the fibrous tissue will support the whole length of the anal canal (Bellomo).

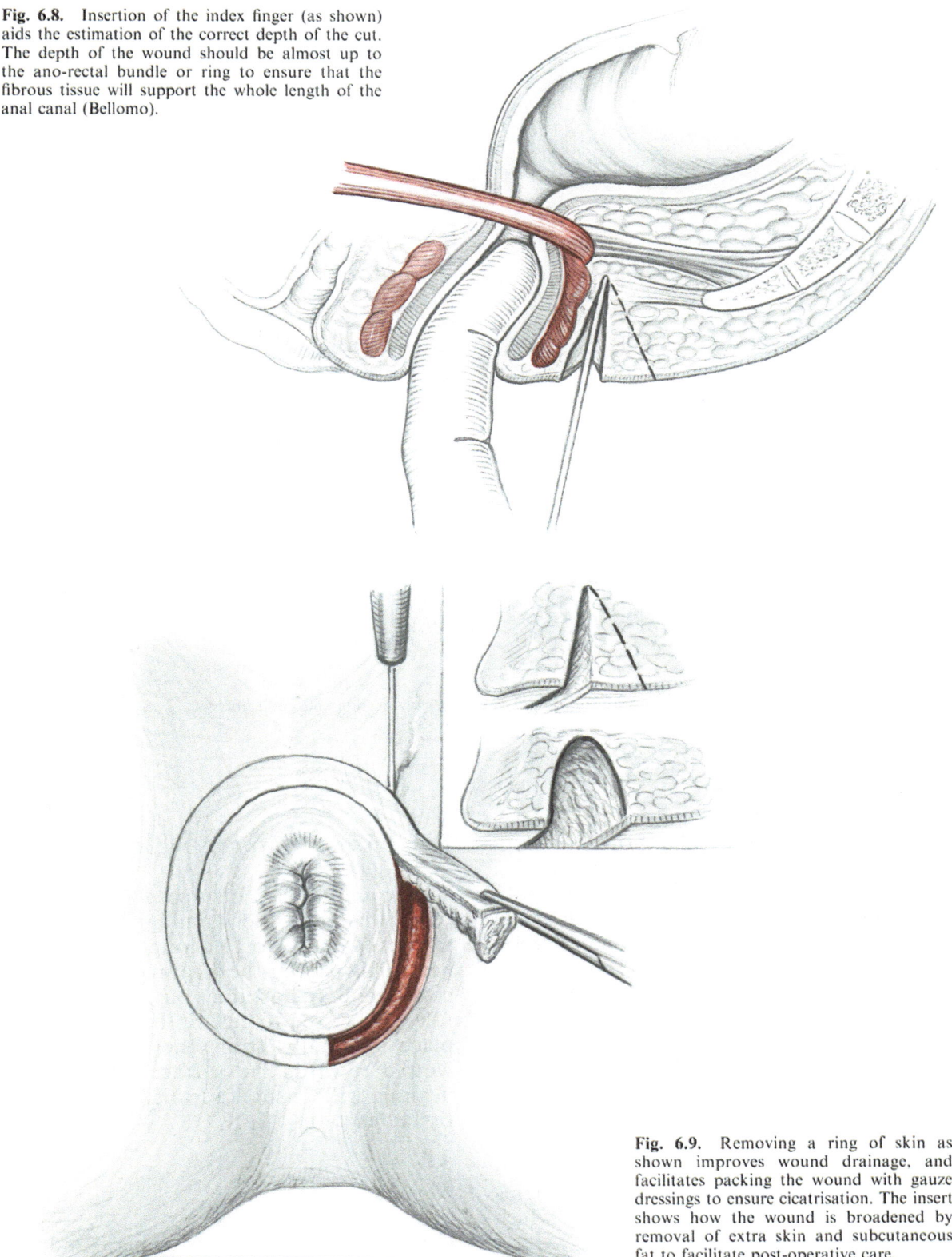

Fig. 6.9. Removing a ring of skin as shown improves wound drainage, and facilitates packing the wound with gauze dressings to ensure cicatrisation. The insert shows how the wound is broadened by removal of extra skin and subcutaneous fat to facilitate post-operative care.

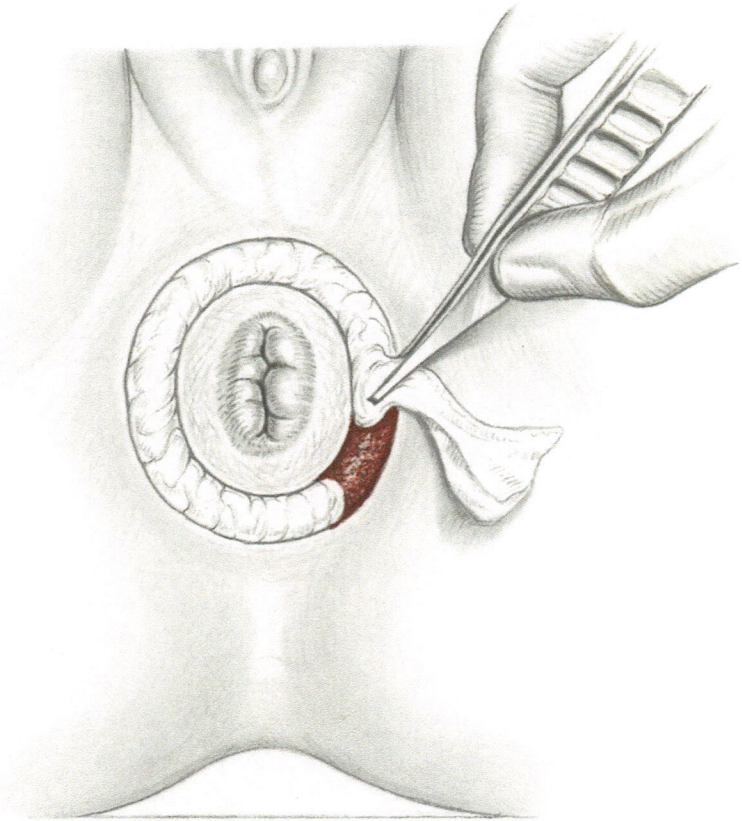

Fig. 6.10. Packing the wound to ensure slow healing and good fibrosis.

incision, which should be not less than 3.0 cm but not more than 5.0 cm deep i.e. it should extend up to the level of the ano-rectal bundle at the top end of the anal canal (Fig. 6.8). Providing the surgeon deliberately proceeds with extreme slowness, haemostasis is achieved without difficulty. Once the required depth has been reached, the wound is broadened by removal of a ring of skin and deeper tissues to allow for easy insertion of packs [both immediately and during the healing period (Fig. 6.9)].

At the end of the operation, the wound is lined by petroleum-jelly gauze strips ("Jelonet", Smith and Nephew) upon which other antiseptic-soaked ("Proflavine") gauze strips are packed (Fig. 6.10).

Post-operative Management

The wound is not disturbed for 48 hours. After this time the wound is dressed and re-packed daily for as long as it takes to heal. This part of the treatment need not be conducted in hospital, but must be carefully supervised to ensure that healing takes place gradually from the depths of the wound towards the surface. Only *delayed* healing will ensure a satisfactory fibrous tissue reaction.

Results

Good results for incontinence (and pro-lapse control if one is present) have been reported in up to 80% of cases, but few surgeons (including the authors) have large enough series to be certain of how this operation compares with others done for comparable cases. For surgeons who work in countries where patients cannot spend long in or near hospitals for socio-economic reasons, or who would be unable to re-attend frequently for potential complications, the operation is a good alternative to other similar perineal procedures (e.g. Thiersch or post-anal repair) which are not only also subject to failure but also have a higher need for skilled post-operative management.

Gracilis Muscle Sling Procedure (Syn. Pickrell-von Rapport Technique) [2,3,4,9,143]

Introduction

Very few colo-proctological surgeons have more than minimal experience of this procedure. Where circum-anal support is indicated, most surgeons prefer to use a Thiersch or Notaras type of operation for reasons of simplicity and predictability (with "reversibility" as an additional bonus). The fact that the Thiersch procedure fails so often has not persuaded the majority of surgeons to substitute for the passive prosthetic ring the active living contractions of somatic muscle (gracilis or adductor longus). The reasons for this reluctance are as follows:

1. Somatic muscle does not possess the ability of smooth muscle to maintain continuous tonic activity sufficient to provide continuous closure of the anal canal.
2. The muscular sling often suffers ischaemic degeneration after it has been inserted, and becomes an inert fibrous band.

3. The procedure is neither simple nor free of complications.
4. Even "successful" transpositions fail to provide any degree of symptomatic improvement because the patient is unable to learn how to "use" the muscle.
5. large individual experience has to be built up to enable a surgeon to perfect his selection for, and technique of, the operation; suitable cases do not present often enough for most surgeons to acquire the necessary experience.

Because most patients who undergo the gracilis sling operation have congenitally defective sphincters, the great majority of these operations are carried out in children. Such patients are most likely to have an acceptable result because their tissues are supple and well vascularised, and the ability to adapt to an abnormal physiological requirement is greatest in infancy and early childhood. However, a few patients reach adult life with an established colostomy because no attempt has been made to reconstruct a deficient or absent anal canal. In such mainly young patients, the prospect of continuing problems over many years can motivate them to accept the chance of some degree (at least) of defaecatory control that is offered by a gracilis sling. Such patients are also sufficiently determined to overcome initial problems after the operation, and to work through any complications towards an acceptable result.

Because spinally innervated somatic muscle can only be relied upon to produce intermittent, short-lived "bursts" of increased tonus, and such contractions can be repeated only a certain number of times (10–12) before muscle fatigue sets in, there are limits to the usefulness of the procedure unless some degree of adaptation of function takes place. This adaptation undoubtedly occurs in some patients (especially when they are young) who can then be fully continent at all times. Adaptation can be encouraged by a long course of pre-operative gracilis exercises. More usually, some degree of nocturnal incontinence

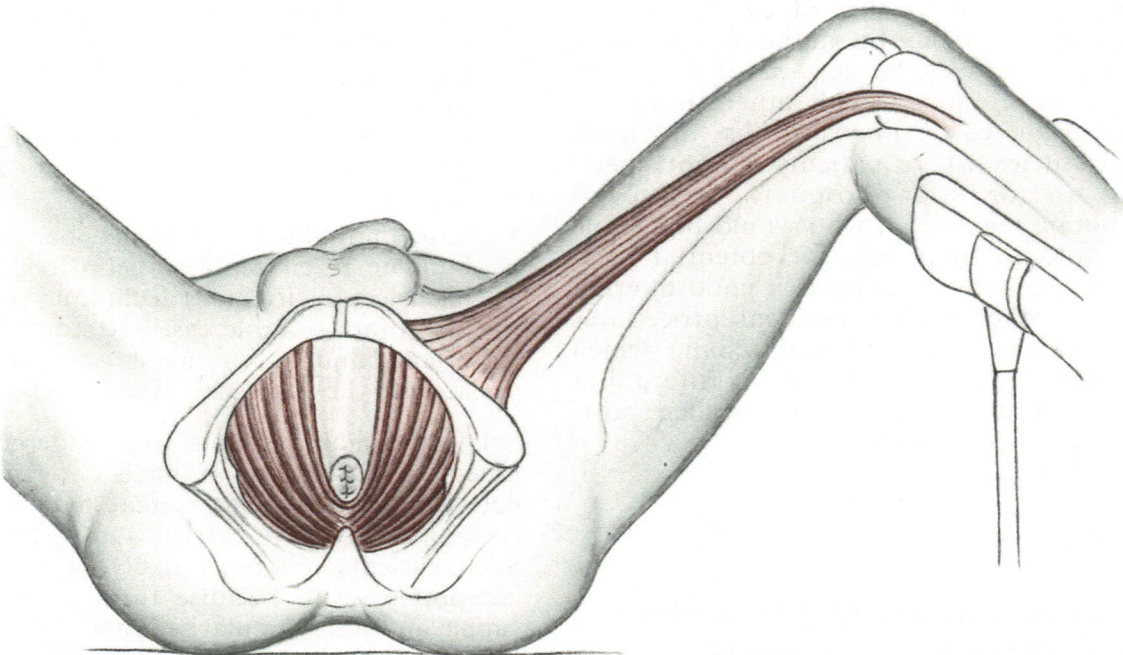

Fig. 6.11. With the patient in lithotomy position, the position of each gracilis muscle can be envisaged, and the "wrap-around" procedure planned. Access to the gracilis muscles is easiest in the lithotomy position, with the legs held in Lloyd-Davies supports.

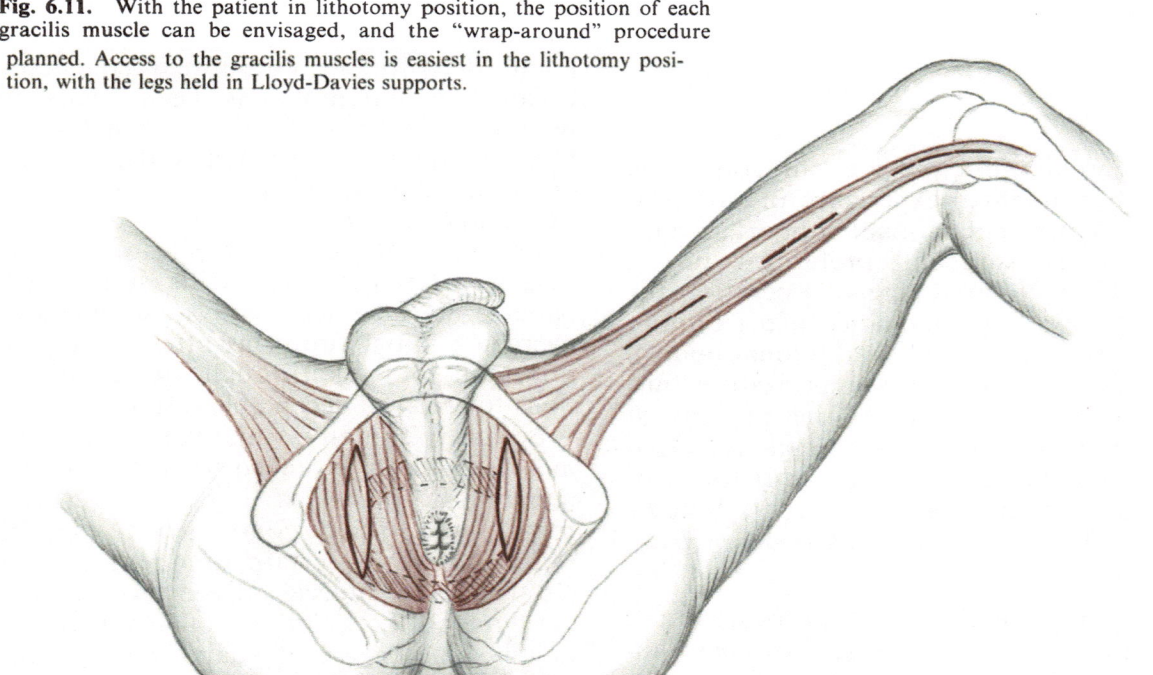

Fig. 6.12. Each (or only one) gracilis muscle is freed, if necessary through several small skin incisions along its length. The incisions into the ischiorectal fossae on each side of the anus should be generous. The authors recommend a generous ischiorectal incision rather than a separate incision for reattachment of gracilis at the end of the operation. The tendinous attachment of gracilis is divided as near as possible to the tibia in order to preserve its entire length: pulling the tendon taut before it is cut is essential. Many surgeons use anterior and posterior incisions rather than lateral incisions, but this is a matter of preference.

persists after a gracilis sling insertion, and patients usually require a pad at all times. Recently, in an attempt to achieve sustained muscle contraction (and possibly also to speed up adaptation) implanted portable nerve stimulators have been developed, with encouraging early results (Williams) [18]. This most interesting development is fully described later (pp. 95–100).

Indications and Selection of Patients

The operation does best in young patients with a congenitally defective or absent anal sphincter. If the perineal tissues are scarred to more than a minimal degree (by trauma or sepsis) it is difficult to put in the muscle graft so that it can contract freely postoperatively. Needless to say, the integrity of the gracilis muscle(s) and its nerve supply must be guaranteed before the procedure is initiated. A young, highly motivated patient is a major factor promoting a successful outcome.

Preparation

Because most patients are young, there is little preparation needed. *However, the ability to control gracilis muscle contraction should be built up by careful supervised exercises for several months before surgery in order to obtain the best possible result.* Most adult patients already have a colostomy, but if not, the usual measures (see pp. 25, 62) to ensure a clean empty rectum are given. Per-operative antibiotic prophylaxis by weight-related intravenous gentamicin, ampicillin and metronidazole is mandatory. Because a wound haematoma followed by infection will destroy the repair, no pre- or per-operative anticoagulants should be used, but graduated compression stockings are recommended because a prolonged post-operative period of bed rest is required. Because there is always the possibility of ischaemia and necrosis of the gracilis muscle, tetanus toxoid should have

been given at a suitable time beforehand to ensure a high degree of immunity over the operative period.

Operative Technique

An indwelling catheter is not usually required. Digital examination confirms that the ano-rectum is empty before the patient is brought into the operating theatre, and if there is any residual faecal contamination an immediate rectal wash-out is given.

The operation is carried out in either the lithotomy or the prone position, according to the surgeon's preference. Draping is done in such a way as to allow proper skin preparation and the draping should allow satisfactory access to the back and inner sides of the whole of both upper legs; it is the authors' experience that this is easier to achieve in the lithotomy position with the legs in Lloyd-Davies supports. This position enables the operator to envisage the anatomy of the gracilis muscle (Fig. 6.11) and to plan appropriate incisions (Fig. 6.12). After putting on the drapes, the anus is cleaned out with "Betadine" (Napp) solution. The authors recommend a "double sling" using both gracilis muscles (rather than the technique using only one) because the "sling" effect is enhanced by using both muscles: however, it is occasionally necessary to use one muscle, and both techniques are illustrated. if only one muscle is used, it can be employed as an encircling anal sphincter, as shown (Fig. 6.17).

Deep incisions are made on each side of the anus, and tunnels are created by combined blunt and sharp dissection around the anus so that the deep extensions can be joined in front of and behind the anal canal (Fig. 6.12). All tunnels should be generous, and show allow the passage of at least two fingers in a vertical direction (Fig. 6.13). *Unless the tunnels are wide enough to allow for easy passage of the gracilis slings, the muscle may be damaged by excessive traction at the time of the operation, or throttled by compression-ischaemia afterwards. It is particularly important that any fibrous scar*

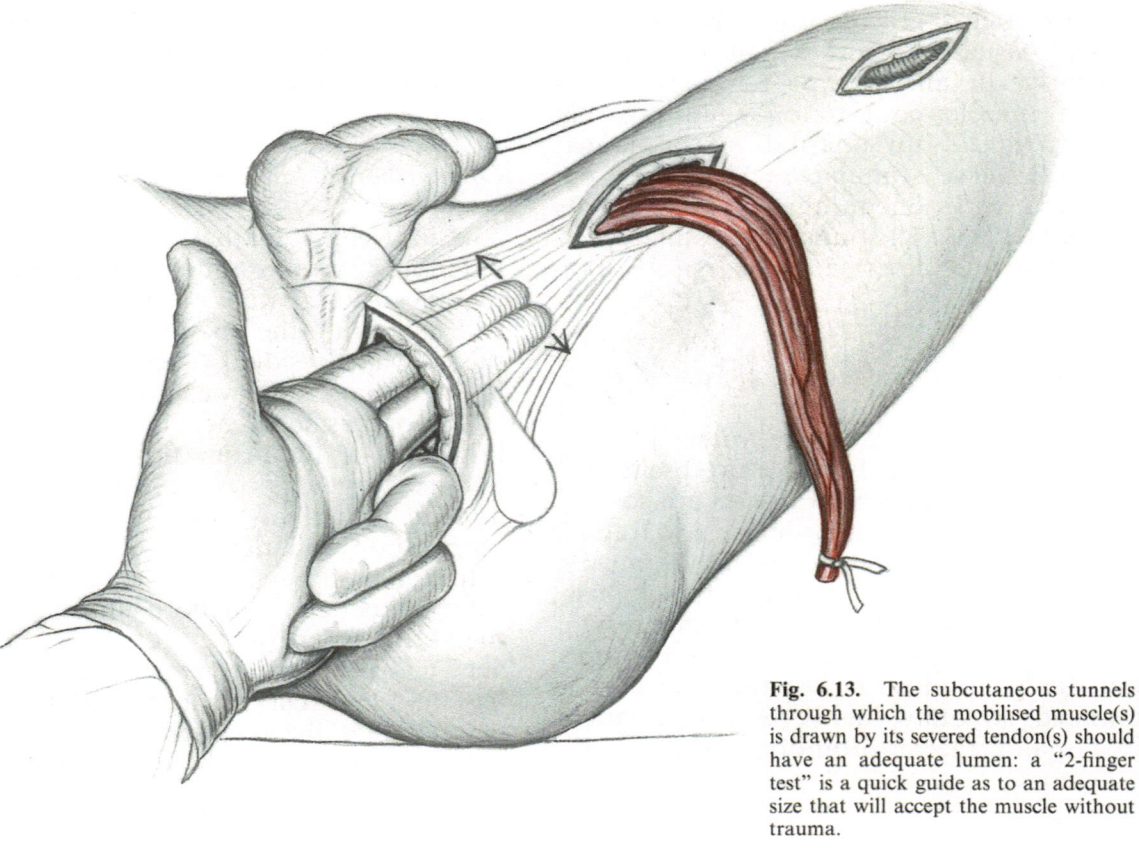

Fig. 6.13. The subcutaneous tunnels through which the mobilised muscle(s) is drawn by its severed tendon(s) should have an adequate lumen: a "2-finger test" is a quick guide as to an adequate size that will accept the muscle without trauma.

Fig. 6.14. One gracilis muscle is being drawn around the anus in the tunnels that have been created.

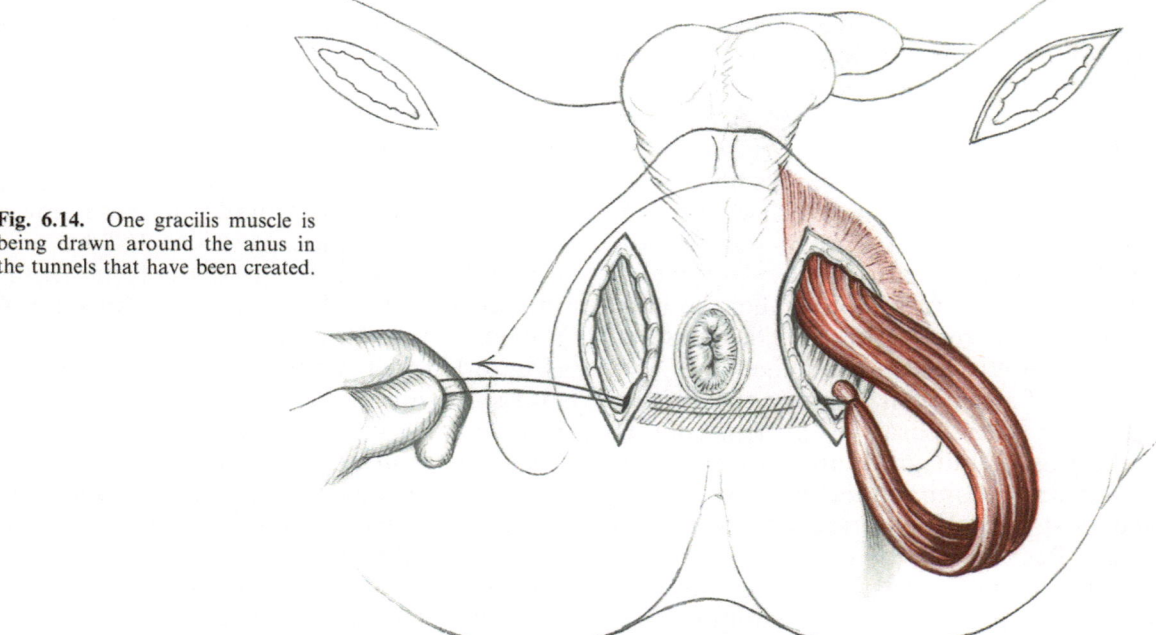

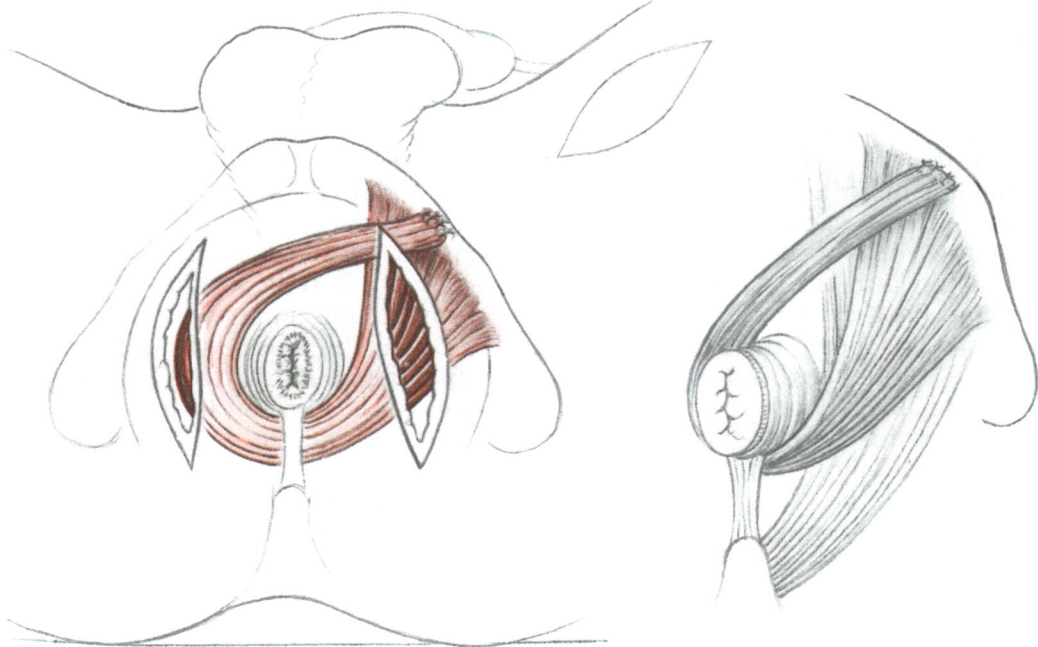

Fig. 6.15. The sling fastened (by strong unabsorbable sutures stitches) to the ischial tuberosity or (as shown here) the inferior pubic ramus. Before attachment to the periosteum, the gracilis transplant is drawn taut by adduction of the thighs, and any redundant muscle is discarded. It is clear from the illustrations that attachment to the ischial tuberosity is preferable (if the muscle is long enough) as the encirclement is then complete.

Fig. 6.16. The completion of a "double-sling" technique.

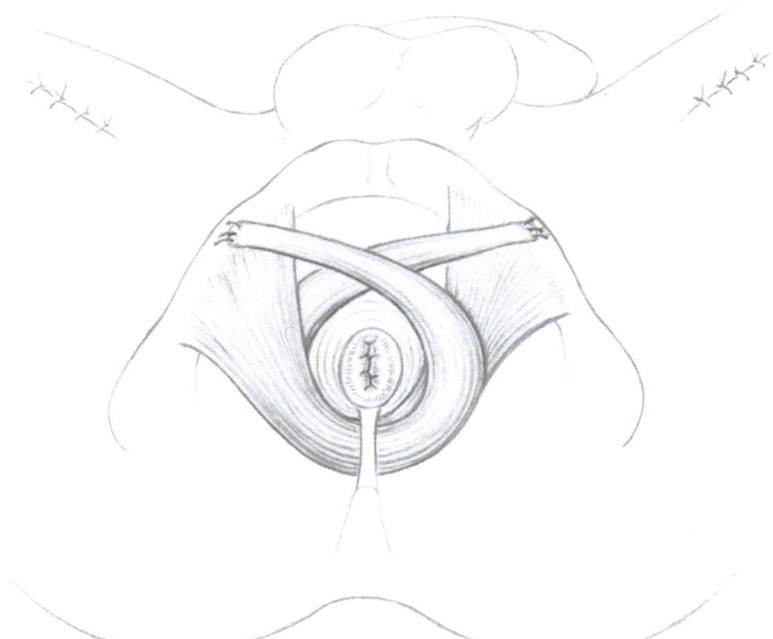

tissue should be cut back generously so that there is reduced likelihood that the slings will be tethered by post-operative adhesions.

Through separate short longitudinal incisions down the thigh, and another cut close to its attachment to the tibia (Fig. 6.12), a suitable length of each gracilis muscle is freed to allow for it to be withdrawn by its severed tendon into the peri-anal tunnel at the sides and back of the ano-rectum. After each muscle has been threaded forwards through the tunnel around the posterior aspect of the anal canal (Fig. 6.14), it is forcibly drawn forwards again to be reattached by silk stitches to periosteum of the lower surface of the ischial tuberosity or the inferior pubic ramus (Fig. 6.15). The thighs are adducted and the muscle is drawn tight before it is attached; any excess muscle is discarded once suitable tension has been achieved. If both muscles are used, a reassuringly strong, wide posterior band

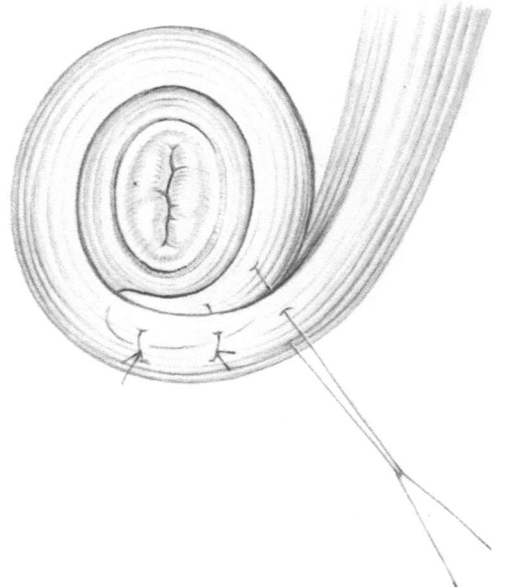

Fig. 6.17. In some cases, the muscle can be wrapped fully round the anus (as shown) and secured by an overlapping suture technique to itself (cf. technique of sphincter repair: Chap. 8). If a double-sling technique has been employed, fastening the ends of the muscles to each other may be the most desirable method of anchoring the transposed muscles.

of muscular support is provided to the back and sides of the anal tube (Fig. 6.16). Because the muscles are pulled through under some tension, the anal canal is kept closed "passively" by a mechanical squeezing effect, as well as by the usual voluntary contractile efforts for enhanced short-lived effects to keep the anus closed. If a single muscle of short length is used, it is better to wrap it fully around the anal canal to provide circumferential support, and to refasten the muscle to itself by overlapping stitching as illustrated (Fig. 6.17) (N.B. the muscle is almost always long enough to wrap around the anus and be attached to the ischial tuberosity). During all the manoeuvres to bring the mobilised lengths of muscle through the wounds and around the anal tube, the muscle must not be twisted or necrosis is inevitable. Digital examination on the operating table after the slings have been completed should confirm that a finger can be inserted easily up to the second knuckle and has the sensation of being firmly gripped. If the anal lumen feels restricted, gentle daily anal dilation by the finger will be immediately required (i.e. starting the day after surgery) to ensure an adequate lumen. The continued integrity of the sutures should be carefully conserved when this is necessary, by graduating the degree of dilatation, starting with the 5th finger.

Meticulous haemostasis should be confirmed prior to wound closure. No drains are required. The wounds should be sprayed with topical povidone iodine solution and closed in layers by fine (00) chromic catgut sutures. Skin closure is by fine (00) silk or monofilament nylon stitches, but skin clips can also be used (Fig. 6.18). A light gauze dressing is applied utilising an Op-Site spray.

Despite every precaution to preserve the blood supply to the gracilis muscle during its mobilisation, necrosis can occur when it is transferred. For this reason, some surgeons now advocate mobilisation of the muscle as a separate preliminary manoevre and perform the transposition in a separate final stage (see p. 96, stage 1).

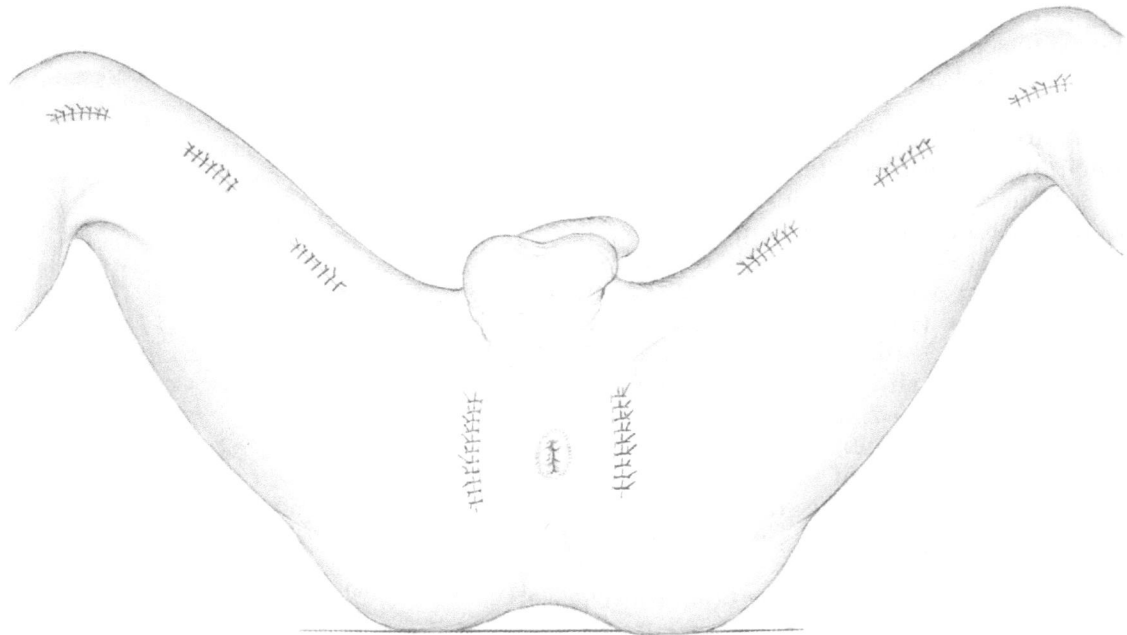

Fig. 6.18. Procedure completed and the incisions closed.

Post-operative Management

In order to avoid premature forcible contractions of the gracilis muscle in response to moving the legs (or worse still, walking) before the repair has had time to gain some strength, the patient is kept in bed for 7 post-operative days, and active leg movements are *discouraged* during this time (foot and ankle movement is *encouraged* to keep the calf-veins free of clots). Antibiotic cover is continued for 24 hours, but is not necessary thereafter unless the wound becomes inflamed, or a pyrexia develops. The patient's bowels are not confined if a colostomy is in place, but otherwise the stools are kept semi-solid by giving Milpar, 25 ml two or three times daily, for the first 7 days, and continued thereafter in doses as required to keep the stools soft and the rectum empty. Early faecal impaction will ruin the result of the procedure and must be prevented by additional enemas if indicated. Stitches are removed on the 7th and 8th post-operative days when skin healing is firm. The patient is gradually mobilised from the 8th day onward, but is not allowed to leave hospital until rectal evacuation is being achieved.

If a colostomy has been put up prior to the operation, this can be closed before the patient leaves hospital (or at a later date if the surgeon feels that extra time is desirable before the sling is tested by restoring the faecal stream). If the patient is young, and the operation has caused considerable pain, it is better to wait until digital examination is entirely painless, and the child's confidence has returned, before closing the colostomy.

Results

These are unpredictable but Corman has had very respectable results in his series (8 out of 14 patients had "good" or "excellent" results). In the case of a child with unscarred peri-anal tissues and some remnant of sphincter muscle, the gracilis sling operation can restore continence. Meticulous post-operative care and the support of an intelligent and dominant mother can make success more likely. In young adults, physiological pelvic floor and other exercises to promote gracilis contraction combined with bio-feedback programmes, can also materially improve an early result that is "disappointing". The "funnel anus" deformity (see p. 9) is a type of case where a reasonable result can be expected with confidence. For patients with considerable scarring as a result of trauma or infection, or who have no normal anal sphincter muscle (e.g. the "high" anal congenital deformity), disappointment is usual after the gracilis sling operation. Overall, no more than 50% of such cases will experience any improvement, and fewer than 20% will have control of semi-solid or fluid stools. It is rare for flatus incontinence to be restored in any patient by a gracilis sling carried out in adult life.

In a few patients in whom the muscle transplant clearly fails (in that no actively contracting gracilis sling muscle can be detected post-operatively) a fibrous narrowing of the anal canal develops. Some patients are able to "hold" an enema as a result of such stenosis, and can then keep themselves clean by using a distal wash-out technique on a daily or thrice-weekly basis: such patients may prefer this to a colostomy, and be satisfied that some positive help has been obtained from the operation.

References and Further Reading

1. Bellomo R (1988) Sphincter incontinence: a personal technique. Colo-Proctology 10: 383
2. Corman ML (1980) Follow-up evaluation of gracilis muscle transposition for faecal incontinence. Dis Colon Rectum 23: 552
3. Corman ML (1983) The management of anal incontinence. Surg Clin North Am 63: 177
4. Corman ML (1985) Gracilis muscle transposition for anal incontinence: late results. Br J Surg 72: (Suppl) pp 21–22
5. Corman ML (1989) Colon and rectal surgery, 2nd edn. Lippincott, Philadelphia, pp 192–200
6. Gabriel WB (1963) The principles and practice of rectal surgery, 5th edn. HK Lewis, London, pp 106–132
7. Goligher J (1985) Surgery of the anus, rectum and colon, 5th edn. Ballière Tindall, London, pp 257–260
8. Horn HR, Schoetz DJ Jr, Coller JA, Veidenheimer MC (1985) Sphincter repair with a silastic sling for anal incontinence and rectal procidentia. Dis Colon Rectum 28: 868
9. Kalisman M, Sharzer LA (1981) Anal sphincter reconstruction and perineal resurfacing with a gracilis myocutaneous flap. Dis Colon Rectum 24: 529
10. Labow SB, Rubin RJ, Hoexter B, Salvati EP (1980) Perineal repair of rectal procidentia with an elastic fabric sling. Dis Colon Rectum 23: 467
11. Labow SB, Hoexter B, Moseson MD et al. (1985) Modification of silastic sling repair for rectal procidentia and anal incontinence. Dis Colon Rectum 28: 684
12. Mann A (1970) Gracilis anoplasty: report of a successful case. Aust NZ J Surg 39: 405
13. Mann CV, Hoffman C (1988) Complete rectal prolapse: the anatomical and functional results of treatment by an extended abdominal rectopexy. Br J Surg 175: 34
14. Pickrell K, Broadbent TR, Masters FW, Metzger JJ (1952) Construction of a rectal sphincter and restoration of anal continence by transplanting gracilis muscle: a report of 4 cases in children. Ann Surg 135: 853
15. Plumley P (1966) A modification to Thiersch's operation for rectal prolapse. Br J Surg 53: 624
16. Saraffof D (1937) Ein einfaches ungerfahrliches Verfahren zur operativen Behandlung des Mastdarnvorfalles. Arch Klin Chir 190: 219
17. Thiersch K (1891) quoted by Carrasoo AB (1934) Contribution à l'étude du prolapse du rectum. Masson, Paris
18. Williams NS, Hallan RI, Koeze TH, Watkins ES (1989) Construction of a neo-rectum and neo-anal sphincter following previous proctocolectomy. Br J Surg 76: 1191

Stimulated Graciloplasty

by B.J. Mander and N.S. Williams

General Introduction

Pickrell first described the technique of unstimulated graciloplasty in man[1]. It is unlikely that the unstimulated graciloplasty functions in any way other than as a biological Thiersch wire. It is impossible for the majority of patients to maintain appropriate voluntary contraction and thus to control the function of the sphincter muscle. It is also the case that the gracilis muscle contains predominantly type II muscle fibres[2] which characteristically fatigue rapidly and consequently sustained muscle contraction is not possible. Pioneering studies in the 1970's indicated that the application of chronic electrical stimulation (CES) to skeletal muscle converts it to a predominantly type 1 muscle capable of sustained contraction without fatigue[3]. In addition the incorporation of CES provides a mechanism to achieve continuous involuntary muscle contraction. Two groups, Baeten in Holland and Williams in England, simultaneously set about investigating the feasibility of constructing an electrically stimulated gracilis neosphincter. Baeten *et al.* reported a case of a young woman who had previously had an unsuccessful Pickrell-type gracilis sling for congenital faecal incontinence[4]. Williams *et al.* reported a preliminary series of six patients with faecal incontinence[5]. They also used the technique in two patients as part of a reconstruction procedure with a coloperineal anastomosis in one[6] and an ileal pouch-perineal anastomosis in the other[7]. These preliminary studies established the feasibility of using the procedure to treat patients with incontinence arising from a variety of aetiologies. However the results were inconsistent and there was considerable morbidity. The technique has undergone a variety of modifications to make it more reliable.

Indications and Selection of Patients

The electrically stimulated gracilis neoanal sphincter can be used for:

1. Incontinence patients with a damaged or denervated sphincter mechanism but who have an intact anorectum. Construction of a neosphincter is indicated if a conventional operation has failed or is contraindicated
2. Patients with anorectal agenesis who have undergone pull-through procedures and suffer from incontinence
3. A selected group of patients who have undergone abdominoperineal excision of the rectum for cancer, in whom there should be no evidence of local recurrence or distant metastases. In these patients a coloperineal anastomosis is constructed prior to neosphincter construction

The technique should not be used for:

1. Patients whose gracilis muscle is damaged or not normally innervated. If there is any doubt preoperative electromyography should be performed to establish that the gracilis muscle is normal
2. Patients with disseminated malignancy or local pelvic recurrence
3. Patients lacking the manual dexterity to control the stimulator with a magnet
4. Persistent perineal sepsis or Crohn's disease
5. The presence of a cardiac pacemaker

Care should be taken before undertaking the procedure in patients with coexistent severe evacuatory difficulties as these may prevent a satisfactory result.

Preparation

All patients require extensive counseling before undergoing the procedure. The technique is performed in stages and this, together with the muscle training protocol, places considerable demands on the patient and their relatives. The principles of the technique, the postoperative regime and any potential complications are fully discussed prior to surgery. All patients are warned that they may end up with a permanent stoma. The patients are shown the stimulators and provided with appropriate literature. After a period of reflection the patient should be encouraged to return for further discussion and where possible they should meet a patient of a similar age who has undergone the procedure.

Once the decision has been made a site is chosen for the stimulator. This is usually placed in a subcutaneous pocket overlying the lower ribs anteriorly. The exact site will depend on patient shape and to some degree patient preference. The stimulator is invariably placed on the opposite side to the covering stoma. Both sites are then marked with indelible ink.

Patients should receive thromboembolic prophylaxis during all stages of the procedure in the form of subcutaneous heparin, 5000 units twice daily. Full bowel preparation is required for Stages 2 and 3. Prior to the procedure patients are restricted to fluids for 48 h and given two sachets of picolax the day prior to surgery. Antibiotic prophylaxis is provided by metronidazole and cefuroxime sodium for Stage 1 and metronidazole, ampicillin and gentamicin for Stages 2 and 3. For Stages 1 and 3 one dose is given at induction and two further doses postoperatively. For Stage 2 antibiotic cover should continue for 5 days.

No muscle relaxation should be used by the anaesthetist during Stage 2 of the procedure. Such agents make it impossible to observe muscle contraction during nerve stimulation and will make it extremely difficult to reliably identify the nerve to the gracilis.

Operative Technique

Stage 1. The patient is placed in the modified Lloyd-Davies position with both hips abducted. The contralateral leg to the covering stoma is prepared using povidone–iodine.

A 10 cm longitudinal incision is made on the medial aspect of the thigh along a line connecting the medial femoral condyle to the inferior public ramus. The distal limit of the incision should be 2 cm above the medial femoral condyle. The skin incision is deepened, the fascia lata incised and the gracilis muscle identified. The muscle is the most superficial of the abductors and has a posterior tendon at its distal end. The sartorius muscle arches over the distal part of the gracilis prior to its insertion on the tibia further aiding identification. The distal third of the gracilis muscle is then mobilised by ligating the two or three distal vessels that enter the muscle on its lateral surface. The wound is closed using a continuous 2/0 chromic catgut suture for the fascia lata and a continuous subcuticular 3/0 polypropylene suture for the skin. A covering stoma is usually created at this stage. The authors' preference is for a laparoscopically assisted right iliac fossa loop ileostomy.

The vascular delay procedure was introduced to reduce the likelihood of perineal sepsis associated with distal muscle ischaemia which was a problem in the early stages of the development of the procedure. The small distal vessels are inevitably sacrificed at transposition. Their ligation opens up arterio–arterial communicating channels from the main proximal vascular pedicle thereby ensuring good distal muscle perfusion following transposition. Since the introduction of the delay technique we have not experienced further problems with muscle ischaemia. Other groups undertake transposition without pre-preparing the muscle and it may be that the complications related to ischaemia were part of the learning curve associated with the technique. Current research is being undertaken to determine if this additional step is still necessary.

Stage 2 is undertaken 6–8 weeks after Stage 1 with the patient in the modified Lloyd-Davies position. The patient is catheterised and the thigh, abdomen and perineum are shaved and disinfected with povidone–iodine. The previous thigh incision is opened and extended proximally and laterally to curve over the tendinous origin of adductor longus. The tendon of the gracilis muscle is traced distally and divided with strong scissors as close as possible to its insertion on the tibia. The tendon is then clamped with a pair of artery forceps which are then used to exert some distraction on the muscle facilitating proximal mobilisation towards the main vascular pedicle. Any peripheral vessels not divided at the delay procedure are ligated and all the areolar tissue overlying the muscle and attaching it to the deeper muscles is divided. The main vascular pedicle is identified as it enters the lateral border of the muscle, usually at the junction of the proximal third and distal two-thirds of the muscle. It consists of an artery and two venae commitantes. Once identified the pedicle is mobilised back to its point of exit from the adductor longus muscle with great care. The peripheral branches of the nerve to the gracilis muscle lying directly on top of the main vascular pedicle can be identified by means of a nerve stimulator to ensure their preservation. The muscle is then mobilised proximally to its origin on the lower half of the body of the pubic symphysis and the inferior pubic ramus.

The main nerve to the gracilis is sought by entering the plane between the adductor longus and the adductor brevis approximately 3 cm proximal to the main vascular pedicle. The nerve is a continuation of the anterior division of the obturator nerve and crosses the adductor brevis from lateral to medial (Fig. 6.19). Identification of the nerve is confirmed by eliciting a contraction of the gracilis using a disposable nerve stimulator (set at 0.5 V). The areolar tissue on either side of the nerve is carefully cleared and the site for electrode implantation chosen before the nerve divides into its terminal branches.

A 2 cm incision is then made approximately 5 cm above the mid-inguinal point on the side on which the muscle has been

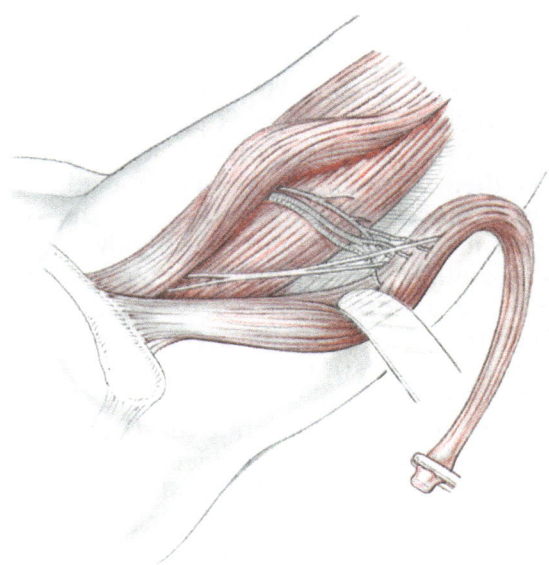

Fig. 6.19. The main vascular pedicle of the gracilis muscle and the main nerve supply which crosses the adductor brevis muscle from lateral to medial.

mobilised. A pair of long artery forceps is passed under the adductor longus and carefully tunneled subcutaneously until its tip emerges through the skin incision. The tip of the electrode (NICE) is grasped between the jaws of the artery forceps and gently drawn down the subcutaneous tunnel so that it emerges parallel to the main nerve.

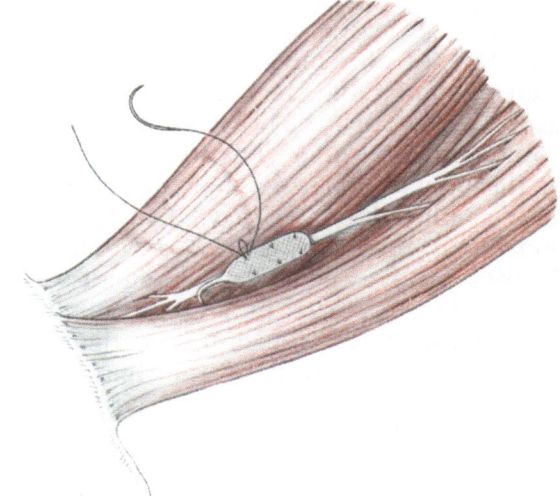

Fig. 6.20. The attachment of the stimulating electrode to the main nerve to gracilis muscle parallel to its long axis.

The electrode plate is sutured over the main nerve parallel to the long axis of the nerve using six interrupted 3/0 silk sutures (Fig. 6.20). Each suture is passed through a hole on the periphery of the electrode plate and then through the underlying adductor brevis muscle and back through the plate to ensure that the knots lie on the surface of the plate. Great care is taken to ensure that the underlying nerve is not damaged. Once the position of the electrode is correct all the sutures are tied.

A transverse incision is made approximately 5 cm in length over the anterior lower ribs in the mid-clavicular line at the position previously marked. The incision is then dissected inferiorly to create a pocket for the purpose designed implant (NICE). A tunneller with the trocar *in situ* is introduced through the lower incision above the groin and advanced superficially to emerge into the pocket. The trocar is removed from its covering tube and the proximal end of the lead is threaded through the tube to emerge in the upper incision (Fig. 6.21). The tube is then withdrawn and the proximal end of the electrode connected to the stimulator as follows.

The connector part of the lead is first threaded through a silicon boot which is everted to expose the connections. The four screws on the superior surface of the stimulator are then released and the connector part of the lead is then fully pushed into the port of the implant. The screws are then tightened and the silicone boot levered over the top of the implant and pressed home with the roller. The implant is placed in the pocket ensuring that any redundant lead is placed posteriorly. The transverse incision is then closed with a subcuticular 3/0 polypropylene stitch. The small wound in the groin is closed in a similar manner.

Two curvilinear incisions are then made approximately 2 cm from the right and left margins of the anal verge. A circumferential subcutaneous tunnel around the anal canal, lateral to any remaining sphincter, is created and deepened to accommodate the gracilis. The skin bridges anteriorly and posteriorly are preserved. Care must be

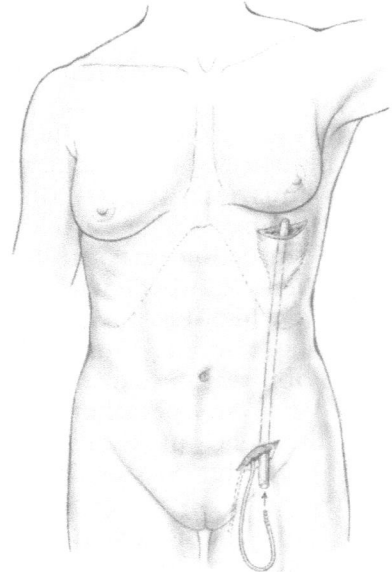

Fig. 6.21. The trochar being threaded from the groin incision to the upper incision over the chest. Once in place, the electrical leads from the stimulator are passed through the trochar. Once in place, the stimulator can be switched "on" and "off" using a surface magnet. During the periods when anal closure is required, the stimulator is set at the required level to maintain continence by persistent subtetanic impulses.

exercised when making the anterior dissection in women. There is often considerable scarring between the vagina and rectum. The dissection is aided by infiltrating the plane with a weak solution of adrenaline (ephedrin) in saline (1:300 000).

Using careful sharp dissection with scissors the plane is opened anterior to the rectum sufficient to pass a Jacques catheter which can then be used as a retractor. The dissection is then deepened under direct vision. A headlight may facilitate vision at this stage. Meticulous care is taken to ensure haemostasis.

A further incision is made in the skin crease between the thigh and buttock on the same side as the prepared muscle. A tunnel is then created via this incision to emerge close to the upper part of the mobilised gracilis muscle. It is necessary to divide Scarpa's fascia with scissors. The tunnel is widened until it accommodates at least three figures. A similar tunnel is then created from this incision to that on the lateral side of the anal verge.

Using a pair of long artery forceps attached to the distal tendon of the gracilis muscle the muscle is then transposed to the perineum through the carefully created tunnels (Fig. 6.22). Care is taken to ensure it does not become twisted during its transposition. The muscle is then brought around the anal canal in a gamma configuration (Fig. 6.23). A small incision is then made over the contralateral ischial tuberosity and deepened to periosteum. Three interrupted 0 ethibond sutures on a J-shaped needle are then passed through the periosteum and clipped.

The ipsilateral leg is then abducted to the midline and the muscle pulled through its tunnels until it sufficient tight around the anal canal i.e. it should allow the insertion of the tip of the index finger. The tendon

of the gracilis is then sutured to the ischial tuberosity using ethibond sutures.

The stimulator is then programmed using telemetry to check that contraction effects occlusion of the anal orifice. All wounds are sprayed with an antibiotic spray (Tribiotic). The leg would is closed in layers, continuous 2/0 chromic catgut to the fascia lata and 3/0 subcuticular polypropylene for the skin.

Postoperative Care Following Stage 2

The patient is nursed with the legs together for the first 3 days and is then encouraged to mobilise. Electrical stimulation commences on approximately the 10th postoperative day once all the wounds have healed. The muscle is "trained" using a gradually increasing duty cycle over the fol-

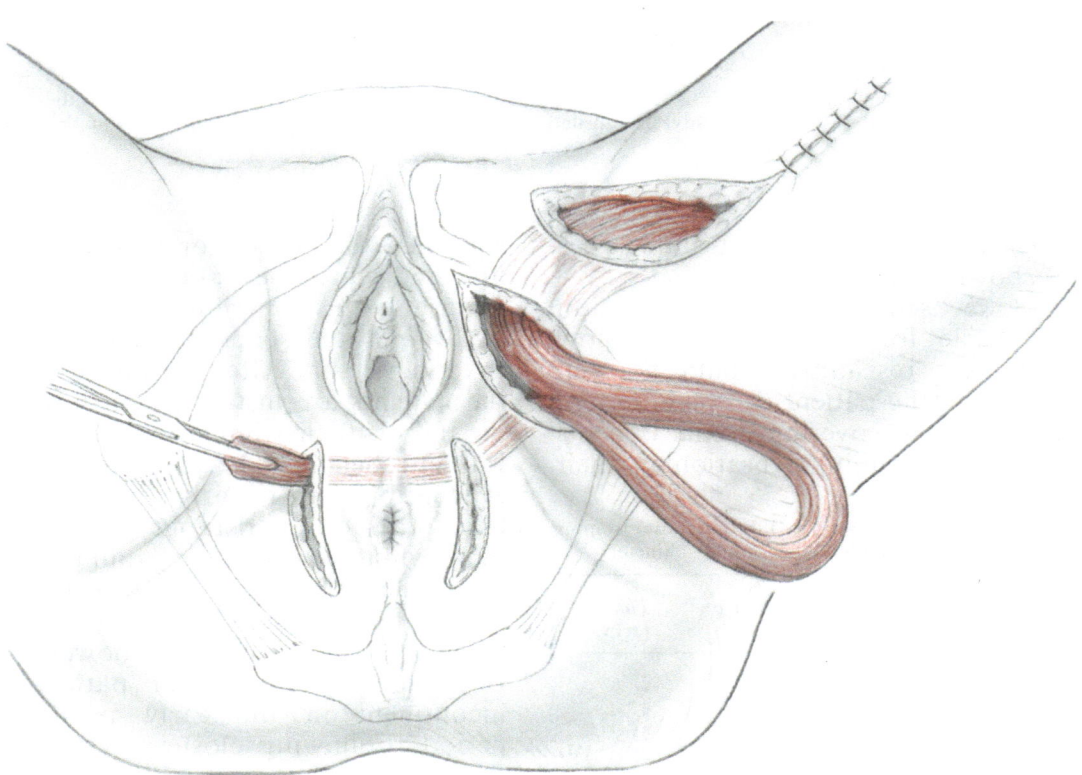

Fig. 6.22. During transposition of the gracilis muscle through the perineal tunnels, great care must be taken to preserve the alignment of the muscle and to prevent traction damage to the vascular pedicle and/or to the nerve of the muscle.

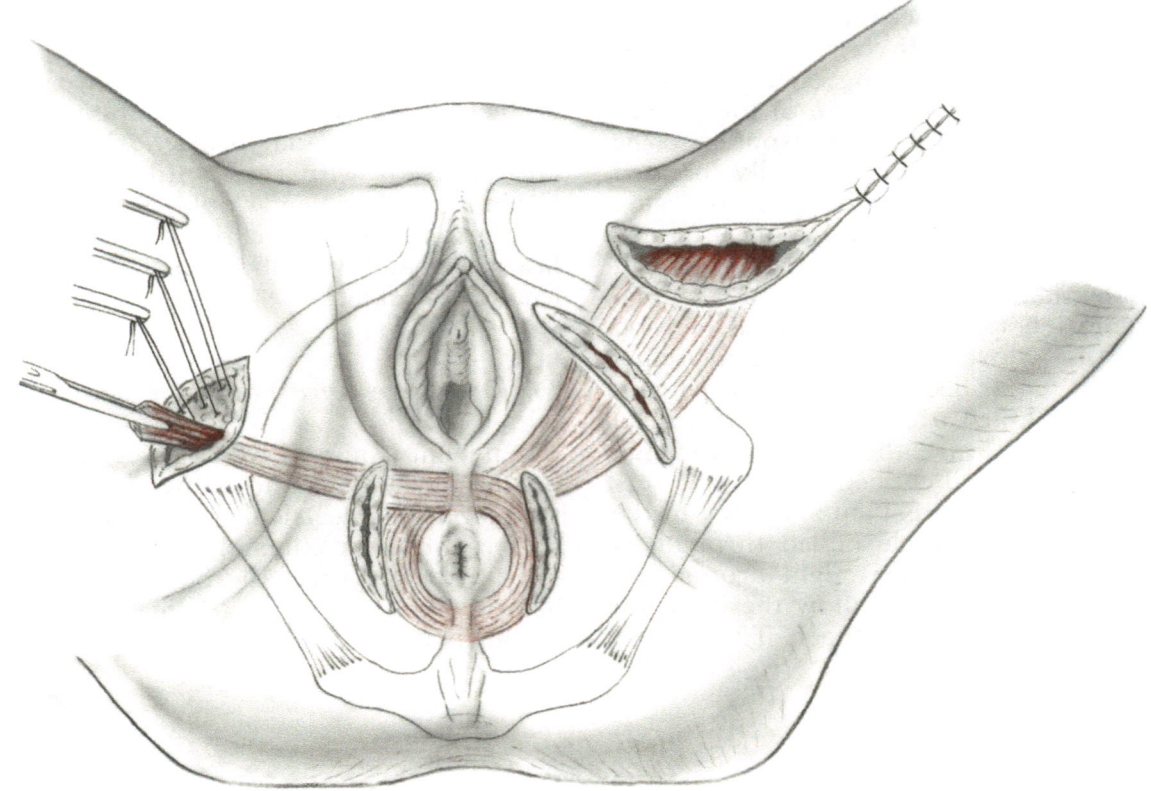

Fig. 6.23. The gamma configuration that is used to surround the anus, and the muscle is then tightened to the appropriate degree prior to fixation to the ischial tuberosity. The ipsilateral leg is adducted (not shown) before the muscle is sutured to the ischial tuberosity.

lowing 12 weeks. The current training protocol is shown in Table 6.1.

After 8 weeks the process of conversion of the muscle form fast-twitch to slow twitch (fatigue resistant) should be well under way and the patient can be admitted for closure of their covering stoma. Patients usually report a pulling sensation in their

leg when the stimulator is switched on at first and when the parameters are altered. Invariably this consciousness is short lived.

Stage 3. This consists of closure of the covering stoma. After closure of the stoma the patients are instructed on how to turn on and off their stimulators with a magnet. Initially their may be problems with rectal evacuation, particularly in patients who have previously undergone post-anal repair or in whom a history of straining predated their incontinence. Such problems can usually be overcome with a combination of suppositories, enemas and bowel training. It is not uncommon for patients to be incontinent in the early post-operative period. Following closure of their stoma stool consistency is usually very loose but they should be reassured that this is likely to be temporary.

Table 6.1 Electrical parameters used during initial training of the electrically stimulated gracilis neoanal sphincter

Weeks	Pulse width (ms)	Frequency (Hz)	Time on (secs)	Time off (secs)
0–2	210	9	1	6
2–4	210	12	2	4
4–6	210	12	4	4
6–8	210	12	4	2
8–10	210	12	4	1
10 onwards	210	12	continuous	

Results

Physiological and histochemical studies on the patients confirm that the neosphincter acts as a truly dynamic sphincter capable of sustained contraction[8]. This adaptation of the muscle is a consequence of long-term stimulation and reverses if stimulation ceases. Sustained sphincter pressures of greater than 60 cm H_2O are reported after 18 months of stimulation. The results of this technique depend enormously on the aetiology of the underlying incontinence. Williams has reported a series of 20 patients with incontinence arising as a consequence of a deficient sphincter mechanisms[9]. In six of the patients the operation was unsuccessful but in 60% good levels of continence were achieved. The results in patients with a congenital aetiology or following abdominoperineal excision are less good. There is undoubtedly a learning curve associated with the procedure. Baeten's group in Maastricht have reported overall continence rates of 73% in 52 patients followed-up for a median of 2.1 years[10]. In patients with a pure sphincter defect good continence was achieved in 92%. Continence rates were less good in patients with associated abnormalities of anorectal sensation, those with congenital incontinence and cauda equina lesions. It is our experience that in patients with impaired sensitivity, although good closure of the anal canal can be achieved with a neosphincter, the inability to sense impending egress of faeces may result in overflow incontinence.

The procedure of the electrically stimulated gracilis neoanal sphincter has provided relief from incontinence for a significant number of patients who would otherwise have ended up with a permanent stoma. Approximately 65% of patients have a good result. At present the published series are small and the length of follow-up short. Questions regarding the long-term efficacy of the procedure and the robustness of the electronic hardware will only be answered with longer follow-up.

References

1. Pickrell KL, Broadbent TR, Masters FW, Metzger J.J. (1952) Construction of a rectal sphincter and restoration of anal continence by transplanting the gracilis muscle in four cases in children. Annals of Surgery 135: 835

2. Schwartz MS, Swash M, Ryan J (1991) Why is the gracilis muscle relatively uninvolved in neuromuscular disorders? Neuromusc Dis 1: 365

3. Salmons S, Vrbova G (1969) The influence of activity on the contractile characteristics of mammalian fast and slow muscle. J Physiol 201: 535–549

4. Baeten C, Spaans F, Fluks A (1988) An implanted neuromuscular stimulator for fecal continence following previously implanted gracilis muscle. Report of a case. Dis Colon Rectum 31: 134

5. Williams NS, Hallan RI, Koeze TH, Pilot MA, Watkins ES (1990) Construction of a Neoanal Sphincter By Transposition of the Gracilis Muscle and Prolonged Neuromuscular Stimulation For the Treatment of Fecal Incontinence. Ann Roy Coll Surge Engl 72: 108

6. Williams NS, Hallan RI, Koeze TH, Watkins ES (1990) Restoration of gastrointestinal continuity and continence after abdominoperineal excision of the rectum using an electrically stimulated neoanal sphincter. Dis Colon Rectum 33: 561

7. Williams NS, Hallan RI, Koeze TH, Watkins ES (1989) Construction of a neorectum and neoanal sphincter following previous proctocolectomy [see comments]. Br J Surg 76: 1191

8. George BD, Williams NS, Patel J, Swash M, Watkins ES (1993) Physiological and Histochemical Adaptation of the Electrically Stimulated Gracilis Muscle to Neoanal Sphincter Function. Br J Surg 80: 1342

9. Williams NS, Patel J, George BD, Hallan RI, Watkins ES (1991) Development of an electrically stimulated neoanal sphincter. Lancet 338 (8776): 1166

10. Baeten CG, Geerdes BP, Adang EM, Heineman E, Konsten J, Engel GL, et al. (1995) Anal dynamic graciloplasty in the treatment of intractable fecal incontinence. New Engl J Med 332: 1600

CHAPTER 7

Per-anal Techniques

General Introduction

There are very few per-anal techniques for the treatment of faecal incontinence that have withstood long-term scrutiny of the results [8,13]. If the causes of the incontinence combine not only the presence of an ano-rectal abnormality but also a weak anal sphincter (e.g. as in many patients with rectal mucosal prolapse or third degree haemorrhoids) *a per-anal technique that involves forcible dilation of the anal orifice may be contra-indicated.*

However, some per-anal techniques for incontinence have proved useful for special situations. Mucous leakage can be caused by anterior mucosal prolapse (or a rectocele) and this can be alleviated by the operation of *mucosectomy*. In some of these patients the prolonged straining that is produced by the presence of the mucosal bolus (which impacts in the upper anal canal) can aggravate anal sphincter inhibition, and this also will be helped by removing the redundant tissue and so further diminishing the tendency to mucous seepage. In addition to mucous leakage, a rectocele can

divert a faecal bolus into its "pouch", to be subsequently leaked independently of defaecation: a situation of "after-defeacation" very similar to "after-micturition". In cases of complete rectal prolapse associated with incontinence, *The Delorme procedure* [3,5] has proved itself a highly successful technique especially suited to elderly patients judged unfit for a major abdominal procedure: this operation removes the prolapsing mucus-secreting excess epithelium as well as providing the opportunity to plicate and thicken the muscularis propria of the rectal wall.

The operation of per-anal removal of the rectum and associated lower sigmoid colon ("*rectosigmoidectomy*") was once popular for the cure of rectal prolapse associated with faecal incontinence. When it was realised that the operation was followed by recurrence of the prolapse in almost all cases [8,13], the procedure was largely abandoned; however, there have been some favourable reports recently in specially selected patients [6]. As with the Delorme procedure, the prime indication for using the technique is the frailty of the patient. If incontinence is associated with the prolapse, combination per-anal techniques for treating the prolapse and at the same time strengthening the ano-rectal musculature are possible. It is probable that with modern anaesthetic techniques, the length of bowel that can be excised per anum is greater than in previous times when muscle relaxants, epidural anaesthesia and controlled respiration were not available; modern suture materials are also greatly superior to catgut in their ability to provide long-term anastomotic security. Therefore, although the authors have reservations about the resurrection of the rectosigmoidectomy procedure that has proved a failure in the past, they feel that the good reports currently being published from some centres justify retaining the technique in the colo-rectal armamentarium.

Anterior (Rectal) Mucosectomy [11]

Introduction

This procedure is of benefit for those patients in whom there is excessive endoluminal protrusion of the anterior rectal wall and mucosa which is symptomatic. This may occur specifically at defaecation but in many patients the protrusion is only to be found by visual inspection of the anterior rectal wall through a proctoscope. Occasionally an associated "solitary ulcer" [14] is seen with the proctoscope. The condition is more common in women probably because the anterior wall of the rectum and anus is less supported than in male patients, and if degenerative changes develop in the muscles of the pelvic floor, prolapse of the anterior rectal wall and ano-rectal mucosa may result. This is espe-cially likely in patients who strain excessively to defaecate. At first the prolapse is mucosal and produces symptoms of minor mucous leakage with moistness and irritation of the peri-anal skin, often with a secondary fungal infection. At first the condition may be alleviated by a number of conservative measures, singly or in combination. These are stool softeners, avoidance of straining at stool, sphincter exercises, the use of evacuant suppositories and protecting the perineal skin by a barrier cream. Sub-mucosal injections of phenol may help by fixing the redundant mucosa to the underlying muscle tube but improvement is usually very transient. Rubber band ligation of the excessive mucosa may similarly be of value in less severe cases.

There remains, however, a group of patients in whom the condition of anterior rectal prolapse is associated with pronounced pelvic floor weakness, disturbance of rectal function and pronounced loss of continence. In these patients excessive protrusion of the anterior rectal wall frequently blocks the upper anal canal and impedes efficient emptying. The patients complain of a sensation of obstruction and incomplete evacuation of stool as well as mucous leakage and soiling; frequent visits to the toilet are made and excessive straining merely exacerbates the symptoms. The patients may admit to digital evacuation of retained faeces as they find passing a finger into the anal canal helps to ease defaecation. Whether such digital interference reduces the prolapsed anterior mucosa or whether it relaxes paradoxical puborectalis and anal sphincter contraction on straining is a matter of debate.

The condition is often associated with other changes consequent upon the diffuse pelvic floor weakness: uterine prolapse, cystocele and bladder dysfunction. Patients often exhibit the descending perineum [12] associated with a weak pelvic floor and obstructed defaecation. Haemorrhoids are often present and a "solitary rectal ulcer" is found sometimes (see p. 20) at the apex of the prolapsing mucosal or rectal wall. There is some evidence to suggest that the initial anterior mucosal prolapse progresses to full rectal procidentia in a few cases.

Indications and Selection of Patients

Before considering anterior mucosectomy it is essential that both the surgeon and the patient realise that they are treating mainly the consequence of long-standing diffuse pelvic floor weakness frequently associated with habitual straining to defaecate [10] and that long-term precautions must be taken to minimise recurrence and progression of the disorder. Indeed the patient may require additional surgery (such as an anterior buttress repair, see pp. 49–53) to reinforce the weak and attenuated recto-vaginal septum. It is wise to explain to patients that the feelings of urgency of defaecation and of incomplete evacuation may be misleading in that they are interpreting the bolus symptoms arising from redundant mucosa and internal rectal wall prolapse as the presence of faeces; these feelings will often be accentuated in the immediate post-operative period due to oedema and tissue reaction to the internal stitches.

If a patient's main complaint is one of mucous discharge which has already failed to respond to less severe measures e.g. submucosal injections of phenol and/or rubber band ligation, anterior mucosectomy should be performed. The results of mucosectomy in this group of patients are good. The results of mucosectomy in patients who are habitual strainers with an associated obsessional psyche are much less satisfactory and the procedure should be offered with great caution as recurrence of symptoms and/or prolapse are to be expected.

Preparation

Preparation for anterior mucosectomy is the same as for a haemorrhoidectomy. The lower bowel should be emptied with a disposable phosphate enema 2 hours before surgery. Per-operative antibiotics are not required. Early ambulation is recommended post-operatively. Compression stockings should be worn to prevent thrombo-embolism.

Operative Technique

The patient is placed in the lithotomy position with the hips well flexed. The perineum is shaved and cleaned with aqueous chlorhexidine (1:200) solution. The mucosal prolapse is demonstrated by traction with two tissue forceps on the anterior and verge. By combined traction, and upward and forward pressure with the forceps, the anterior anal canal and rectal wall will come into view. Access to the anterior rectal wall is aided by insertion of an Eisenhammer rectal speculum and the prolapsing mucosa is easily seen. The anterior anal canal and rectal walls are infiltrated submucosally with a weak solution of ephedrine (adrenaline) and saline (1:300 000) (Fig. 7.1). With an assistant holding the forceps and applying traction as shown (Fig. 7.1), the mucosa

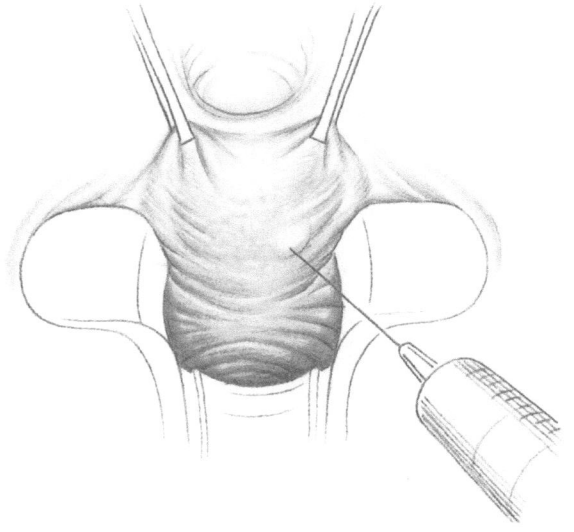

Fig. 7.1. Traction on the anterior anal verge and an Eisenhammer speculum are used to display the prolapsing tissue. A submucosal infiltration of ephedrine (1:300 000) in physiological saline is helpful to control bleeding.

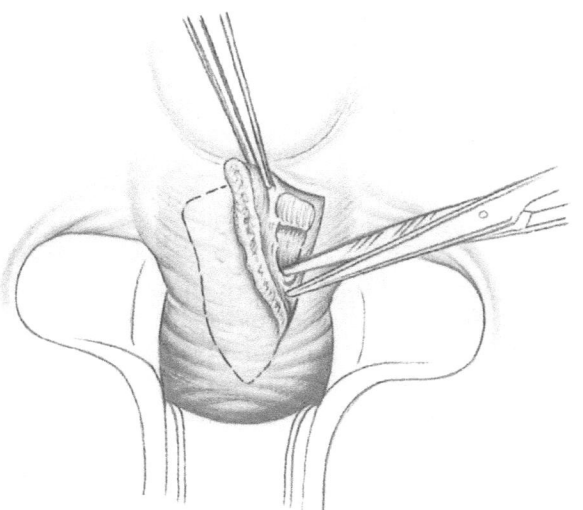

Fig. 7.2. A wide sheet of mucosa is stripped from the underlying muscularis propria of the anterior rectal wall up to high vaginal (female) or mid-prostatic (male) levels.

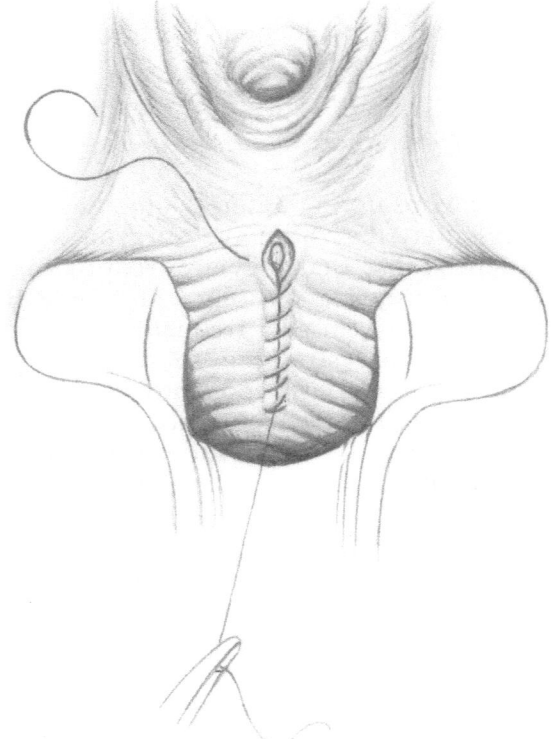

Fig. 7.4. The mucosal defect being closed with a running stitch of 00 chromic catgut. In some patients the authors additionally plicate the underlying muscularis propria of the rectal wall before the mucosal suturing is carried out.

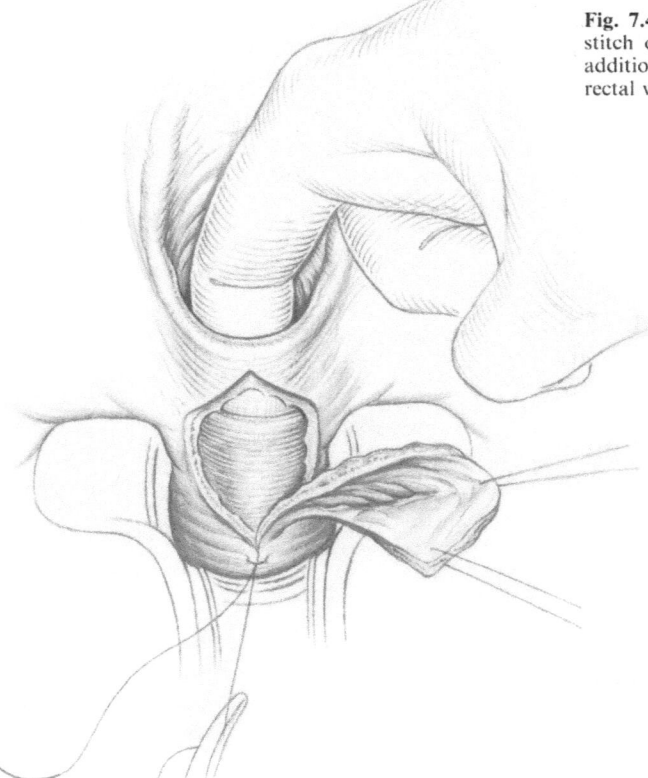

Fig. 7.3. Per-vaginal downward finger pressure can assist display of the mucosal prolapse, as shown. Note the use of a suture in the rectal wall above the apical point of the dissection to prevent retraction of the apex.

from the upper anal canal and lower rectum is stripped from the underlying circular muscle by sharp dissection (Fig. 7.2). A wide mucosal strip is freed and dissected up to approximately the upper vaginal level in females and mid prostate in males. In females a finger can be placed in the vagina and downward finger pressure on the posterior vaginal wall can help exposure by displacing the recto-vaginal septum posteriorly (Fig. 7.3). As the dissection continues the mucosal strip narrows to an apex but before amputating the mucosal strip a 00 chromic catgut stitch is put into the muscularis propria of the rectal wall just above the apical point (Fig. 7.3). This steadies and prevents retraction of the top of the dissection. The mucosa is now excised and the raw defect closed by mucosal apposition using a continuous 00 chromic catgut stitch (Fig. 7.4) after which the traction stitch can be removed. If the mucosal excision is extensive it may not be possible to close the defect, but closure is not essential as re-epithelialisation is rapid; haemostasis is better, however, if the mucosal defect can be closed. A flat pad is applied to the anus and secured by a "T" bandage to soak up any immediate post-operative discharges of blood, mucus or faeces.

Post-operative Management

Pain is usually mild after this procedure. The surgeon must remember that the patient has an underlying disorder of pelvic floor function and aperients should be prescribed as soon as the patient can take oral fluids and should be continued as needed to ensure the patient passes semi-solid or liquid stool without straining. A gentle rectal examination is performed on the fifth or sixth day to ensure the completeness of rectal evacuation and to check that stenosis will not be a problem. Evacuant suppositories may be needed to encourage normal defaecation and occasionally a disposable enema is required. Once a satisfactory bowel habit is established the patient may be discharged home. Follow-up is recom-

mended, especially in those patients with an underlying problem of a weak pelvic floor plus habitual straining. Long-term medication with stool softeners and evacuant suppositories may be required to prevent a return to a straining/prolapse sequence.

Rectal Wall Plication (Syn. Delorme Technique) [3,4,5]

Introduction

Delorme's procedure was first described in 1900 as a method of treating patients with complete rectal prolapse. Recently the Delorme technique has regained popularity and has shown itself to be an operation particularly suited to the frail patient with both complete prolapse and incontinence. It is effective in repairing rectal prolapse in a high percentage of cases and results to date show that recurrent rectal prolapse is unusual in patients who have undergone the procedure. Post-operative constipation and/or incontinence is well known in patients who undergo Ripstein or Wells procedures, and although many regain continence within 4–6 months a proportion require a second-stage perineal repair. Reports so far suggest that patients who undergo the Delorme procedure rarely suffer incontinence postoperatively, and many patients with pre-operative incontinence are cured by the operation; this may be due to the effects of stiffening the rectal wall and preventing intussusception. But the plicated rectum also sits on the ano-rectum as an easily palpable "lump" which may assist in resisting inadvertent faecal leakage.

The principle of the operation is to remove the mucosal lining of the rectal prolapse and to plicate the exposed redundant rectal muscle wall, thus reducing and fixing the prolapsed rectal intussusception. The operation (which does not open the abdominal cavity) is well tolerated by the elderly patient and can be performed under general anaesthesia or regional nerve block.

Indications and Selection of Patients

Although the Delorme procedure theoretically can be used for all patients with rectal prolapse, it is particularly suitable for very frail elderly patients who would not tolerate an abdominal rectopexy. Because post-operative nursing care is minimal, patients with mild to moderate senile dementia are also able to undergo a Delorme operation. Habitual strainers must be cured of this trait whenever possible before the operation because forcible straining in the post-operative period can disrupt the plication sutures in the rectal wall and cause early recurrence of the prolapse. The Delorme procedure is also well established for treatment of persisting incontinence after abdominal rectopexy.

Preparation

Although the operation is well-tolerated, every effort must be made to make the

patients as fit as possible to undergo a procedure which usually involves a general anaesthetic. Although the operation is possible under spinal nerve blocking analgesic anaesthesia, it has disadvantages viz: control can be lost if the patient moves or strains and the prolapse can only be pulled down to its fullest extent from below if the patient is totally relaxed. The bowel must be thoroughly cleaned out pre-operatively by combined purgatives and enemas. Per-operative antibiotics are not indicated for the operation, although they may be needed for other reasons (e.g. chronic bronchitis). Blood loss is usually minimal but it is wise to have the patient grouped and serum saved in case an unexpected haemorrhage occurs.

Operative Technique

The patient is positioned in the lithotomy position with the hips well flexed and a

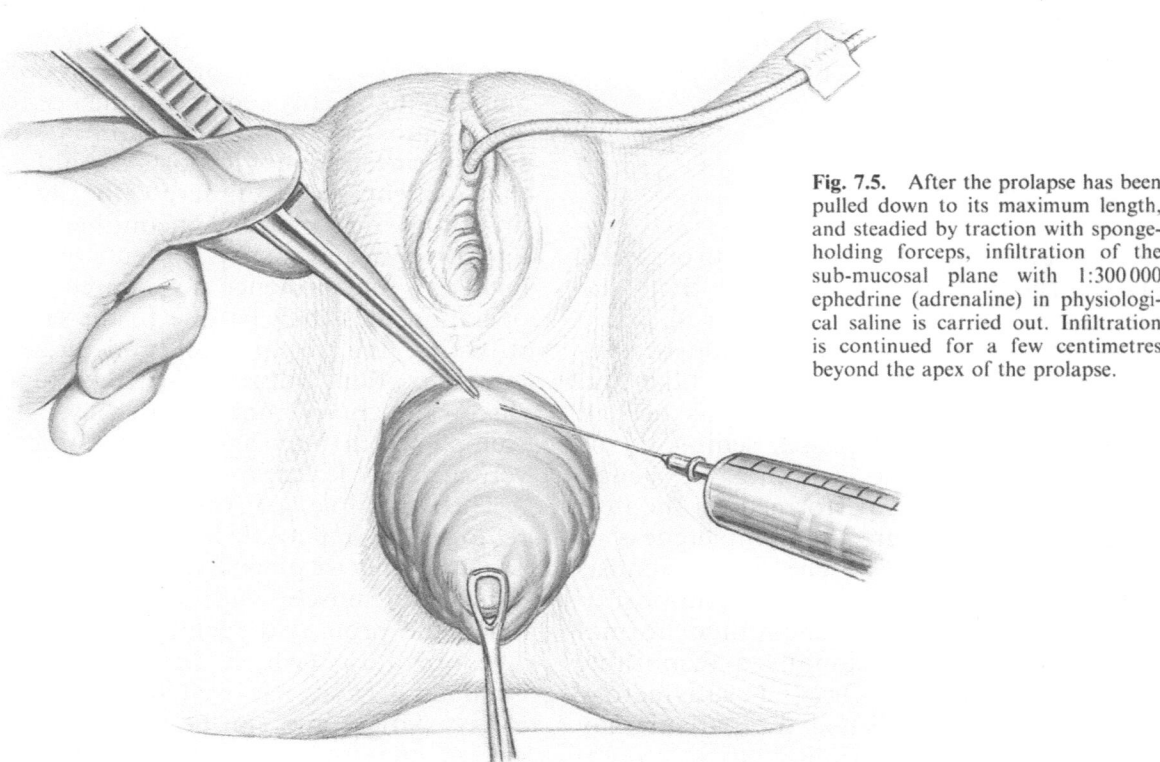

Fig. 7.5. After the prolapse has been pulled down to its maximum length, and steadied by traction with sponge-holding forceps, infiltration of the sub-mucosal plane with 1:300 000 ephedrine (adrenaline) in physiological saline is carried out. Infiltration is continued for a few centimetres beyond the apex of the prolapse.

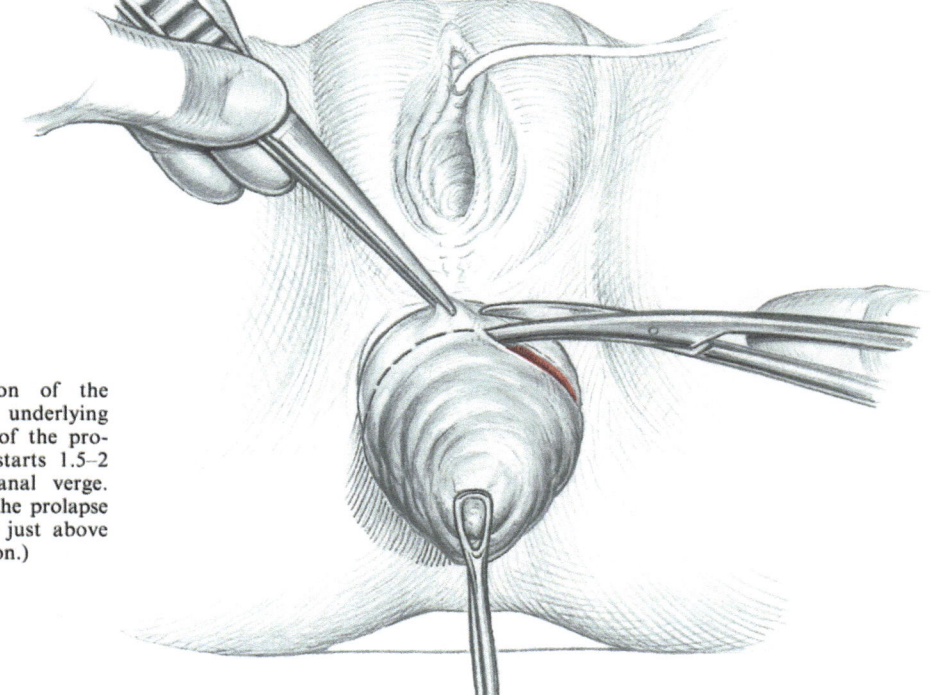

Fig. 7.6. Separation of the mucosa from the underlying muscularis propria of the prolapse (rectal wall) starts 1.5–2 cm distal to the anal verge. (After reduction of the prolapse this level lies at or just above the ano-rectal junction.)

urinary catheter is placed in the bladder. The patient is draped in the usual manner. Under general or regional anaesthesia the rectal prolapse often reduces itself and it is important to recreate the prolapse which is pulled well down (Fig. 7.5) before the operation starts; this is best done with sponge-holding forceps as toothed forceps tend to tear the mucosa. With the prolapse produced and steadied, the mucosa is lifted off the underlying muscle wall by an infiltration of weak solution of adrenaline (ephedrine) (1:300 000) in saline (Fig. 7.5). The infiltration is made from the anal verge to the apex of the prolapse and is continued beyond the apex for a further 1–2 cm. Additional infiltration may be necessary as the dissection proceeds, with the agreement of the anaesthetist.

A circumferential incision approximately 1.5–2.0 cm from the anal verge is made through the mucosa to enter the submucosal space (Fig. 7.6). The mucosa is now stripped off by a sharp dissection from the underlying circular muscle of the rectum.

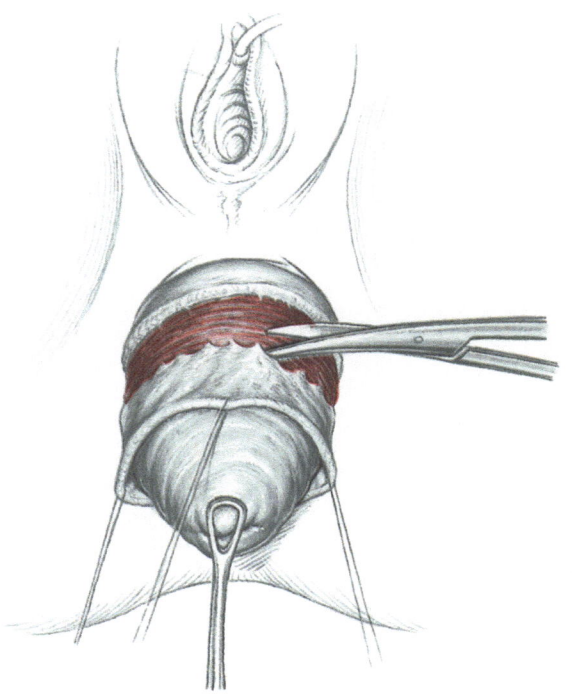

Fig. 7.7. As the mucosal tube is stripped off traction is maintained by stay sutures or ring-forceps.

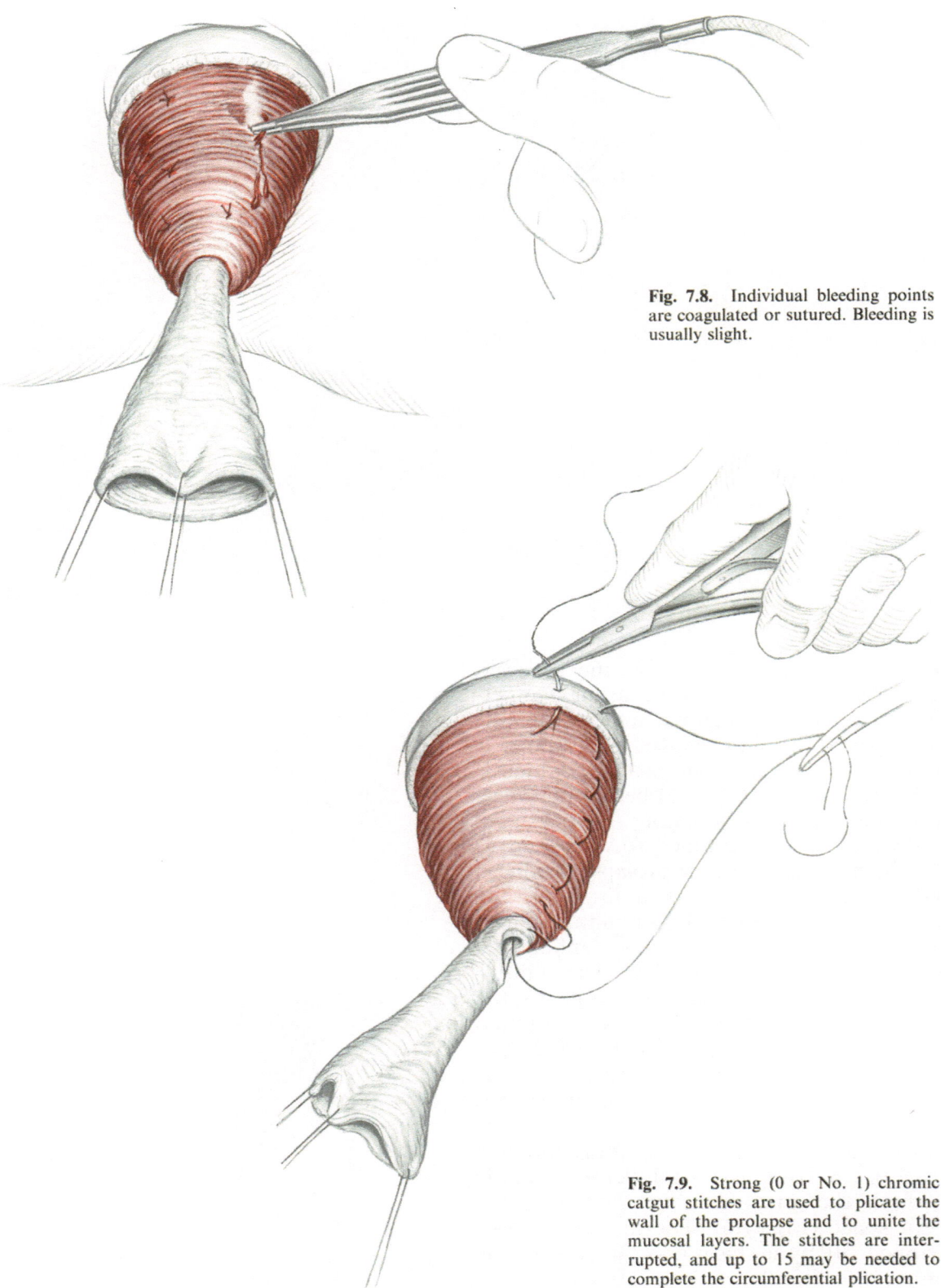

Fig. 7.8. Individual bleeding points are coagulated or sutured. Bleeding is usually slight.

Fig. 7.9. Strong (0 or No. 1) chromic catgut stitches are used to plicate the wall of the prolapse and to unite the mucosal layers. The stitches are interrupted, and up to 15 may be needed to complete the circumferential plication.

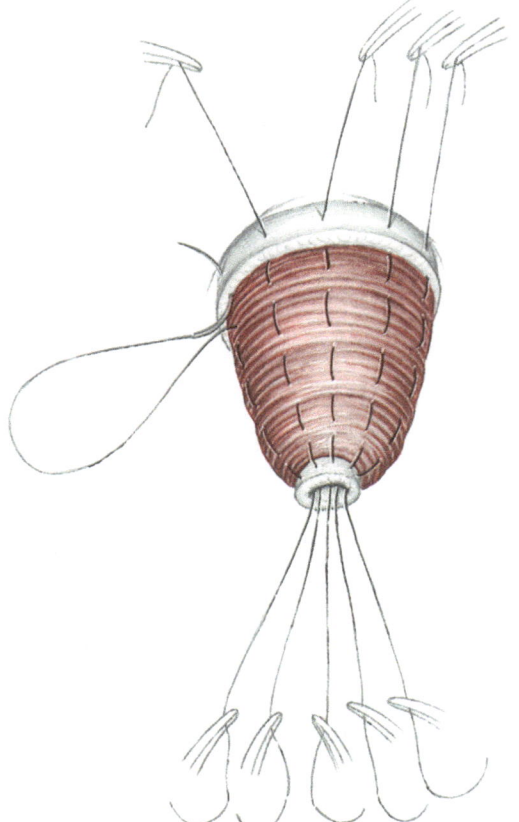

Fig. 7.10. Once the circumferential stitches are in place, traction will concertina the prolapse and appose the mucosal edges.

As the mucosa is lifted up it should be pulled down with tissue-holding forceps or stay sutures (Fig. 7.7). Small blood vessels which are encountered in the submucosal space need to be either coagulated or, with larger vessels, under-run with catgut stitches. If the dissection is kept carefully in the submucosal plane, bleeding is usually minimal (Fig. 7.8). Eventually the mucosa is dissected away as far as the top of the rectal prolapse and discarded. It is important, however, to continue the mucosal resection for a few centimetres beyond this point. Additional submucosal infiltration, as necessary, with adrenaline in saline is used to facilitate the upper reaches of the mucosal dissection. The next stage is to plicate the rectal prolapse. Using 0 or No. 1 chromic catgut, vertical plication stitches are placed first in the anal mucosal

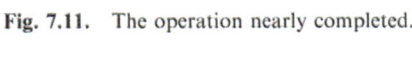

Fig. 7.11. The operation nearly completed.

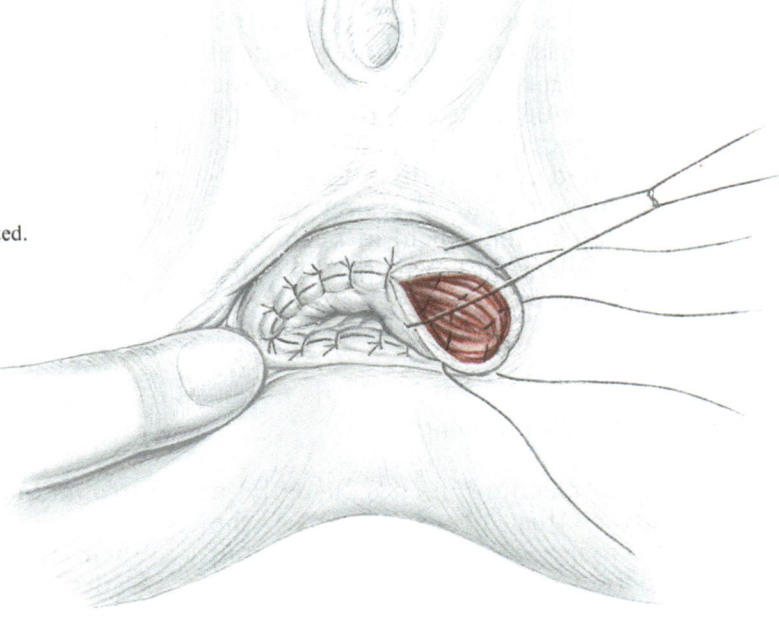

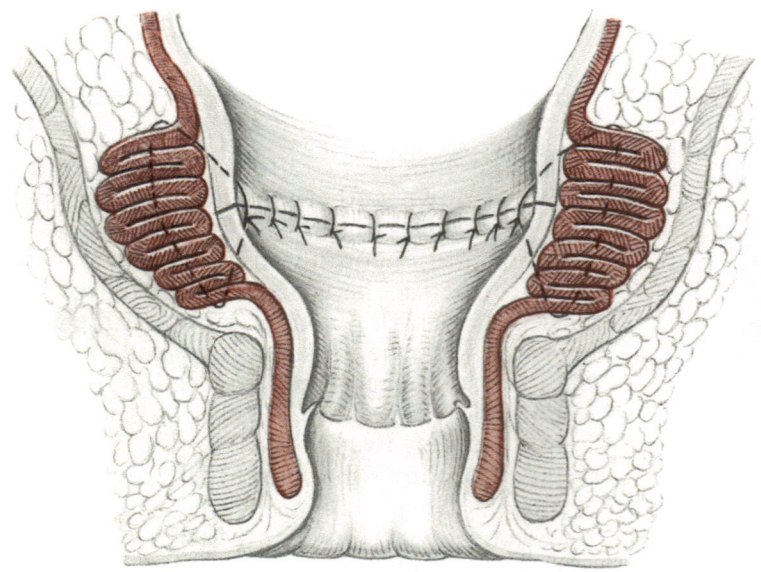

Fig. 7.12. The final position. Note how the level of the mucosal repair has "ascended" with reduction of the prolapse and lies just beyond the ano-rectal junction. The concertinad muscle is felt digitally as a bulky muscular ring.

cuff and then through the exposed circular muscle coat of the rectal wall, finally ending by taking the mucosal cuff beyond the apex of the prolapse (Fig. 7.9). Each stitch is left long and held. Approximately 10–15 sutures are required to complete circumferential plication of the prolapse. When all sutures are in place (Fig. 7.10) gentle traction on the stitches will concertina the circular muscle and reduce the rectal prolapse. Stitches are tied in turn as the prolapse is reduced (Fig. 7.11). After the final stitch has been tied the inverted anus and rectum have been returned to the pelvis. The plicated muscle now sits just above the ano-rectal junction and can be felt as a narrowed ring on digital examination (Fig. 7.12). A flat dressing pad is placed over the perineum held in place by a T bandage to collect the post-operative discharges of mucus and faeces which may be profuse at first.

Post-operative Management

Post-operative bleeding is not usually a problem after this procedure. As the abdominal cavity has not been entered patients are free to eat and drink as soon as they have recovered from the anaesthetic. The patient should be prescribed an osmotic laxative such as magnesium sulphate, Milpar or Cremaffin (Boots), to be taken 3–4 times a day immediately they can tolerate oral intake. This should ensure that bowel movements will be soft and semisolid. By the 6th or 7th post-operative day the patient usually has a satisfactory bowel habit but care should be taken to ensure that neither diarrhoea nor faecal impaction occur. Early mobilisation is essential to prevent thrombo-embolic risks. After discharge the surgeon must continue to see the patient regularly to ensure that defaecation remains satisfactory and that the patient does not revert to a straining habit of defaecation.

Rectosigmoidectomy (Syn. Altemeier Technique) [1,6,7,8,9]

Introduction

When the results of perineal rectosigmoidectomy were published by Hughes

(1949), it was found that not only did more than half the patients have recurrence of the prolapse but more than half the patients remained incontinent. Attempts to improve these results by a coincidental strengthening of the muscles of the pelvic floor have had variable success, but Altemeier seems to have obtained better results by combining anterior resection or rectosigmoidectomy with anterior suture of the inferior levator muscles. Most recently, Goldberg [6] has produced very respectable figures for this operation which he uses when he has been unable to justify an abdominal procedure because of the patient's poor general condition. However, most surgeons faced with an incontinent patient with rectal prolapse will continue to use an abdominal rectopexy as their method of choice, and will only have recourse to rectosigmoidectomy in exceptional cases. When compared with the Delorme technique, which incorporates stitches that plicate and shorten the rectal wall proper (and thus prevent intussusception), the operation of rectosigmoidectomy does not do anything to strengthen the muscles of the ano-rectum unless the Altemeier modification [1,2] [which can be achieved through the perineal (per-anal) approach] is used in every case. Because of this defect in the technique, the authors recommend that if rectosigmoidectomy is used, the Altemeier modification should be employed wherever possible in view of (a) the historically proven high risks for recurrence, and (b) persisting incontinence if only amputation of the prolapsed rectum is performed [7].

Indications and Selection of Patients

Some patients with rectal prolapse are unfit for an abdominal procedure. The operation of rectosigmoidectomy is a possible alternative technique, especially for patients whose life-expectancy is short because of cardio-respiratory disease. Fewer than 5% of cases fall into this category, and many of these will be treated better by the Delorme oper-

ation, which is equally safe and incorporates rectal wall plication as an additional defence against recurrence. For patients who are known to have an exceptionally long length of prolapsing bowel, rectosigmoidectomy will allow removal of the lower sigmoid colon in addition to the rectum itself, and is preferred for these rare cases.

Preparation

The general preparation of these patients is the same as for any major operation, but special precautions are needed for the conditions of ill-health that have decided the surgeon to use the technique. If cardiovascular problems have been the prime indication, then extra care must be taken to prevent complications of thrombosis by the use of suitable anticoagulant regimens over the operative period: the authors favour subcutaneous calcium heparin for this purpose. Frail patients are sensitive to the effects of opiates and ganglion-blocking agents, and both can produce excessive falls of systolic blood pressure unless used circumspectly; drug-induced respiratory depression must also be guarded against. Fluid overload during and after surgery must be avoided, and the fluid balance regulated with extreme care: most patients can dispense with i.v. fluids at an early stage after surgery providing an ileus is not present; a nasogastric tube is not required routinely because ileus is not precipitated by the operation. If respiratory diseases (chronic bronchitis or emphysema) are present, in addition to eliminating any chronic lung infection with antibiotics, a stringent pre-operative course of chest physiotherapy is indicated. The anaesthetist should assess each patient pre-operatively since post-operative ventilatory support may be needed for a period of hours before extubation is safe.

A full bowel preparation is indicated. Because the patients are frequently incontinent, and have a prolapsed rectum, they are usually unable to retain an enema and the surgeon must rely on oral preparation with Picolax (1 sachet 24 hours before operation followed by a second sachet 8 hours later.) The patient should have no solids for 48 hours before operation, and may require the stools to be softened initially by the use of oral magnesium sulphate mixture (25 ml every 6 hours) for 48 hours prior to the Picolax. If renal disease is present, gentamicin should not be used for antibiotic preparation: instead the authors recommend cephradine (500 mg every 8 hours) plus metronidazole (500 mg bd) starting 24 hours before operation and continuing for 2 days post-operatively.

All patients should be fitted with graduated compression stockings pre-operatively, which should be worn continuously during and after the operation until mobilisation is complete and normal activity possible.

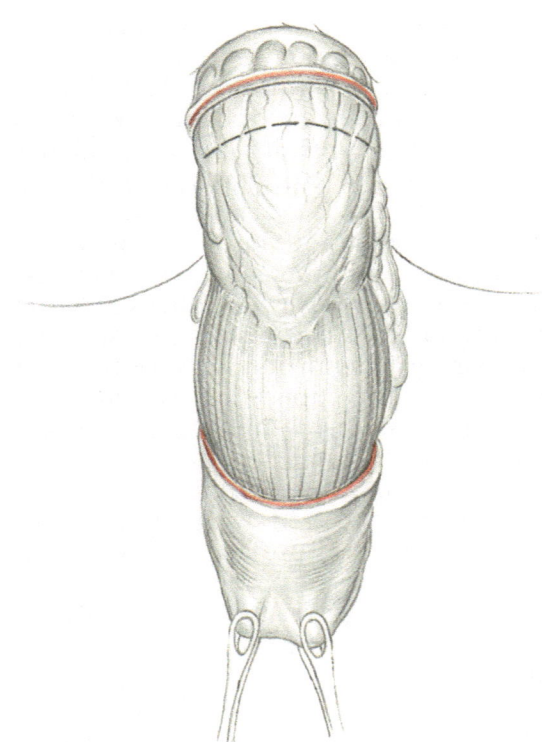

Fig. 7.14. After division of the first layer of bowel wall, traction will bring down the full length of the prolapse. The anterior aspect of the bowel is clothed to a variable extent by a peritoneal sac, which needs to be incised superiorly (---).

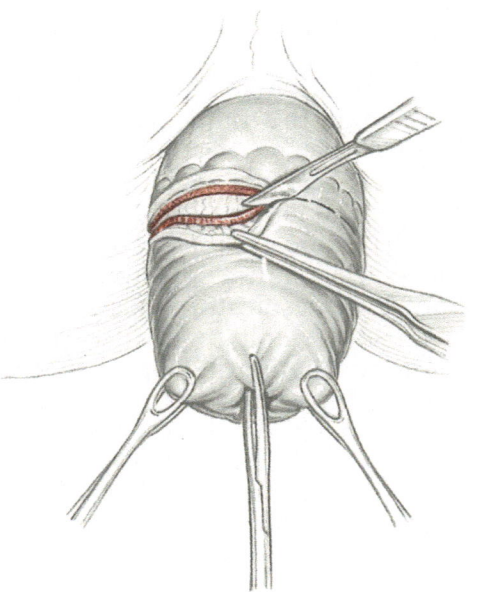

Fig. 7.13. The start of the operation by incising the bowel wall 3–4 cm above the dentate line. The muscularis propria should be divided at a slightly higher level than the mucosa to allow for muscle contraction.

Operative Technique

The patient is catheterised pre-operatively. This operation is more difficult in the jack-knife position (which tends to reduce a prolapse) and is best performed in an acute lithotomy position with the buttocks pulled well down. The table is adjusted to the proper height with a modest "head-down" tilt.

As the patient usually has an atonic sphincter, an anal dilation is not necessary. If the prolapse has reduced itself prior to surgery it is pulled back down again by sponge-holding ring forceps placed around the rectal lumen: a Volsellum forceps can also help to maintain the prolapse as its teeth and angulation are ideal for obtaining a proper grip on the rectal wall.

Once the prolapse has been fully exposed, the operation starts with a circumferential incision around the rectal wall 1–2 cm above the dentate line, i.e. around the most distal part of the ano-rectum (Fig. 7.13). The incision bleeds readily, and arterial "spurters" must be controlled by fine sutures. Goligher advises that the musculais propria should be divided at a slightly higher level than the mucosa to allow for muscle contraction after division. Once the full thickness of the bowel wall has been divided all around, the gut tube is bought down and with slight traction the full length of the prolapse can be displayed (Fig. 7.14).

The anterior surface of the prolapse is covered superiorly by a peritoneal pouch, and this should now be entered and the sac

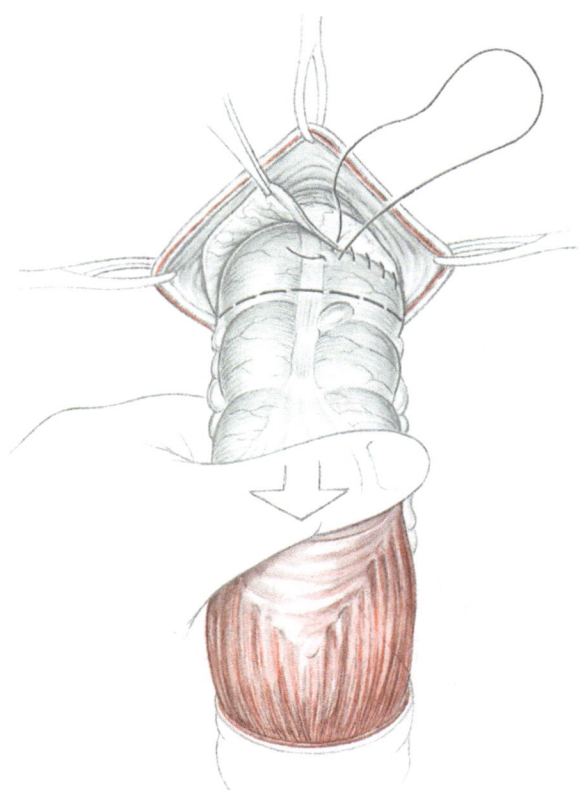

Fig. 7.16. The upper limit of the peritoneal sac is closed off, and the level for bowel division, which is always a few centimetres below the line of sac closure, is selected (---).

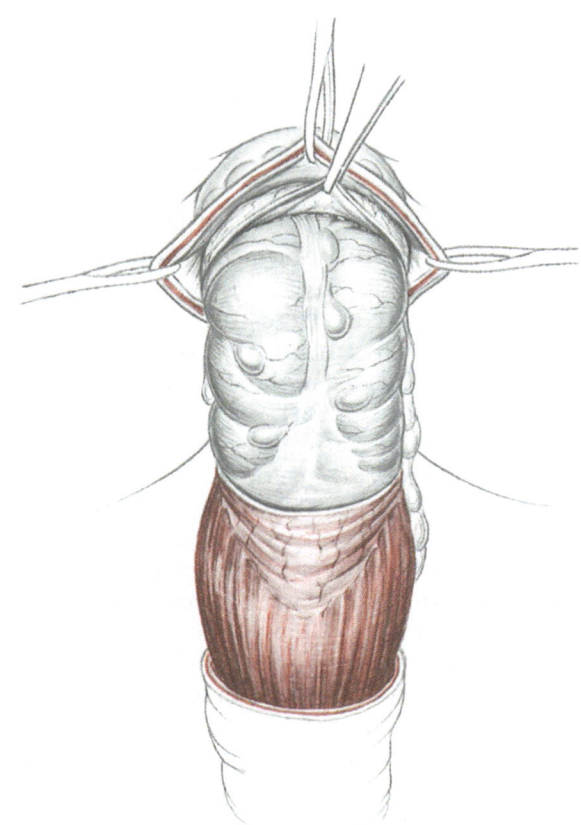

Fig. 7.15. The peritoneal sac is identified, and is cut back.

cut back (Fig. 7.15): the peritoneum is immediately re-closed by a continuous 00 chromic catgut stitch at the highest possible level (Fig. 7.16). In the Altemeir modification (Fig. 7.23) once the peritoneal sac has been closed, the prolapse surface is meticulously cleaned with aqueous Hibitane solution (1/400) and a retractor inserted anteriorly (or posteriorly) to lift the rectum and sigmoid colon forward (or backward) to expose the peri-rectal space. The space can be developed without difficulty by gentle blunt and sharp dissection to expose the muscular limbs of the puborectalis and lower portions of the levator ani muscle. The muscular limbs on each side of the rectum are drawn together by sutures of monofilament nylon (0 strength), which can

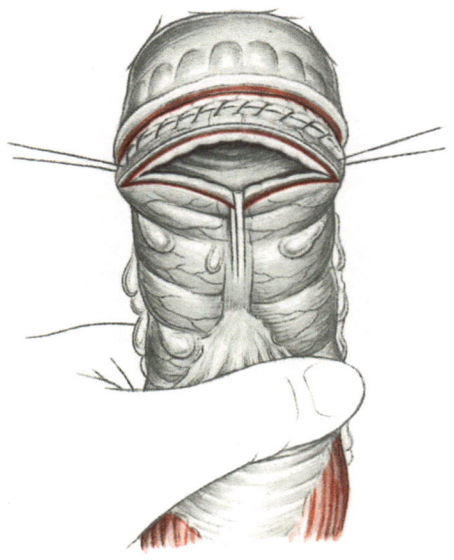

Fig. 7.17. Removal of the prolapsed length of bowel is now continued by division of the proximal bowel. This starts by cutting through the anterior quadrants of the bowel wall as shown, with the corners steadied and secured by stay sutures.

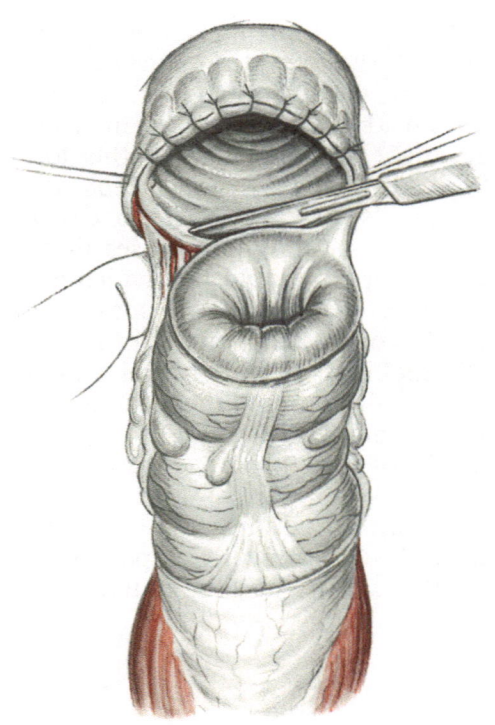

Fig. 7.19. The whole of the redundant prolapsed bowel can now be cut off, leaving only the mesorectum (with its blood vessels) attaching the specimen to the patient.

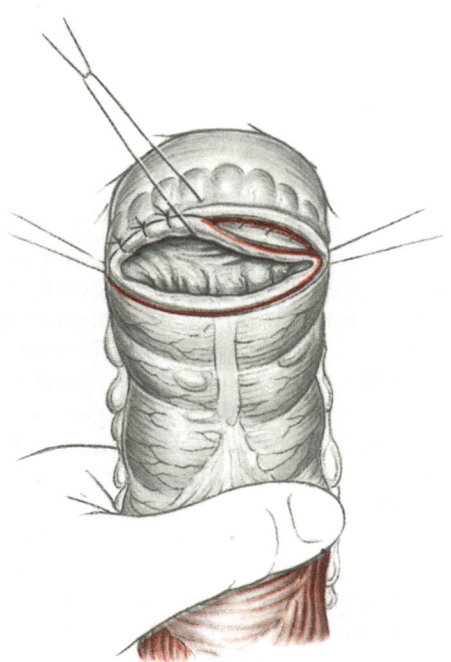

Fig. 7.18. As the anterior layer of the bowel is divided, it is immediately anastomosed seriatim to the distal (ano-rectal) edge of division by interrupted full-thickness stitches of 0 Dexon or Vicryl.

be placed as a latticework if the muscles are atrophic. The authors believe that posterior buttressing (Fig. 7.23b) is preferable to an anterior repair as it restores the ano-rectal angle, but an anterior repair is just as easy and is used in the classical Altemeier operation (Fig. 7.23a).

Whether or not the Altemeier modification has been used, the surgeon must now decide the level at which to divide the upper end of the prolapsed bowel. This should not be at the extreme end of control (because this may make manipulation of the upper end difficult once the prolapse has been removed), and should be below the closed end of the peritoneal sac (Fig. 7.16). The bowel should be steadied by stay sutures placed through each lateral corner of the bowel (Fig. 7.17) before incision of the bowel wall commences. The incision through the bowel wall is best started anteriorly near one corner and is made with

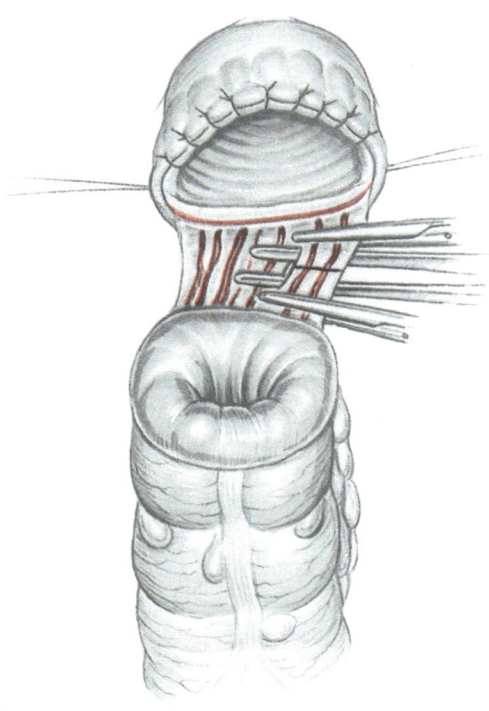

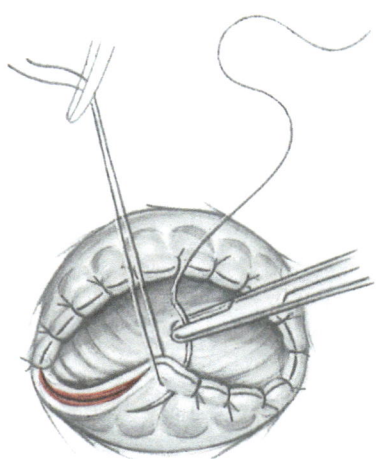

Fig. 7.22. Posterior layer of the anastomosis being completed.

Fig. 7.20. The blood vessels in the mesorectum are large and must be secured by careful individual ligation with unabsorbable suture material (silk or linen).

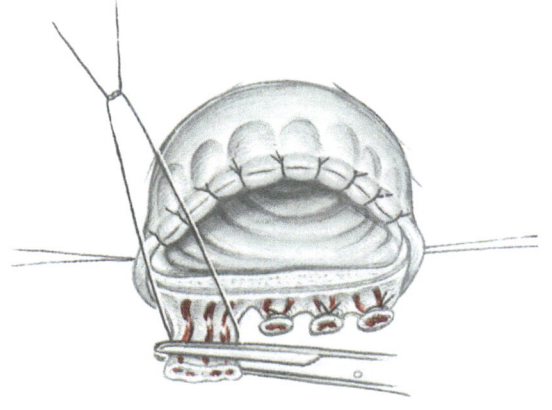

Fig. 7.21. Once the blood vessels have been tied off (as shown) the stumps of the vessels promptly retract and reveal the posterior bowel edges that need to be joined to complete the anastomosis.

sharp-pointed stout curved scissors; as the edges are developed it is possible to insert interrupted full-thickness stitches between the edges of the proximal and distal edges of the incisions to construct the anastomosis (Fig. 7.18). The tissue bites for each separate stitch should be deep, and the material stout: 0 Dexon or Prolene are very suitable. The stitches should be inserted as each centimetre of the circumference of the incisions is developed as this will effectively control bleeding, which can be profuse.

As the dissection reaches the lateral edges of the lumen, the stay sutures can be removed but substituted for by the corner stitches of the anastomosis which are left long and held in forceps under traction.

After completion of the union of the anterior layers, the posterior wall of the colon is now incised (Fig. 7.19) with bleeding from the bowel edges controlled by coagulation or fine sutures. The entire length of the bowel wall is divided fully, at which point the mesorectum containing large blood vessels (the inferior rectal artery and its branches) is the only tissue retaining contact with the upper end of the divided bowel (Fig. 7.20). The mesorectum is divided sequentially between forceps (Fig. 7.21), and each bite of tissue is care-

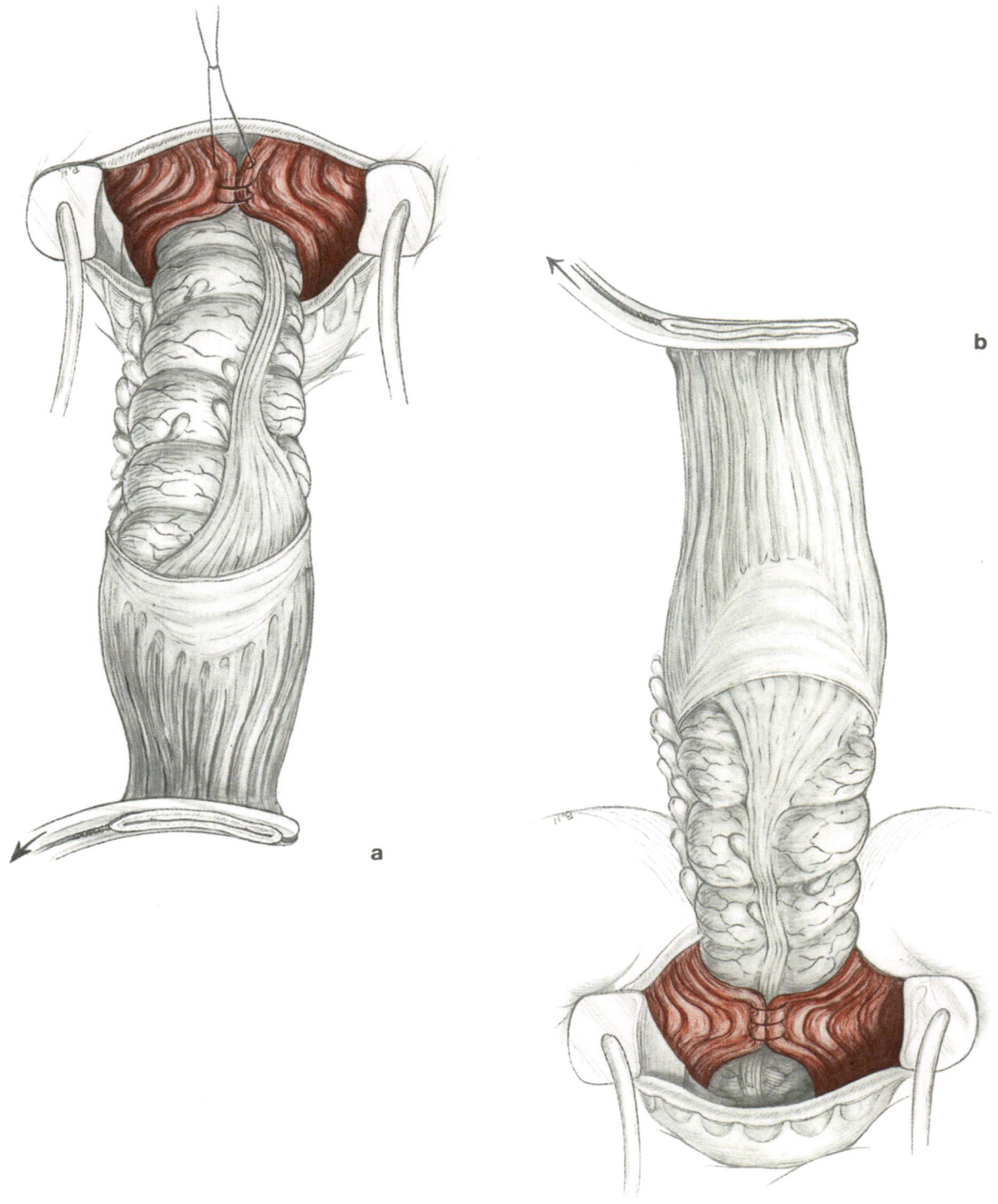

Fig. 7.23. a,b The Altemeier variation of the classical procedure of rectosigmoidectomy. **a** The iliococcygeus and puborectalis muscles can be joined together snugly across the front of the colon before bowel division is commenced. **b** Alternatively (as is preferred by the authors) the levator muscle buttress can be done posteriorly. The authors recommend the use of the Altemeier modification whenever possible.

fully ligated with vinyl sutures (00) before the cut ends are allowed to retract upwards into the pelvis. After the mesorectum has been cut through, the prolapsed bowel is free and can be discarded.

Providing due care has been taken not to divide the posterior wall of the colon at too high a level, the edge of the divided bowel should not retract beyond the field of vision and the anastomosis can be easily completed by further interrupted stitches through the full thickness of each edge of the proximal and distal incisions (Fig. 8.22). The stitches should be close (not more than 5 mm apart) so that gaps do not ensue, and should include deep bites of the anal sphincter muscle.

Once the full circumference of the anastomosis has been closed, the corner stitches are cut and the bowel is allowed to retract.

No drains are used, and no dressings (other than a perineal pad) are required.

Post-operative Management

Most patients make excellent progress once they have recovered from the effects of the anesthetic. Pain is minimal and there is usually no post-operative ileus. Ambulation can be encouraged from the second post-operative day. The stools are kept semi-liquid initially by a mild aperient (liquid paraffin, one spoonful once or twice daily, is very suitable for these patients) and a fluid or low residue diet is advisable until defaecation is established. Once proper stools are being passed, these should be rendered soft (but given proper bulk) by daily use of bran (2 spoonsful) or hydrophilic colloid (Normacol Special, two spoonsful daily) because, if the stools do not have some bulk after the immediate post-operative period is over, the suture line can narrow down to a stricture.

If the anus remains patulous, and incontinence persists after surgery, vigorous anal sphincter exercises should be instituted.

Results

The early results are usually excellent, but with time both incontinence and prolapse are prone to recur. The operation is not a real alternative to other and better procedures (e.g. abdominal rectopexy) but is a substitute for them which is dicated by the poor health of the patient. Most surgeons remain suspicious that the long-term results will be unsatisfactory and associated with a high rate of recurrence.

References and Further Reading

1. Altemeier WA, Giuseppi J, Hoxworth P (1952) Treatment of extensive prolapse of the rectum in aged or debilitated patients. Arch Surg 65: 72
2. Altemeier WA, Culbertson WR, Schowengerdt C et al. (1971) Nineteen years experience with the one-stage perineal repair of rectal prolapse. Ann Surg 173: 993
3. Christiansen J, Kirkegaard P (1981) Delorme's operation for complete rectal prolapse. Br J Surg 68: 537
4. Corman ML (1989) Colon and rectal surgery. Lippincott, Philadelphia, pp 225–229
5. Delorme RL (1900) Communication sur le traitement des prolapsus du rectum totale par l'excision de la muqueuse rectale ou recto-colique. Translated in Dis Colon Rectum (1985) 28: 544–553
6. Goldberg SM, Gordon PH, Nivatvongs S (1980) Essentials of ano-rectal surgery. Lippincott, Philadelphia
7. Gopal KA, Amshel AL, Shonberg IL, Eftaiha M (1984) Rectal procidentia in elderly and debilitated patients: experience with the Altemeier procedure. Dis Colon Rectum 27: 376
8. Hughes ESR (1949) Discussion on rectal prolapse. Proc R Soc Med 42: 1007
9. Miles WE (1933) Recto-sigmoidoscopy as a method of treatment for procidentia recti. Proc R Soc Med 26: 1445
10. Neil ME, Parks AG, Swash M (1981) Physiological studies of the anal sphincter musculature in faecal incontinence and rectal prolapse. Br J Surg 68: 531
11. Nicholls J, Glass R (1985) Coloproctology, diagnosis and out-patient management. Springer, Heidelberg and New York, Chap. 6
12. Parks AG, Porter NH, Hardcastle J (1966) The syndrome of the descending perineum. Proc R Soc Med 59: 477
13. Porter NH (1962) Collective results of operations for rectal prolapse (at St. Mark's Hospital 1948–1960). Proc R Soc Med 55: 1087
14. Rutter KRP, Riddell RH (1975) The solitary ulcer syndrome of the rectum. Clin Gastroenterol 4: 505

CHAPTER 8

Technique of Anal Sphincter Repair
(Syn. Overlap Technique)

Introduction

The commonest injury to the sphincter complex is obstetric [3]; by disruption at traumatic (forceps) delivery, tearing, or by misplaced episiotomy. If not recognised by the attending obstetrician and properly and promptly repaired, the wound will heal by secondary intention. This will result in a deficient anal canal with poor function. The young patient, however, may withstand serious disruption of the external anal sphincter if the puborectalis muscle remains intact, frequently accepting poor control of flatus and faecal soiling as a required sacrifice to the Gods for safe vaginal delivery of her baby. Subsequent childbirth may further stretch the pelvic floor and puborectalis muscles, and the patient may then present with socially unacceptable faecal incontinence (although only too frequently she tries to conceal her "shame"). Development of faecal incontinence may be delayed in other cases until middle age when the pelvic floor muscles naturally begin to dete-

riorate [2]. This deterioration is accelerated in those patients who are habitual strainers. A few patients present as a result of trauma, either from vehicles or missiles: these patients always have extra tissue damage and scarring, especially after high-velocity injury or explosions.

The majority of patients who come to sphincter repair will, therefore, present at a late stage to the specialist surgeon. The wound will have healed, often with considerable scarring, and the patient may have been given a defunctioning stoma. After traumatic rupture the divided anal sphincter retracts to about half its normal circumference, the gap being bridged by dense fibrous tissue. The edges of the retracted anal sphincter can be located often by palpation, or by direct muscle stimulation with a nerve stimulator [7]. Pre-operative sphincter mapping either electromyographically or by ultrasonography may be advantageous if the injury is complex. In recent years it has been commonplace to perform primary sphincter repair without a covering colostomy. Excellent results have been recorded from specialist centres without the employment of a diverting stoma [1,3,5, 6,8,10].

Indications and Selection of Patients

The results of sphincter repair can be very rewarding and most patients should be favourably considered for reconstruction if their symptoms merit it. The patient must be fit to withstand a general anaesthetic, and as with all operations for incontinence, should be encouraged to have a positive mental attitude towards the operation and its outcome.

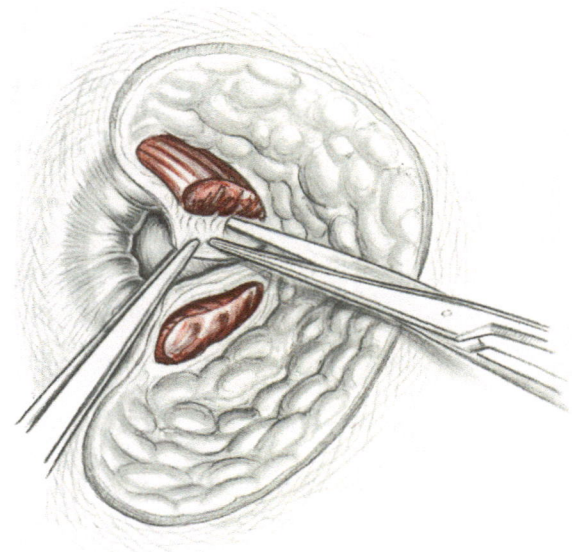

Fig. 8.2. The ends of the divided sphincter muscles, after identification, are dissected up as one unit. Too great mobilisation can produce ischaemia and denervation.

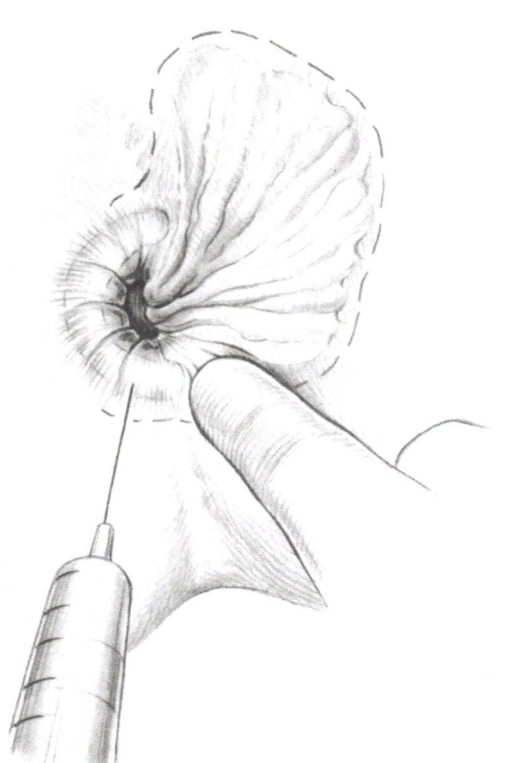

Fig. 8.1. A generous infiltration of 1:300 000 ephedrine in physiological saline is of priceless assistance to proper display of the tissues, especially the sphincter muscles.

Preparation

If the patient has serious health problems, these should be corrected before surgery if at all possible. This is not usually the case. If the perineal skin is excoriated the use of a barrier cream (Vasogen) to clear up surface inflammation is required. The patient may, however, require skilled nursing to initiate epidermal healing. All sources of infection should be eradicated with particular attention to the lungs, urinary tract, vagina and cervix. The patient should have pre-operative oral and mechanical bowel cleansing and per-operative antibiotics are routinely given against aerobes and anaerobes. Pre-operative physiotherapy and graduated compression stockings should be given to reduce the risk of thromboembolism. Anticoagulants are best avoided, although subcutaneous heparin may be given if indicated for patients who are at exceptional risk.

Operative Technique

With the patient in the lithotomy position the skin and subcutaneous tissues around the sphincter and the entire site of injury are generously infiltrated with a weak solution of 1:300 000 ephedrine (adrenaline) in saline (Fig. 8.1). All surrounding scar tissue must now be excised by sharp dissection, which can create a large wound, but this is crucial if the sphincter edges are to be opposed. The use of a nerve/muscle stimulator may be of help.

The mucosa from the anal canal and lower rectum is now mobilised, freeing a 1.0 cm fringe from the underlying muscle so that it can be sutured without tension (Fig. 8.2). This epithelium is immediately closed with continuous 00 chromic catgut (Fig. 8.3). The edges of the divided sphincter muscle are next identified. *It is important to realise that it is not necessary to identify internal from external anal sphincter, and that they should be displayed and repaired as one muscle.* The sphincter muscle on each side of the injury must be

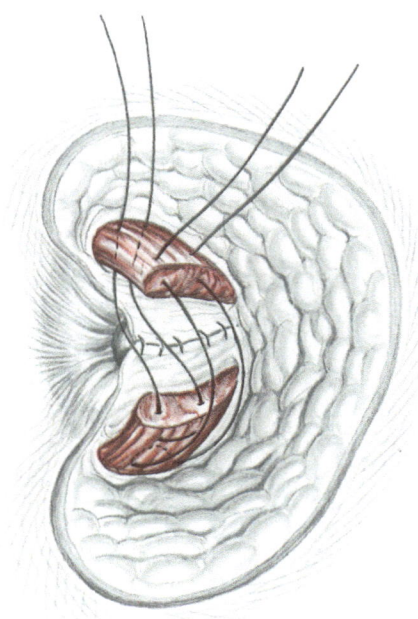

Fig. 8.4. The divided ends of muscle are united by an overlap technique, using 00 Prolene interrupted sutures. It is important to leave fibrous tissue on the ends of the sphincter to provide secure anchoring of the sutures.

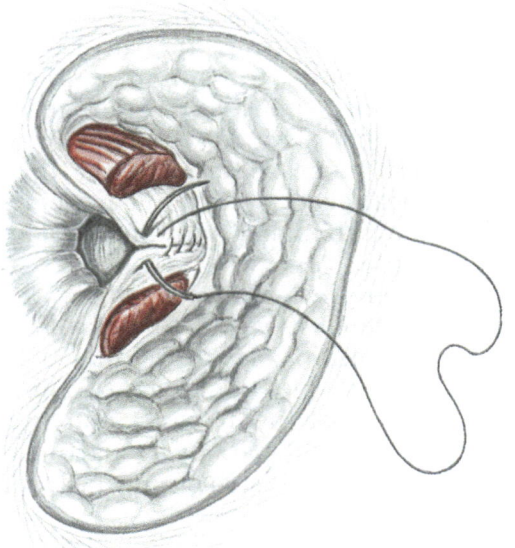

Fig. 8.3. The epithelial layer is repaired at an early stage with a continuous running stitch of 00 chromic catgut.

dissected back for a short distance; great judgement is required to mobilise enough sphincter, *but to preserve some fibrous tissue to hold stitches for subsequent repair and to avoid ischaemia of the ends* [4,7]. Excessive mobilisation will render the muscle ischaemic or cause denervation. It is important, however, to free the sphincter mass on its external aspect where it is usually adherent to the scar tissue of the ischiorectal fossa unless the surgeon has already cut it away.

The ends of the mobilised sphincter are now brought together with an overlap (Fig. 8.4). Horizontal mattress sutures of 00 Prolene are used, creating a solidly interlocked buttress of muscle (Fig. 8.5). This muscular repair lies directly in the cavity of the anal wound, but no attempt should be made to close the perineal skin over this defect if this involves undue tension. Skin

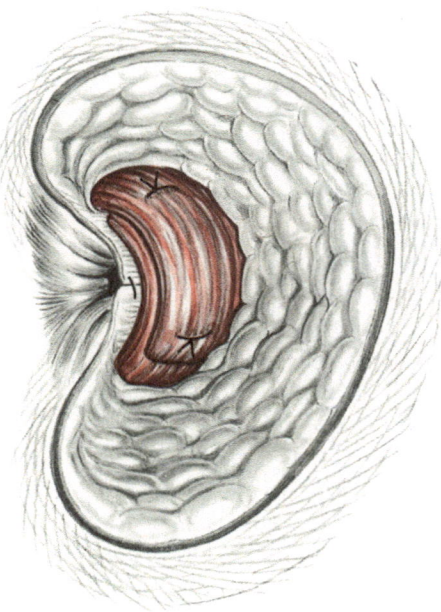

Fig. 8.5. An "ideal" overlapped sphincter repair. In many patients such a result is not practical without increased risks of ischaemia and denervation. In such circumstances, a solid abutment is better than over-ambitious mobilisation.

cover is desirable, but not essential. The "S-plasty" technique is useful to solve many cases when skin is in short-supply but often a simple rotation flap will suffice [4]. A drain is not necessary. The wound can be left safely, however, to heal by granulation if necessary and always does so satisfactorily, provided there is no tension in the edges and adequate drainage. Sometimes the surgeon is faced with a difficult judgement as to the degree of overlap he is prepared to accept. It is better to obtain a good union rather than to risk everything by trying to produce a textbook overlap with undue tension. The resulting repair may narrow the canal to approximately half its normal circumference. This is of no consequence to the final result; indeed, it is better to have a tight anal canal that can always be dilated later, than to end with a repair that is too loose. The wound should be dressed with gauze swabs soaked in hypochlorite solution laid lightly in the cavity. No attempt should be made to pack the dressing forcibly into the wound.

Post-operative Management

The patient should be confined to bed for 24 hours following surgery. Thereafter, the dressings should be separated, either by irrigations, or by allowing the patient to soak in a saline bath. When the dressings have been removed, the wound should be irrigated with saline and hypochlorite solution, and further moist dressings laid in the cavity. This procedure is repeated twice a day, although this may be needed more frequently if the dressings are soiled. Although the open wound may be large and has non-absorbable suture material in its base, it heals quickly. If the patient has a defunctioning colostomy the post-operative management of these cases is undoubtedly easier but with an unprotected repair, by careful supervision of the dressings and of the patient's bowels, the end-results should be identical. In those patients without a colostomy, aperients should be prescribed, starting on the second post-operative day to ensure the patient has soft or liquid motions without straining. A gentle rectal examination may be performed on the sixth or seventh post-operative day to guard against faecal impaction. In a patient with a narrow repair, initial examination should be with the 5th finger. The patient must be freely mobile during the post-operative recovery period to minimise thrombo-embolic risks, and is discouraged from sitting for long periods. The patient may be discharged home as soon as the dressings can be managed on an out-patient basis and require changing only once a day by a skilled nurse.

Post-operative follow-up must be frequent in the early weeks to make sure that no complications are developing. Faecal impaction above a stenosis must be guarded against at all costs, and frequent visits to the Out-patient Department are wise to guard against such a catastrophe.

Results

The results of a technically sound repair are excellent [2]. There is growing realisation that the problem could be favourably influenced by immediate repair of the injured sphincter by a trained colo-rectal surgeon, especially after obstetric damage, as discussed in Chapter 10.

References and Further Reading

1. Blaisdell PC (1940) Repair of the incontinent sphincter ani. Surg Gynecol Obstet 70: 692
2. Browning GCP, Motson RW (1983) Results of Parks' operation for faecal incontinence after anal injury. Br Med J 286: 1873
3. Corman ML (1985) Anal incontinence following obstetrical injury. Dis Colon Rectum 28: 86
4. Corman ML (1989) Colon and rectal surgery, 2nd edn. Lippincott, Philadelphia, pp 186–187
5. Fang DT, Nivatvongs S, Vermuelen FD et al. (1984) Overlapping sphincteroplasty for acquired anal incontinence. Dis Colon Rectum 27: 720
6. Goldberg SM, Gordon PP, Nivatvongs S (1980) Essentials of ano-rectal surgery. Lippincott, Philadelphia
7. Marti MC, Givel JC (1989) Surgery of ano-rectal diseases. Springer, Heidelberg and New York, Chap. 22
8. Motson RW (1985) Sphincter injuries: indications for, and results of sphincter repair. Br J Surg 72 (Suppl): 19–21
9. Parks AG, McPartin JF (1971) Late repairs of the anal sphincter. Proc R Soc Med 64: 1187

CHAPTER 9

Techniques for Congenital Anal Deformity Encountered in Later Life

General Introduction

Most cases of congenital abnormality of the ano-rectum are seen at, and treated soon after, birth [1,4,6,8]. Many of these abnormalities cause immediate problems of obstruction and have to be operated on as emergencies. It is rare nowadays for cases of imperforate anus or Hirschsprung's disease not to undergo definitive operations during the first year(s) of life to correct the underlying abnormalities. However a few children are able to survive in spite of a congenital abnormality when the obstructive element is weak. There are two different routes by which such rare children progress untreated up to adult life. The *first* is following faulty partial surgical correction of a low type of imperforate anus. In these babies, the correct diagnosis is made, but the surgical incision to open the obstructed orifice (usually a "covered-anus" deformity) is placed in the wrong position, so creating in effect a fistulous opening that lies outside the anal ring (usually anterior

to the anal muscles). The *second* is when the anal bud and proctodaeum fail to align correctly with the hind-gut, so that the hind-gut comes to the surface separately from the true site of the anal canal. In this latter case, the ectopic opening may be surrounded by some functioning "sphincter", although it is more common that these muscles (which are derived from the anal bud) are to be found at the proper site on the perineum. Both these contrasting origins lead to situations whereby faeces are discharged onto the surface at sites where the anal sphincter muscles are either deficient or entirely absent. In both cases the ectopic orifice is almost always anterior to the true anal canal, whose site is usually at the midpoint of the perineum (and can be identified frequently by a small surface dimple). Both cases are commoner in female subjects, and are associated with faecal incontinence persisting into adolescent, and even adult, life. In many cases the incontinence can be alleviated or cured by well-judged surgical intervention.

Identification and Assessment of Abnormality [3,4,6,8,9]

In many cases a history of an emergency procedure to relieve meconium obstruction soon after birth will be available. In all cases the patients will have a history of incontinence dating from infancy.

Some patients will have an obvious abnormality of development of the recto-vaginal septum and perineal body. In a few patients the whole of the posterior vaginal wall will be missing, and a cloacal-type deformity is present (Fig. 9.1a). In cases that are not so severe, an ectopic anal opening can be found either low in the posterior vagina (Fig. 9.1b), or at the fourchette, or displaced far forwards on the perineal skin itself. This last position is commonly the result of faulty surgical relief (at, or soon after, birth) of a "covered anus" [1], and the opening is a fistulous track in front of the anus which still lies hidden at its proper site.

Once the possibility of an ectopic opening has been thought of, clinical examination can elicit extra valuable information. An anal dimple should be looked for with great care. In a few cases, in addition to the dimple a minute orifice can be seen: if this is so, then it is virtually certain that functioning anal sphincter muscle is present beneath the dimple and if an opening is seen, judicious graduated probing may eventually open up the orifice sufficiently to re-establish the anal canal. Such a case corresponds to a low ano-cutaneous fistula (Wingspread classification [9]).

Even if an anal dimple is not obvious, it may be possible to demonstrate muscular contractions in response to pin-prick stimulation of the perineal skin. If such contractions are seen, then some anal sphincter muscle is certainly present in the correct position. In such children, as well as those in whom a narrow opening is visible (anal stenosis, Wingspread classification), a meticulous search for an anal orifice must be carried out, if necessary by examination and probing under anaesthesia.

Next, the clinician needs to find out if the levator muscle floor (and particularly the puborectalis muscle) has developed in a normal way. The presence of puborectalis may be confirmed in many cases by digital pressure through the posterior vaginal wall, or with the finger in the ectopic opening. If a cloacal-type deformity is present, the muscular floor of the pelvis is usually maldeveloped, and in severe cases the coccyx and sacrum are also deficient. Every known test must be made to establish the state of development of the muscular floor of the pelvis [8]. Both plain X-rays of the pelvis and ultrasonic radiology are helpful. The former will demonstrate any bony abnormality of the lumbo-sacral spine and pelvis, which will alert the clinician to possible neurological deficit as well as structural deformity. The latter can be used to outline the adnexal structures as well as to demonstrate whether the pelvic organs are maintained in a normal alignment. A CT scan can supplement ultrasonography in building up an accurate picture of the pelvic organs. A "Wangensteen invertogram" can demonstrate the termination of normal bowel above the defect, and its relation to the pelvic floor, which can be confirmed by a distal "loopogram" [3].

If required, special examination by electromyography can be used to map the presence (or absence) of puborectalis and anal sphincter muscles, both in the "correct" position as well as in the vicinity of the ectopic orifice.

At completion of a thorough programme of clinical and laboratory investigation, the patient can be allocated to one of four different categories:

1. *No identifiable muscle,* either around the abnormal opening or in the correct anatomical position. *Puborectalis muscle absent.* Cloacal-type deformity usually present (Fig. 9.1a)

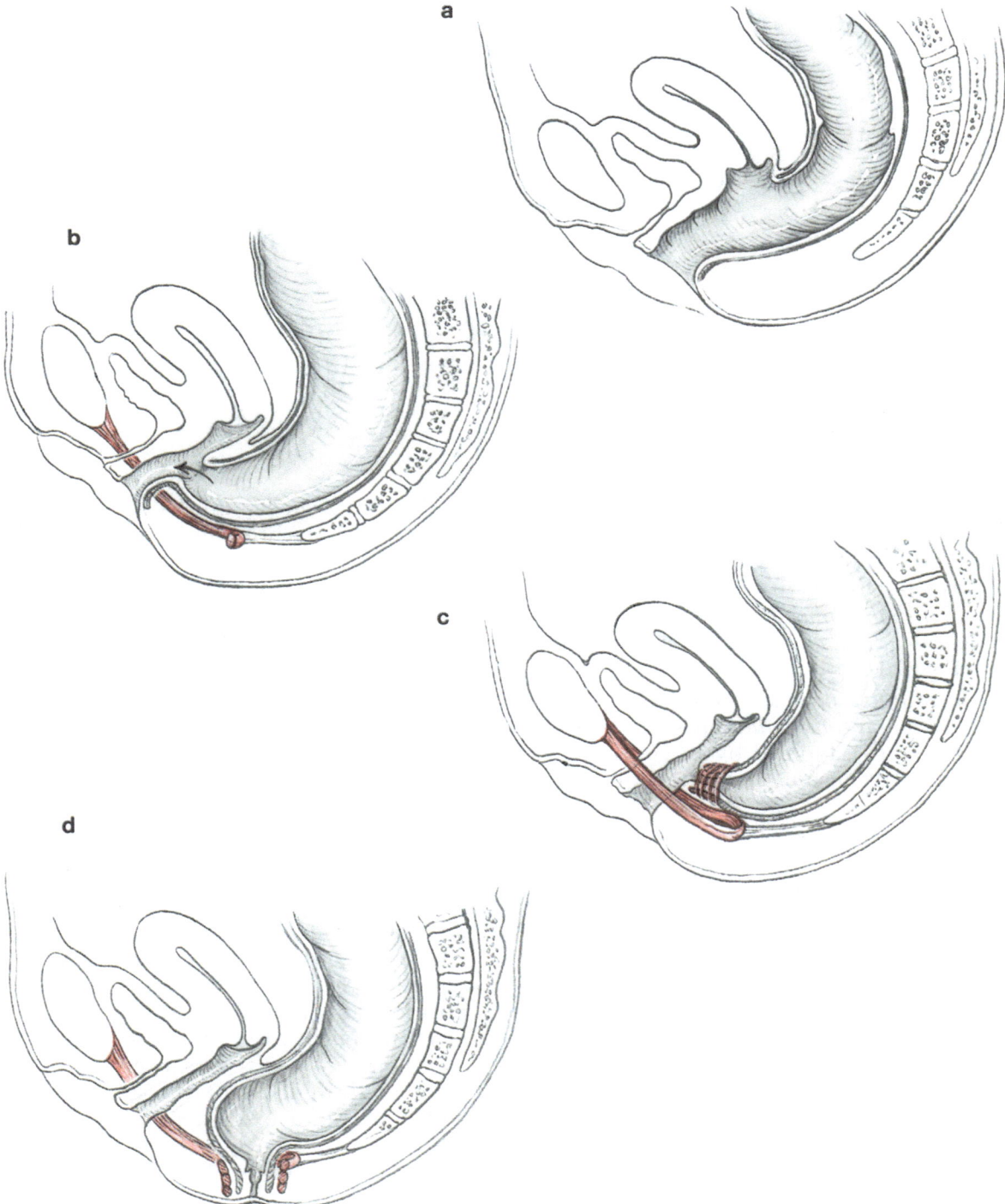

Fig. 9.1. a–d Important variations which can present to the surgeon with faecal incontinence for consideration of surgical cure. **a** Cloacal type deformity. *No repair possible.* **b** Ectopic opening but some development of pelvic floor and puborectalis musculature. *Low chance of correction.* **c** Ectopic opening with some functioning anal muscle, and intact puborectalis. In many patients the anal muscles are in their correct perineal site. *Repair possible.* **d** "Covered anus" deformity. Normal pelvic floor and sphincter muscles. *Excellent chance of correction.*

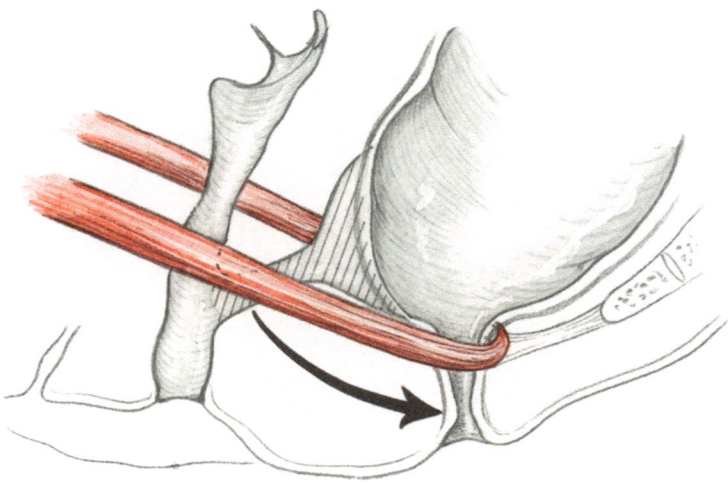

Fig. 9.2. The first and most important principle to be followed if a successful result is to be achieved is that the displaced ano-rectum must be replaced after mobilisation in correct alignment between the limbs of the puborectalis muscle.

2. *No identifiable muscle*, either around the abnormal opening, or in the correct anatomical position. *Puborectalis present* (Fig. 9.1b)

3. *Identifiable muscle at the site of ectopic opening, and an intact puborectalis muscle* (Fig. 9.1c)

4. *Identifiable muscle at the proper perineal position* and *an intact puborectalis muscle* (Fig. 9.1d), typified by a "covered anus" deformity or an "ano-cutaneous fistula" (see text)

For category (1) no surgical procedure for the incontinence is possible. For category (2) the chances of a successful result are very slim, but occasionally a better than expected result can emerge. For categories (3) and (4) a successful result is possible.

General Principles Underlying the Operations [6,8]

It is impossible to define the operation for any case undergoing surgical correction for an ectopic anus: every case needs individual handling, and each operation is as personal to the patient as fitting on a new suit of clothes. However, it is possible to outline certain principles that enhance the chances of a successful outcome.

The first principle must be to ensure that the gut tube is brought down through the pelvic floor between the limbs of the puborectalis muscle whenever this is possible (Fig. 9.2). Achieving correct alignment between the termination of the gut tube and the puborectalis sling can be enough to correct continence in some patients, and can almost always be achieved.

The second principle must be to draw down the ectopic opening *together with any surrounding muscle that has been identified* through the same route onto the perineal skin that is followed during normal development: this will give the best chance for preserving the nerve supply and any residual muscle function (Fig. 9.3).

The third principle is to identify and preserve any sphincter muscle in the "normal" position and *to dissect so that the ectopic anus is brought through the epicentre of this area* (Fig. 9.4). This will bring the gut tube through the middle of the muscular circle and allow it to exert a normal contractile effort.

Certain errors of technique should be avoided:

1. It is not advisable or necessary in all cases to move the ectopic opening posteriorly by carrying out surgical division of all tissue lying between the

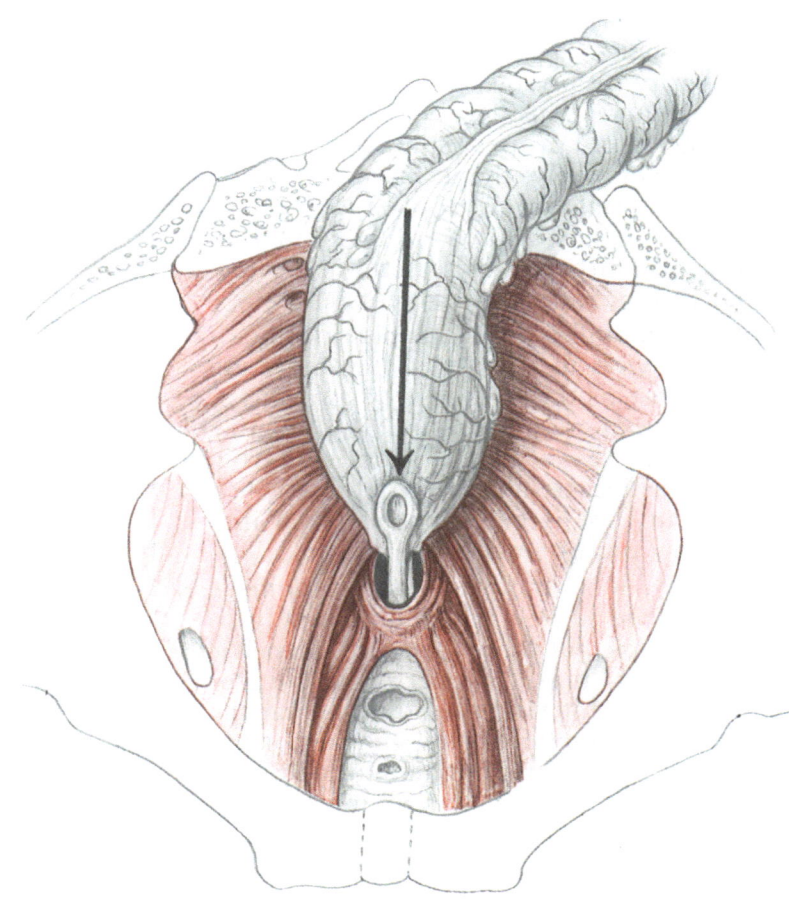

Fig. 9.3. The second important principle to be followed is that the mobilised distal segment must be brought down through the pelvis as closely as possible to the normal developmental route. Rigid adherence to the midline ensures minimal damage to pelvic nerves and blood vessels.

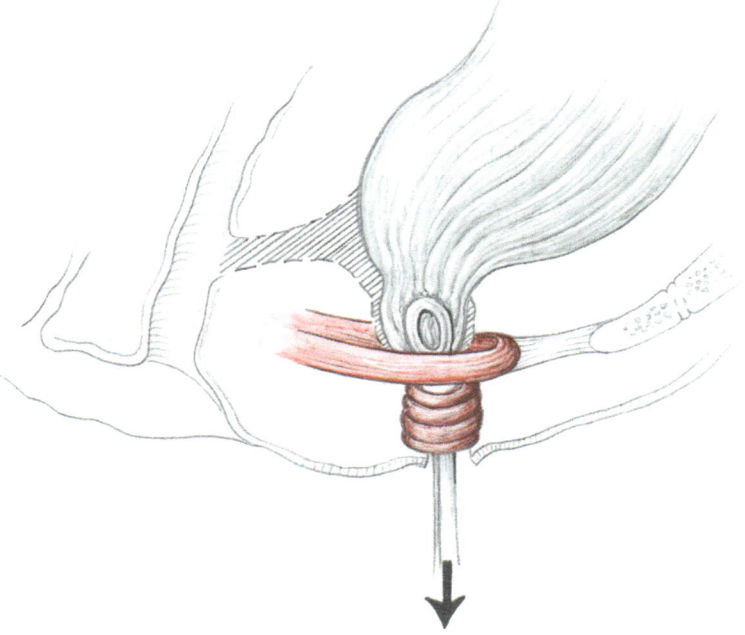

Fig. 9.4. The third important principle is that the ano-rectum should be brought through the exact epicentre of any previously identified anal muscle fibres. The anal dimple (if one is present) is an accurate guide to the central point.

ectopic orifice and the planned new site; such a technique will divide the integrity of any residual circular muscle fibres and considerably diminish the chances of proper sphincter control post-operatively; the technique of posterior sagittal ano-rectoplasty (PSARP) [2,5,7] is best suited to a paediatric practice, although it is useful in particular instances in adult patients as well.

2. When mobilising the ectopic opening, it is not wise to carry out the dissection too close as this will destroy any muscle tissue that may surround the opening and will leave the surgeon with thin and friable tissue to work with when the gut tube is being pulled down into its new position on the perineum.

3. Finally, it is important not to damage the pelvic nerves and blood supply to the ectopic gut tube: therefore the pelvic dissection must be performed under such excellent visual conditions that the parasympathetic nerves and important blood vessels are not damaged during mobilisation: this may require combined abdominal and perineal approaches. All dissection should be carried out as near to the mid-point of the pelvis as possible.

Selection and Preparation of Patients for Surgery

Most patients are usually sent to the surgeon with the diagnosis of congenital abnormality already made. A few patients who have an ectopic opening on the perineum behind the fourchette may not realise that the opening is abnormally situated, although incontinence will date from birth.

After the presence of a congenital abnormality of the anal orifice has been confirmed the special tests already referred to should establish whether or not there is enough puborectalis and sphincter muscle that can be used to restore some control once the anus has been moved to the normal site. The chief responsibility of the

specialist by this stage is to identify cases to whom a repair *should not* be offered. All patients in whom the lower three sacral vertebrae are missing or are seriously deformed suffer from severe abnormalities of the sacral plexus, and are usually unable to respond to appropriate stimulation of the sensori-motor end-organs of the pelvic floor and sphincter muscle remnants; it is usual for these cases to lack entirely the normal appreciation of rectal fullness, and invariably they do not possess intact recto-anal reflex responses. Such cases should not have their hopes raised by an attempt at repair based on sentiment rather than reality. Borderline cases should have urinary outflow control tested and a complete uro-dynamic assessment; if patients possess normal or near-normal urinary detrusor function, this can be taken as an encouraging sign for the presence of a sufficient degree of remaining sacral plexus function to justify an attempt at restoration. Patients in whom an intact puborectalis sling can be found should be regarded as having a reasonable chance of a successful result: in most of these cases, if an assiduous enough search is made, some residual sphincter muscle can be identified either at the ectopic site, or more frequently at the mid-point of the perineum. If the patient has had repeated previous attempts at correction of the deformity, especially if these have been accompanied by serious sepsis, there may be too much scar tissue to allow adequate assessment of the state of the pelvic floor or sphincter muscles: this will be particularly true for those patients (the majority) in whom the ectopic opening is stenosed. Fortunately it is unusual for these patients to have scar tissue that extends up to the level of the puborectalis, and in those with an unscarred pelvic floor (especially puborectalis) an attempt at repair is certainly justified. The unfortunate few in whom the entire lower pelvis has been irreparably destroyed (or is solidly enmeshed by impenetrable fibrosis) should not have yet another "no-hope" procedure inflicted on them with its considerable risks of dangerous trauma to other pelvic structures (especially the ureters).

Those patients who have reached adult years with a "covered anus" (Wingspread "low" type [9]) deformity that has been partially treated by the establishment of an iatrogenic recto-perineal fistula can be identified by finding anal sphincter muscle at the "normal" site, and in some of them by finding a microscopic true anal opening. A few cases will have been born with an already established track, which usually runs forwards from the rectum in a superficial plane to open at or near the fourchette: these cases offer an ideal prospect for cure if they are handled correctly by firstly re-establishing the normal anal canal (by dilatation) and then by subsequent closure of the fistula once the anal canal is opened up sufficiently to allow free passage of the faecal stream. This group also can have a good result from a posterior sagittal ano-rectoplasty [5,6,7].

Before proceeding to surgical reconstruction for patients with congenital anal deformity it must be remembered that such abnormalities are frequently multiple. Not only the genito-urinary, but also the heart and related pulmonary and aortic vessels should be examined for valvular and septal defects. A detailed family history should be taken and the state of health of all siblings should be noted. The psycho-social context in which the patient lives must be assessed, and the difficulties of predicting the outcome should be appreciated by the patient and everybody associated with the operation: parents are inclined to blame the surgeon unless they are prepared for disappointment (even when the surgeon may be inwardly optimistic).

Once operation has been decided upon, preparation differs between those patients who already have a colostomy and those who do not. If the patient has a colostomy, the distal bowel should be cleaned mechanically by daily wash-outs over several days: this may require a preliminary dilation of a stenosed ectopic orifice. Those subjects in whom a colostomy is not already present should have the stools rendered liquid by frequent doses of salts (magnesium sulphate 25 ml every 6 hours) and if the ectopic opening is both accessible and uncontracted twice daily *soap and water* enemas to remove long-standing faecal masses are useful. All patients should have antibiotics for several days before operation because the inactive and dilated reservoir of the distal bowel becomes a home for a wide variety of both anaerobic and aerobic bacteria and in cases with pronounced rectal dilation the enema should contain a weak antiseptic solution (aqueous chlorhexidine 1:2000 is suitable, but providone iodine solution can also be used). A defunctioned rectum not only stenoses but can develop "disuse proctitis" which may need treating prior to surgery.

Covered Anus Deformity with Associated Perineal Fistula ("False Anus")

In these patients (Fig. 9.5) the direction and depth of the fistula track of the false anus are important guides to the site of the true anal canal.

With the patient catheterised and in the lithotomy position, the fistulous track is carefully probed (Fig. 9.6): the operator is looking most especially for the point at which the track ceases to run backwards and changes direction to pass upward into the rectum. Once this point has been established, attention is turned to the perineal skin at its midpoint where, in the usual case, there should be either a visual 'dimple" or a palpable depression (Fig. 9.6). Whenever possible, preliminary electro-stimulation should have been done to confirm the presence of a functioning sphincter at this site. The probe in the false anal track can be moved around like a urinary sound to establish the depth and length of the true anal canal (Fig. 9.7).

A small cruciate incision is now made through the skin over the "true" covered

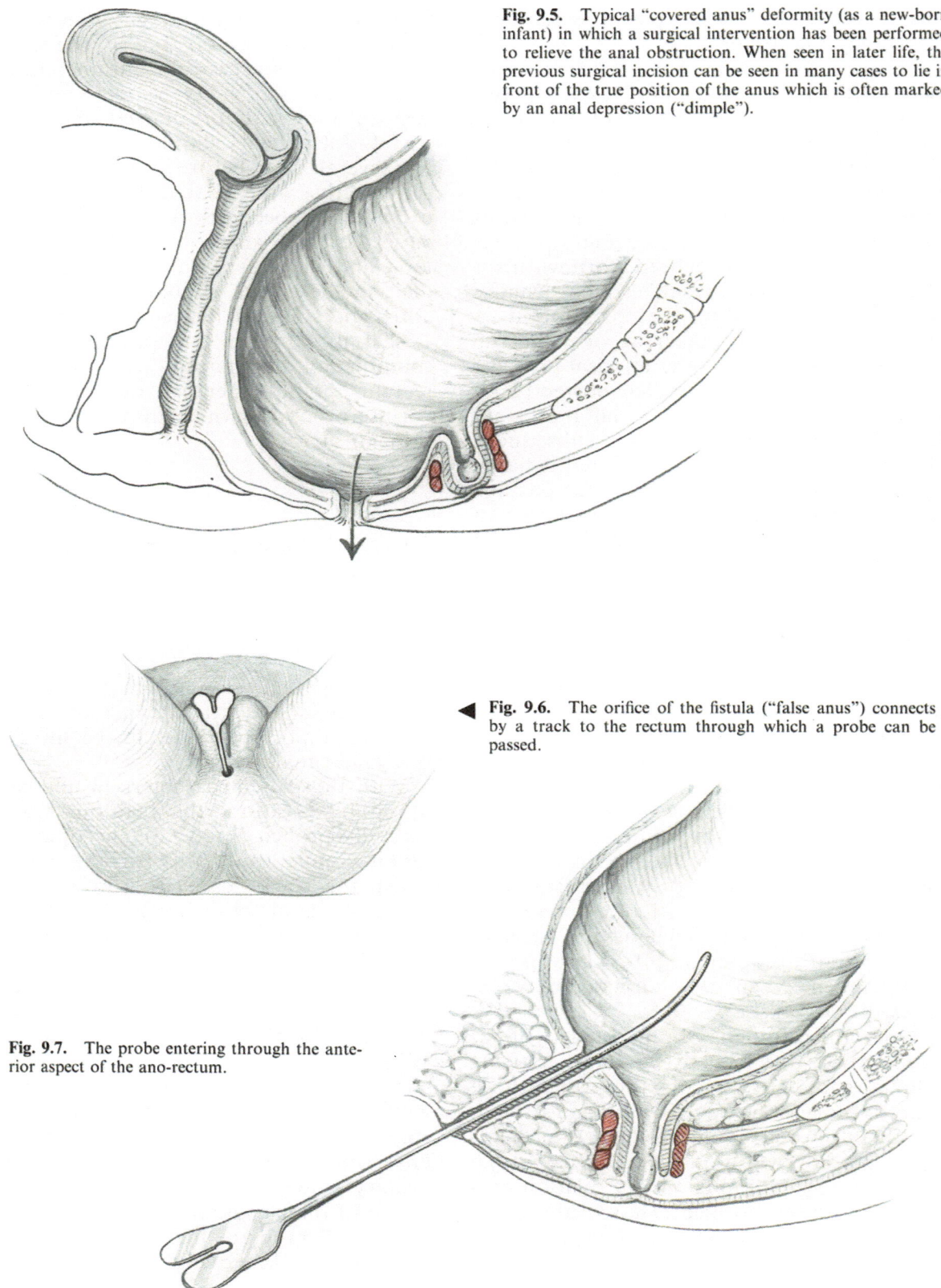

Fig. 9.5. Typical "covered anus" deformity (as a new-born infant) in which a surgical intervention has been performed to relieve the anal obstruction. When seen in later life, the previous surgical incision can be seen in many cases to lie in front of the true position of the anus which is often marked by an anal depression ("dimple").

◀ **Fig. 9.6.** The orifice of the fistula ("false anus") connects by a track to the rectum through which a probe can be passed.

Fig. 9.7. The probe entering through the anterior aspect of the ano-rectum.

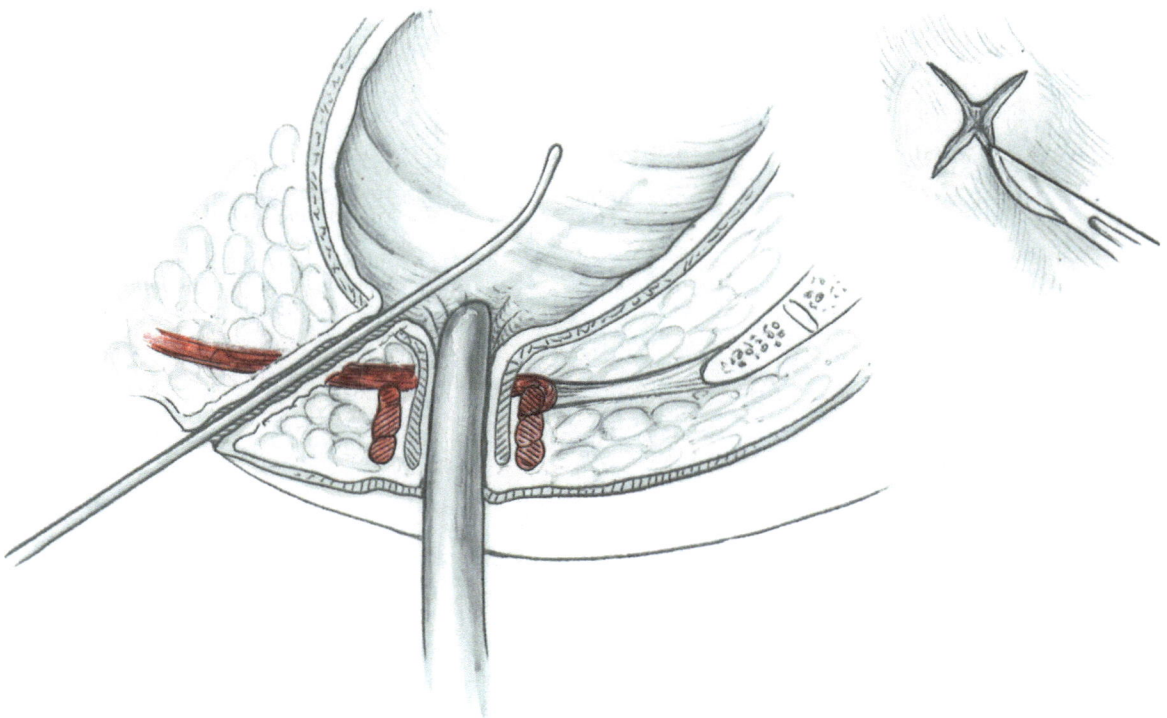

Fig. 9.8. After making a cruciate incision over the anal dimple, the true anal canal can be gently dilated up. Eventually the rectum is reached and opened into. The probe (which has been left in place) can be manipulated and the point at which it enters the rectum identified. The length of the "true" anal canal is assessed.

Fig. 9.9. The anterior fistulous opening ("false anus") is now cored out up to the rectal wall.

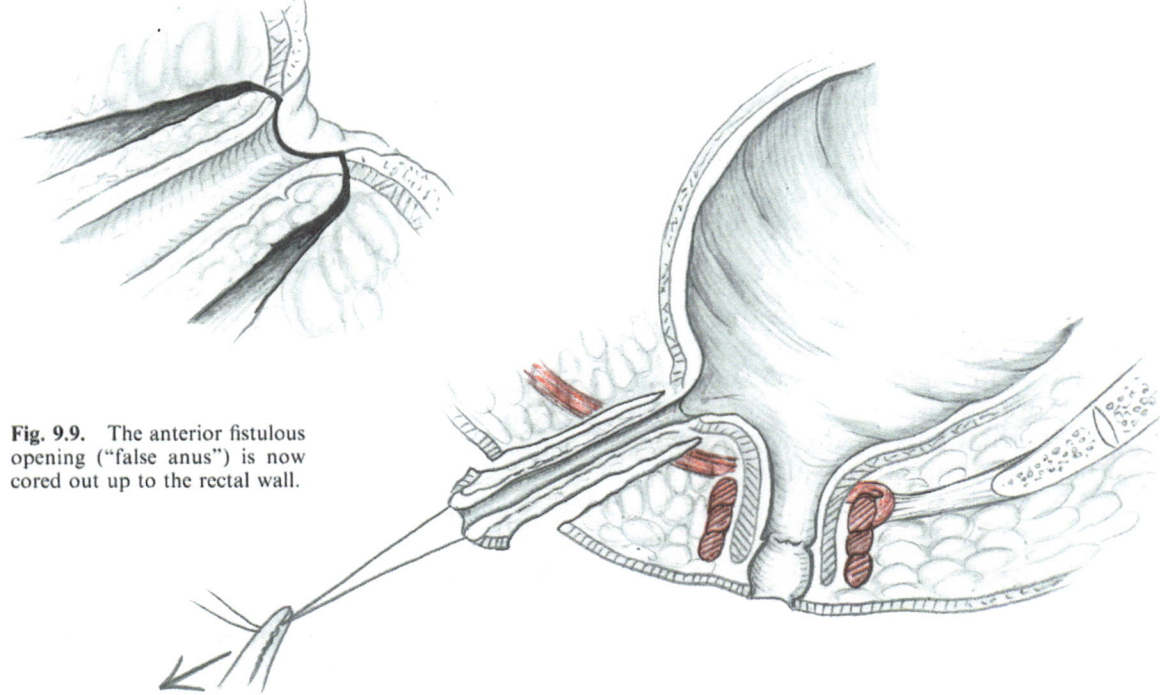

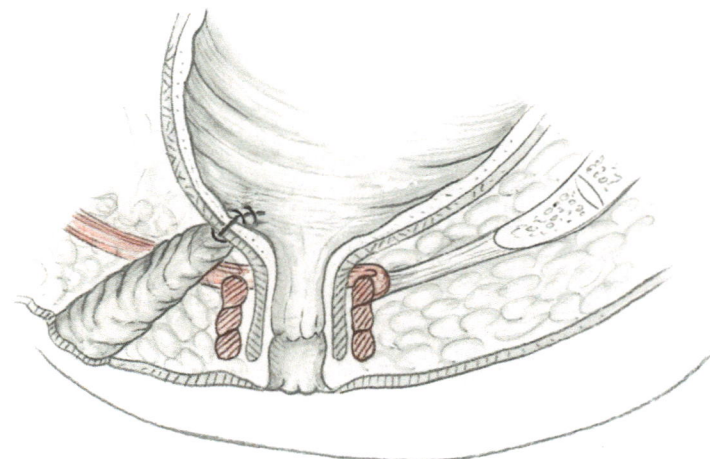

Fig. 9.10. After amputation of the fistula track the rectal wall is closed with interrupted fine (000) sutures of Vicryl. The newly opened anal canal must be kept dilated to an adequate lumen while the wounds heal, and maintained to a proper size when the diverting stoma is closed.

anus, which can now be further verified by identifying gut epithelium. Once it has been found, the anal canal can be opened up by gentle dilation and followed into the lower rectum (Fig. 9.8): initial dilation should be with graduated Hegar's dilators, but subsequently the index finger can be used. In those patients in whom a satisfactory lumen cannot be established a posterior sagittal ano-rectoplasty can be employed [5]. Once the anal canal has been opened up sufficiently it is possible to identify the point at which a probe in the fistula track enters the rectum through its anterior wall (Fig. 9.8). The probe is left in the fistula track, which is now cored out from its external opening as far as its junction with the anterior wall of the gut (Fig. 9.9). This part of the dissection can be made easier by an infiltration of adrenaline (1 part per 300 000 in physiological saline) which will control bleeding. Once the wall of the rectum is reached, the fistula is amputated, and the defect in the wall closed with fine (000) interrupted sutures of Vicryl (Fig. 9.10). The external part of the wound is left open to heal by granulation.

Anterior Ectopic Deformity

Before the patient with anterior ectopic deformity (Figs. 9.11 and 9.12) is premedicated the surgeon is responsible for marking on the perineal skin the "site of election" for the newly transposed anus. If sphincter muscle has been identified preoperatively, the midpoint of the muscle area should have been established by electromyography ("sphincter-mapping") and a clear indication provided to the surgeon as to the site of the muscle fibres. If an anal dimple is present, this point marks the best site for resiting the new anus.

The patient is catheterised before entering the operating room: in a male patient (which is exceedingly rare) a small malleable bougie can be used instead of a catheter in order to aid identification of the urethra during the perineal dissection.

Most adult cases are unsuitable for posterior sagittal ano-rectoplasty (PSARP) because the sphincter muscle, once divided, cannot be rejoined anteriorly. Because these cases are most commonly seen in females, the technique is described as for a woman. For these operations the authors recommend the lithotomy rather than the prone position as this facilitates access to the vagina, and permits simultaneous abdominal dissection if this is necessary. If the

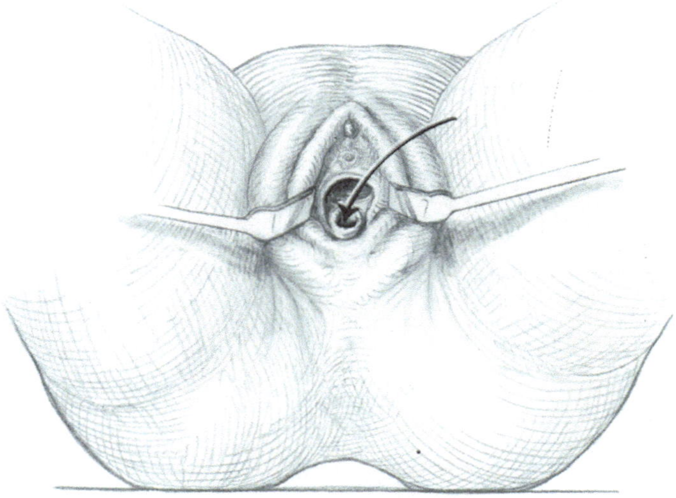

Fig. 9.11. A typical anterior ectopic anal opening presenting low in the posterior vaginal wall.

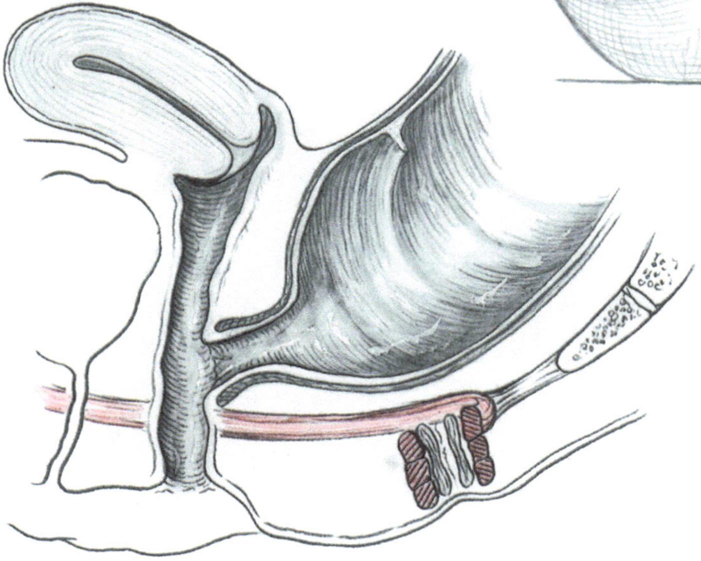

Fig. 9.12. A sagittal view of anterior ectopic anal displacement. In this case, the vaginal opening is higher than in Fig. 9.11, and will need very careful assessment of the pelvic floor muscles before a reconstruction is recommended.

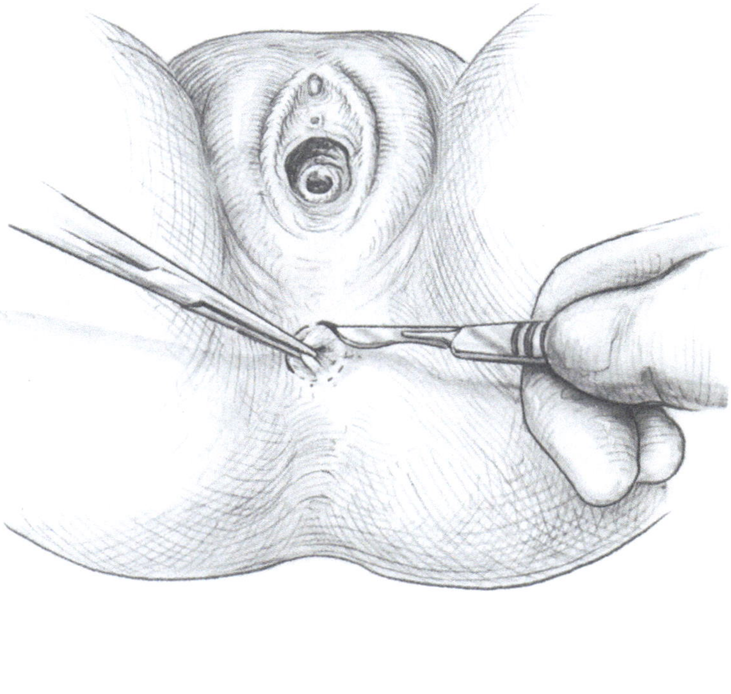

Fig. 9.13. A disc of skin is removed from the point which the surgeon judges to be the "true" site for the anal opening. An anal dimple or electromyographic mapping are of crucial importance for this decision.

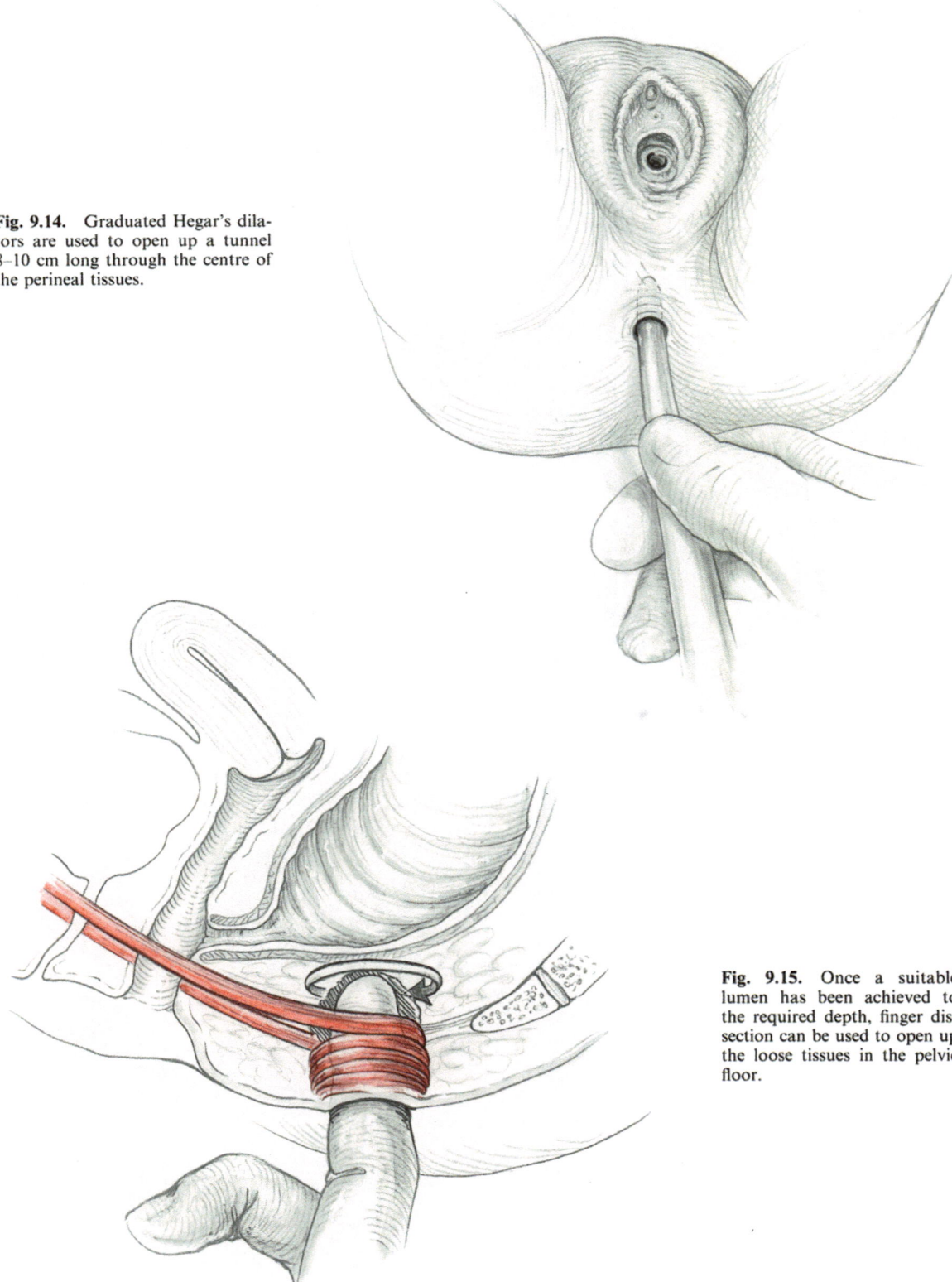

Fig. 9.14. Graduated Hegar's dilators are used to open up a tunnel 8–10 cm long through the centre of the perineal tissues.

Fig. 9.15. Once a suitable lumen has been achieved to the required depth, finger dissection can be used to open up the loose tissues in the pelvic floor.

puborectalis and other parts of the levator ani muscle are definitely present, it is best to start by establishing the new route for the displaced anus and rectum through the pelvic floor. After removing a small disc of skin and subcutaneous tissue (Fig. 9.13), blunt dissection of the anocutaneous tissues using a series of Hegar's gynaecological dilators (Fig. 9.14) will open up a tunnel 8–10 cm long in the midline to reach a level a few centimetres above the muscular floor of the pelvis: this will usually lie opposite the 3rd to the 4th sacral vertebrae. It is now possible to insert one or both index fingers and tunnel out a generous "cave" in the soft tissues of the pelvis surrounding the lower bowel as it descends in the pelvis (Fig. 9.15). If a vaginal anus is present, the fingers can be used to burrow forwards to approach the posterior wall of the vagina on each site of the ectopic anal opening, staying well clear of any midline structures and the rectum itself.

At this point, the operator turns his attention to the ectopic opening which is closed with a purse-string suture (in some cases this is better done at the beginning of the operation). A circumferential incision is made around the ectopic orifice leaving a surrounding margin of tissue at least 0.5 cm wide (Fig. 9.16). This margin will preserve any remnant of sphincter muscle of somatic origin as the dissection is deepened, as well as keeping intact the inner circular unstriped muscle layer of the gut tube. The tissues around the displaced bowel are gradually parted by meticulous blunt and sharp dissection until a large enough length has been mobilised to reach the new site for the anal orifice without tension: during the later stages of this part of the operation the two separate approaches that have been developed should meet in the cavity that has been created in the middle of the floor of the pelvis (Fig. 9.17). The ectopic anus and attached rectum (which has also been mobilised for several centimetres) are now ready for transposition. At this point the surgeon must be absolutely certain of two points:

1. That there is sufficient length of mobilised lower rectum and anus to translocate to the perineum without tension

2. That the newly formed tunnel through the mid-point of the perineum is sufficiently wide to accommodate the ectopic anus when it is drawn through

If the surgeon is not satisfied on these points, consideration should be given to carrying out a posterior sagittal anorectoplasty as an alternative [7].

Providing these two vital considerations have been fulfilled, the ectopic anus should be grasped by a forceps inserted through the neo-anal opening and drawn down to reach beyond the level of the perineal skin (Fig. 9.18). The purse-string suture is now removed, and the mucosal edge of the ectopic anus is joined to the surrounding perineal skin by interrupted sutures of 0 Vicryl, which should include generous bites of tissue on each side at least 5 mm deep (Fig. 9.19).

The area of the pelvic dissection is not closed, but is drained by a soft Latex or Silastic drain which is put through the site of the original ectopic opening and fastened

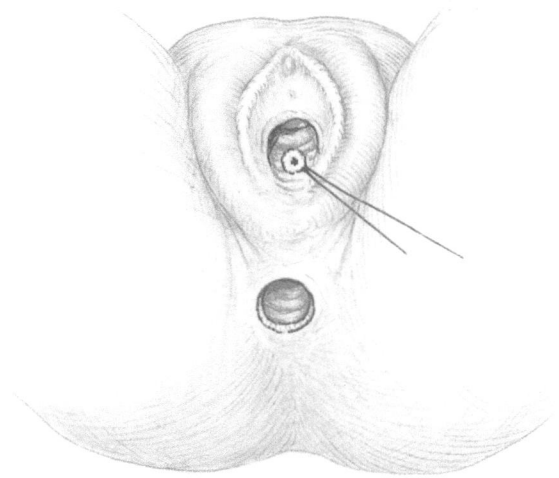

Fig. 9.16. The vaginal ectopic opening is closed with a purse-string suture, which is left long. The dissection of the displaced anus and lower rectum is performed circumferentially leaving a margin of at least 1.0 cm.

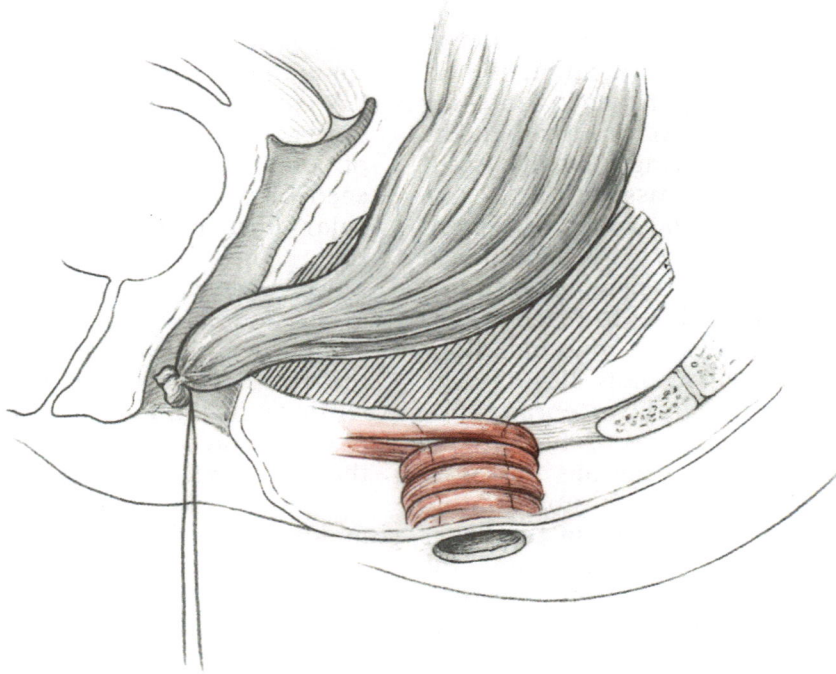

Fig. 9.17. Eventually the trans-vaginal dissection will meet up with the previously excavated cave in the pelvic floor. The mobilised ano-rectal tissues should have sufficient length to reach the perineum without tension.

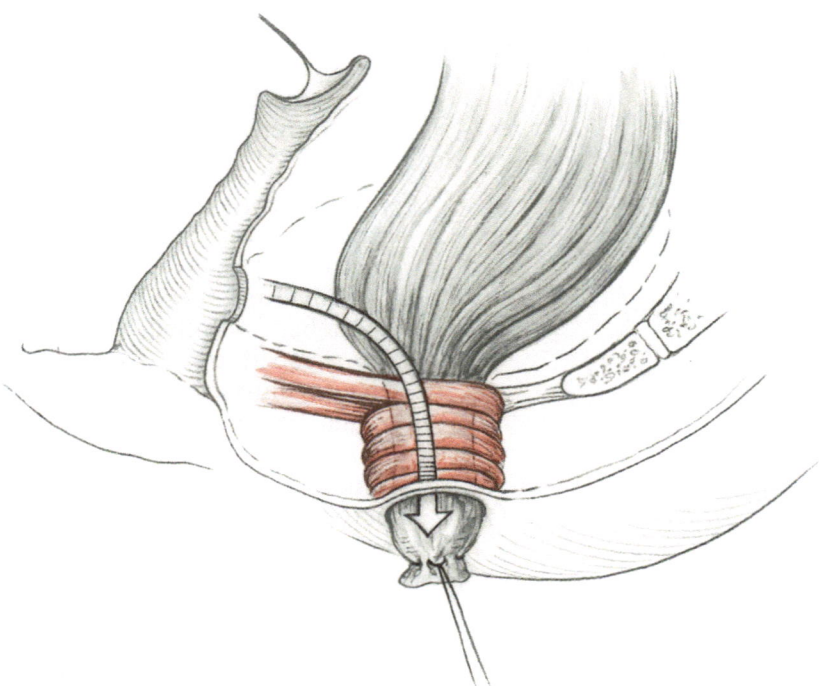

Fig. 9.18. The mobilised distal ano- rectal segment can now be grasped and drawn down through the perineal tunnel. No force should be used and no tension must develop during this manoeuvre. If the bowel will not reach without undue tension the procedure will fail.

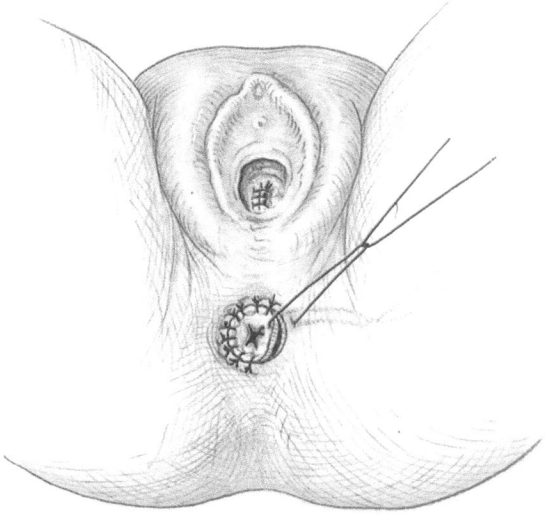

Fig. 9.19. Finally, the purse-string suture is removed, and direct muco-cutaneous suture with interrupted 0 Vicryl stitches is carried out.

with stitches to prevent displacement. The wound edges can be narrowed by a few stitches, providing the cavity continues to drain freely.

Most of these patients will already have an established colostomy which can be closed when sound healing of the wound is complete. If the patient comes to the operating theatre without a diversion, the authors recommend that a temporary diversion should be established to protect the operation both from septic complications and disruptive pressure from the faecal stream which can easily destroy the repair. The protective diverting stoma should not be closed until the surgeon is satisfied that:

1. The ano-rectal wounds are soundly healed
2. The anal lumen is of sufficient size that faecal passage is easy and assured. This usually takes 6–12 weeks. The intervening period prior to colostomy (or ileostomy) closure can be usefully taken up by regular dilation (up to No. 18 Hegar) to open and maintain a good anal lumen

No Definite Anal or Puborectalis Muscle

Most of these patients present with a colostomy already in place. If the sacrum is defective but is intact below S3 and normal micturition is present, it is possible that some development of the proctodaeum and anal bud has occurred even though this cannot be definitely established. As it is the patient's only chance for restoration of defaecation control it is justifiable to carry out an abdominal exploration of the pelvis in order to establish whether some muscles of the pelvic floor are present, and especially to identify puborectalis. This will also establish the true level at which hind-gut descent has terminated, which may be lower than pre-operative radiological investigations (invertogram or loopogram) suggest.

Patients who require such an abdominal exploration will usually have a high abnormality with at best an ectopic opening high up on the posterior vaginal wall or at worst a cloacal-type abnormality. Most of these cases have no useful remnant of pelvic floor muscle, and will require a permanent end-colostomy. If this turns out to be the case after careful exploration of the pelvic anatomy, the ectopic opening should be freed up and the end of the distal bowel used to form a proper terminal stoma in the left iliac fossa.

If, against all the odds, some pelvic floor muscular development has taken place and the iliococcygeus and puborectalis muscles can be identified, the same procedures can be followed as for the patient with an anterior displacement deformity (pp. 136–140), except that placement of the mobilised opening on the perineal skin is made at an arbitrary point selected by the surgeon, with direct mucocutaneous suture-anastomosis.

In these cases, any return of continence is dependent on good function of puborectalis [8]. At best only faecal control can be expected, and flatus, mucus and liquid stool will continue to leak; these cases, even after the best possible result, will continue to

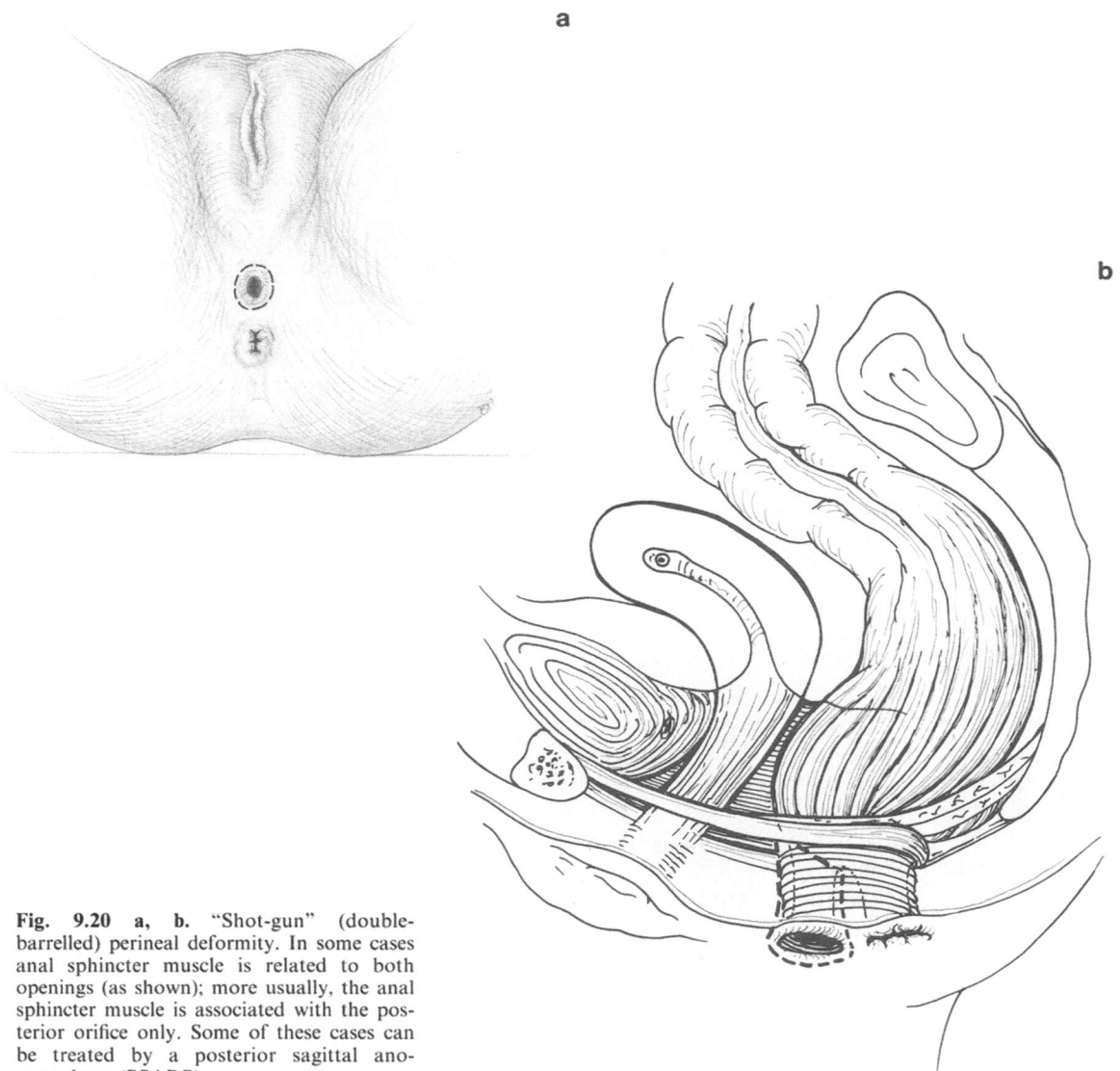

Fig. 9.20 a, b. "Shot-gun" (double-barrelled) perineal deformity. In some cases anal sphincter muscle is related to both openings (as shown); more usually, the anal sphincter muscle is associated with the posterior orifice only. Some of these cases can be treated by a posterior sagittal ano-rectoplasty (PSARP).

need a perineal pad. Many patients will remain faecally incontinent, but some of them can keep themselves clean by using distal washing-out or enema techniques. A surprising number of them will prefer to keep what amounts to a perineal colostomy rather than return to an artificial stoma. A stimulated gracilis sling can be used for some of these patients (see pp. 95–100).

Ectopic Opening Adjacent to an Anal Orifice ("Shot-gun Deformity")

In these patients, the two canals lie parallel to one another, and unite a few centimetres above skin level (Fig. 9.20). It is impossible to mobilise and close the ectopic opening without damaging the anterior fibres of the external sphincter muscle, at least to some

Fig. 9.21. The anterior opening and its connecting tube (which is usually short) are dissected out, and cut back as far as the wall of the ano-rectum, which is repaired by interrupted fine (000) Prolene sutures in at least two layers.

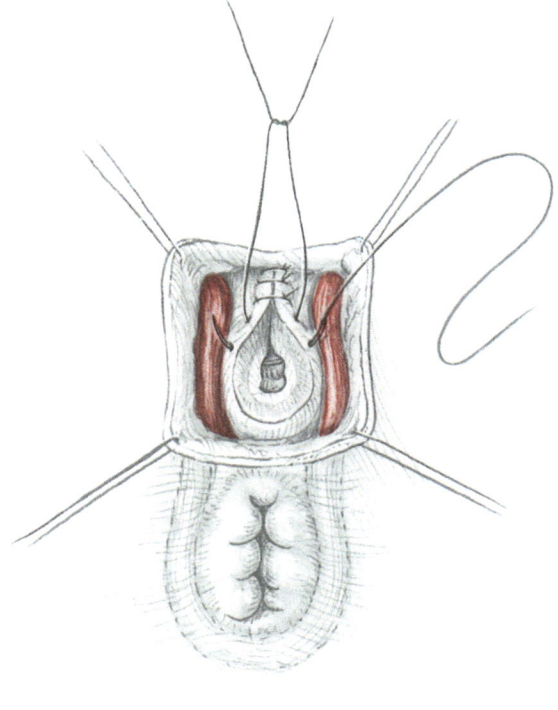

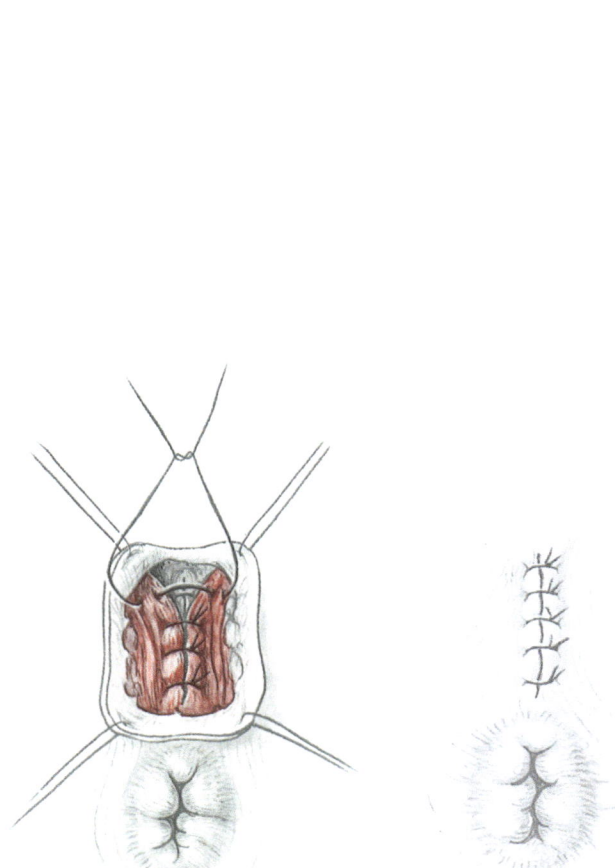

Fig. 9.22. The anterior muscles of the ano-rectum are drawn together over the closure line, if possible by an overlapping technique or a buttress repair.

extent. This can be mitigated by carrying out the dissection of the ectopic canal in a bloodless field achieved by the use of a weak adrenaline infiltration (1 part per 300 000 physiological saline), which allows the operator to see and preserve the muscle fibres.

The ectopic tube is carefully dissected out up to the point where it joins the true anorectum. At this point the ectopic canal is cut away, leaving a good cut of tissue for use in closure of the defect. This part of the procedure closely resembles the technique used for closing the neck of a pharyngeal

diverticulum. The defect is closed in two layers: an inner continuous stitch of 000 Prolene to the mucosa, reinforced by interrupted Vicryl sutures, also 000 size, to the muscle (Fig. 9.21).

Once the defect has been repaired, the surgeon should identify the damaged edges of the anal sphincter. After these have been demonstrated and defined, an immediate direct repair using strong Dexon sutures (0) should be carried out, if possible by a double-overlap method.

In other cases, an anterior buttress procedure, as described on pp. 49–53, is the

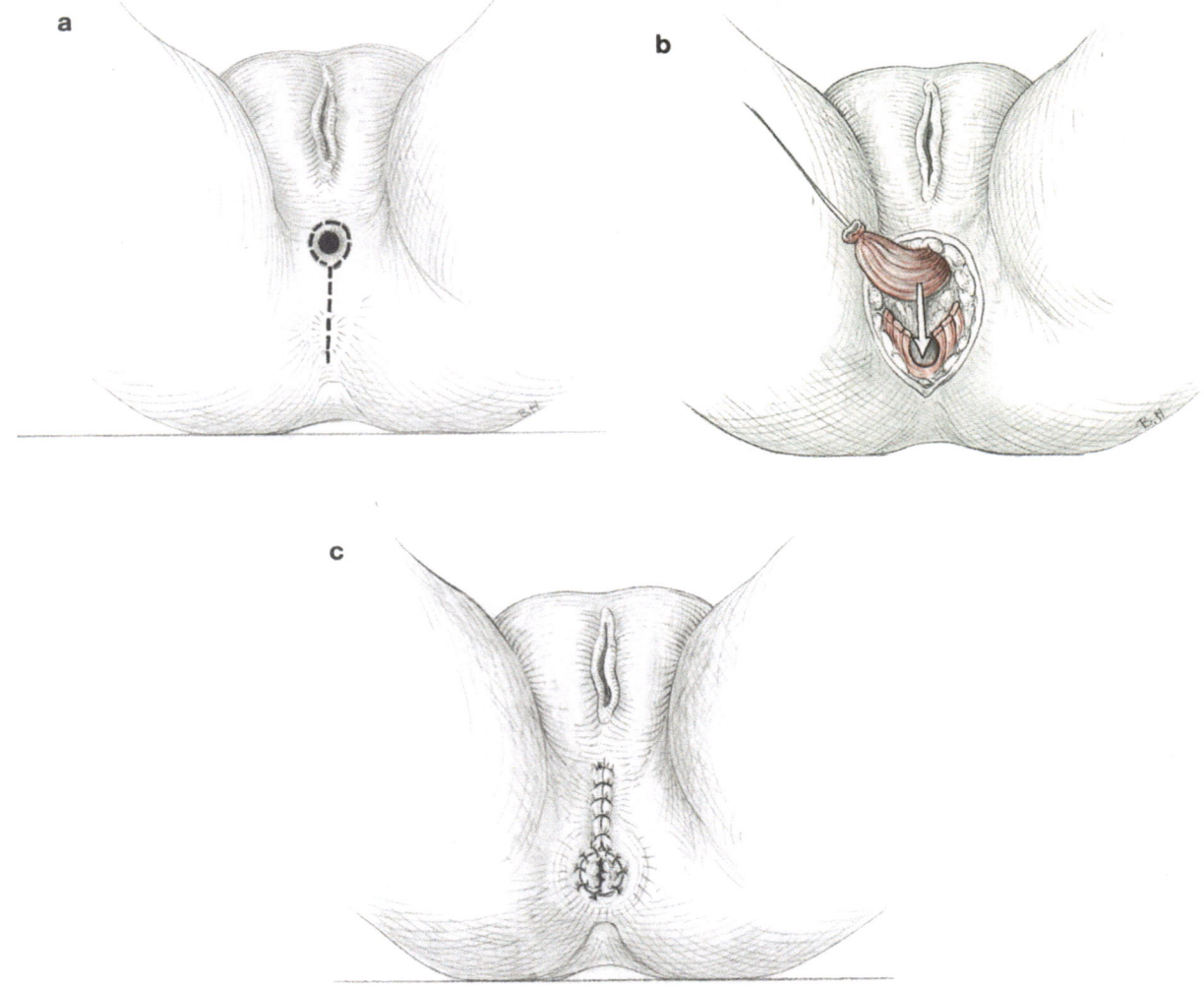

Fig. 9.23 a–c.   Posterior sagittal ano-rectoplasty as described by Pena.

most suitable technique for reinforcing the anterior wall of the anus and lower rectum and tightening of the anal sphincter muscles (Fig. 9.22).

A simple "cut-back" technique should not be employed for these cases as it leaves the patient incontinent. However, a posterior sagittal ano-rectoplasty can be used when a pliant anal canal and good sphincter muscles are present (Fig. 9.23 a–c).

Cloacal-type Deformity

These patients require such a long programme of reconstruction, with multiple operations and long periods of hospital admission, that it is not possible to recommend this type of surgical ordeal of very uncertain outcome to patients who present as adults with incontinence due to this deformity. They should be persuaded that a good colostomy offers them their best chance for a life free of invalidism.

Post-operative Management

The post-operative care of these patients is simplified by the presence of a diversion; either by a colostomy installed previously, or by a stoma (either an ileostomy or a colostomy as seems to be best) established simultaneously with the transposition procedure. This obviates the need to empty the distal bowel post-operatively until the repair has had time to become firm, and any septic complications have subsided.

Because septic complications can interfere with the best possible functional result by creating fibrosis or by destroying stitch lines, great care must be taken to reduce these to a minimum by the following measures:

1. Meticulous surgical technique to reduce intra-operative bleeding
2. Careful haemostasis at the end of the procedure
3. Proper drainage (suction) of potential cavities

But antibiotics are also important for reducing or preventing septic collections which can accumulate during the first days after surgery: both aerobic and anaerobic organisms need to be "hit" by the antibiotic treatment and the authors recommend a 5-day course of cephradine (500 mgm i.m. twice daily) plus metronidazole (200 mg daily), but in younger patients these doses may need to be adjusted.

The usual precautions against venous thrombosis should be taken by:

1. Early mobilisation
2. The use of pressure-graduated stockings at and beyond the time of the operation
3. Frequent physiotherapy to encourage breathing and leg movements.

Heparin is not usually required for these cases.

The catheter should be removed when I.V. fluids are no longer required. In those patients who do not need abdominal exploration, ileus is brief or non-existent and fluids and low-residue, high-calorie oral intake can be started as soon as the patient is conscious.

Pain is not usually a serious problem in these patients, and opiates should not be given unnecessarily: this is particularly important for patients who have undergone multiple operations beforehand.

Although the stitching of the tissues, and especially of the neo-anus, may have been done with delayed but so-called absorbable sutures (e.g. Vicryl or Dexon), these usually do not disappear from the surface union of the perineal skin with the transposed anus. They should not be removed before the eighth to tenth post-operative day, and if, as is often the case, the surgeon wishes to check the state of the repair, removing these sutures can be done optimally at the same time as an examination under anaesthesia around the 10th–14th post-operative day. Post-operative examination under anaesthesia is useful in most of these patients prior to hospital discharge. Not only can any pelvic collections be detected and drained before any damage is done, but the progress of healing can be checked and the adequacy of the lumen of the neo-anus verified. If there is any tendency to anal stenosis (e.g. below a size that will permit comfortable insertion of the index finger to the second knuckle) a programme of regular dilation must be instituted until an adequate lumen is established: only at this point should closure of the diversion stoma be carried out.

The patients must be warned that the first few weeks will be difficult after the faecal stream is re-established. They are virtually in the same position as a new-born babe and need time to "learn" control. It may take up to 12 months of constant encouragement and advice before a substantial degree of continence is established. During this time, management of faecal bulk and consistency may need constant flexibility, and supervision should be frequent and close: any tendency to faecal retention must be treated appropriately by suppositories and enemas (given by a nurse who is both experienced and sympathetic) and the physician must be prepared to make numerous checks that the rectum is able to empty itself. Faecal impaction is the enemy of these repairs by stretching the rectal wall (so that it loses its power to contract) and by destroying the integrity of the newly reconstructed tissues. Once the damage is done, and the patient has experienced the "incontinence" of spurious diarrhoea associated with rectal retention, the patient's loss of morale may be as difficult to restore as the physical damage.

Summary

Careful selection is the key to obtaining satisfying results. In turn, this depends on identification of both the site and quantity of any residual sphincter and pelvic floor muscle. Once the presence of sphincteric contractions has been verified, or a good puborectalis muscle is found, all possible steps must be taken to place the ano-rectal organ into its correct relation with these muscles. During this reconstruction, damage to any muscle should be avoided by careful planning of both the route and the technique of the repair. The correct alignment of the ano-rectum within the arms of the puborectalis is as important as identification of the epicentre of any remnant of sphincter muscle. The presence of a faecal diversion is important to allow the repair to settle in and to prevent unnecessary complications. Once faecal restoration has occurred, careful and constant supervision is indicated for up to 12 months to achieve the best possible results. If all these criteria are met, and both patient and surgeon are prepared to make the required commitment, a satisfactory result is possible.

References and Further Reading

1. Browne D (1955) Congenital deformities of the anus and rectum. Arch Dis Child 30: 42
2. De Vries P, Pena A (1982) Posterior sagittal ano-rectoplasty. J Pediatr Surg 17: 638
3. Marti MC, Givel JC (1989) Surgery of ano-rectal diseases. Springer, Heidelberg and New York, pp 297–304
4. Nixon H, (1985) Congenital deformities of the ano-rectal region. In: Surgery of the anus, rectum and colon, 5th edn. Ballière Tindall, London, pp 285–304
5. Pena A (1985) Posterior sagittal approach for the correction of ano-rectal malformations. Year Book Med Publ Chicago, 19: 69
6. Pena A (1989) Surgical management of ano-rectal malformations. Springer, Heidelberg and New York
7. Pena A (1989) In: Corman ML (ed.) Colon and rectal surgery, 2nd edn. Lippincott, Philadelphia, pp 270–271
8. Smith ED (1976) The identification and management of ano-rectal anomalies. The factors ensuring continence. Prog Pediatr Surg 9: 7
9. Stephens FD, Smith ED (1986) Classification, identification and assessment of surgical treatment of ano-rectal anomalies. Pediatr Surg Int 1: 200

CHAPTER 10

Techniques for Repair of Traumatic Injury of the Anal Sphincters

General Introduction

Traumatic injuries by military projectiles or impalement wounds with spikes or other weapons may result in complete or partial division of the anal sphincter and pelvic floor muscles [1,5]. If the wound is clean and there is minimal tissue disruption, it may be possible to consider a primary repair of the sphincter and pelvic floor musculature, especially if the surgeon has experience in this field. If, however, there is considerable tissue disruption, which may occur in high-speed missile or explosion injury, it is wise to limit initial surgery to cautious minimal debridement, open drainage and a defunctioning colostomy. Later, clinical and laboratory evaluation is used to assess any remnant of functional muscle and to plan reconstruction. If there is much tissue loss, reconstruction will have to be delayed until the wound is clean and totally free of sepsis, which may take 3 months. Sphincter mapping by electromyography may be of use, and the success of surgery relies on accurately locating viable sphincter muscle and its mobilisation for a sound repair. If there is extensive muscle loss, direct repair may not be possible and the surgeon may have to consider muscle transfer procedures such as the gracilis sling (see pp. 87–100).

Another cause of serious traumatic injury to the anal sphincter is during operations for high fistula in ano when excessive sphincter muscle is divided. Faecal incontinence will ensue, and this is particularly so if the ano-rectal ring is divided during the treatment of supra-levator fistulas. It is usually possible to offer late reconstruction in these cases after the fistula has healed and sepsis has been eradicated [9].

Indications and Selection of Patients

All patients with major traumatic division of the anal sphincter muscle should be considered for reconstruction. This is particularly so in female patients who have undergone injury at childbirth. However, these patients should be tested for nerve damage which is common after difficult childbirth [10] as the results of repair are less good in these patients. Major reconstruction following injury from military projectiles or explosives should always be considered optimistically in young patients, but the success of the procedure depends absolutely on the extent of nerve damage as well as tissue loss. Major sphincter and pelvic floor reconstruction in an elderly patient presents a considerable surgical challenge with diminished chances for a good result; if there is extensive tissue loss, a permanent stoma may be an acceptable and sensible alternative.

Preparation

If a patient can be treated by an experienced surgeon within a few hours of injury, and there is no underlying sepsis, a primary repair has many advantages. In particular the divided muscle can be identified and repaired before retraction and subsequent fibrosis develop, which make later reconstruction more difficult.

The patient must be fit to withstand a general anaesthetic, and the extent of any associated injuries must be considered before embarking on what can be a prolonged surgical procedure. Pre-operative antibiotics should be administered, including ampicillin if there is more than minimal muscle damage. It is often extremely difficult to assess the extent of an injury without excellent facilities; general anaesthesia and better than average theatre lighting are essential. A decision to perform primary repair, or to delay formal reconstruction and establish a colostomy, can only be made after complete evaluation and debridement. The labour ward is *never* the right place to carry out a primary sphincter repair.

In the obstetric patient a primary repair is nearly always possible so long as the injury is immediately recognised. Because of medico-legal considerations, primary repair of obstetric injury may become a procedure that always involves a colo-proctological expert and is therefore included in this chapter.

Acute Primary Repair of Traumatised Anal Sphincter and Pelvic Floor [1,5,9]

Introduction

It is impossible to describe repair of a disrupted anal sphincter or pelvic floor except in general terms as each injury is different and the reconstruction will need to vary with the extent of damage. The stages of primary reconstruction, however, are the same, as follows:

1. Thorough cleansing of the wound
2. Assessment of the damage
3. Identification of sphincter muscle (and levator muscles in severe injury)
4. Debridement, *preserving all viable muscle*
5. Reconstruction
6. Colostomy, if required
7. Late closure of colostomy (if present)

It is vital to preserve all viable muscle and to sacrifice only that tissue that is ischaemic or macerated. The fat can be freely sacrificed as it withstands post-operative sepsis poorly, especially if contaminated with organic matter. It is best to remove the fat of the ischiorectal fossa back to clean bleeding tissue. Skin cover is similarly not critical in the primary repair, and the temptation to cover any reconstruction with skin under tension must be resisted. This will only produce areas of dead space which will lead to deep-seated

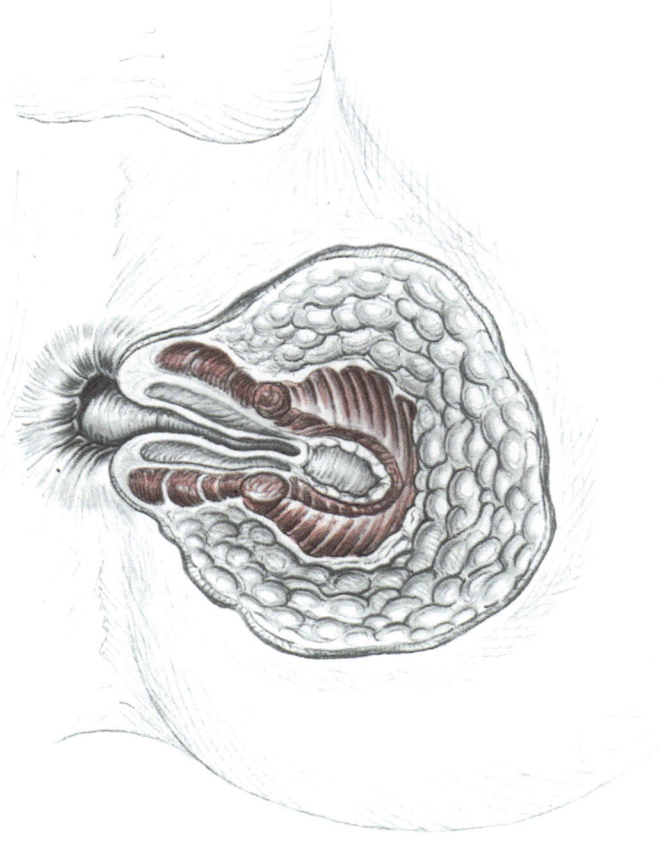

Fig. 10.1. After careful, but adequate, debridement and washing-away of all foreign material in the wound, it may be possible to identify separate muscle groups e.g. external anal sphincter and the lowest parts of the levator muscle.

infection with pocketing of pus. Skin cover can be achieved, later if necessary, by rotation flaps or skin grafting (Fig. 10.10).

Operative Technique

The patient should be placed in the lithotomy position with the hips well flexed. (As the repair is made hip flexion may need to be reduced on the table to relax the perineal floor and musculature and to facilitate apposition of the skin.) A catheter is passed into the bladder and is retained until the patient is mobilised. Perfect illumination is essential to examine the wound, and if the injury is severe, rectoscopy, sigmoidoscopy and cystoscopy may be needed to exclude or evaluate possible additional injury to the bowel, bladder, prostate or urethra.

The perineum should be cleaned with a solution of aqueous chlorhexidine (1:200) and all foreign material removed. It may be possible to identify separate muscle groups, e.g. external anal sphincter, puborectalis and levator muscles (Fig. 10.1). Care should be taken to preserve branches of the inferior haemorrhoidal nerves which lie on the inferior surface of the levator muscles as they approach the sphincter muscles.

After cleansing and debridement, a decision must now be made whether to proceed to a primary repair, or to delay reconstruc-

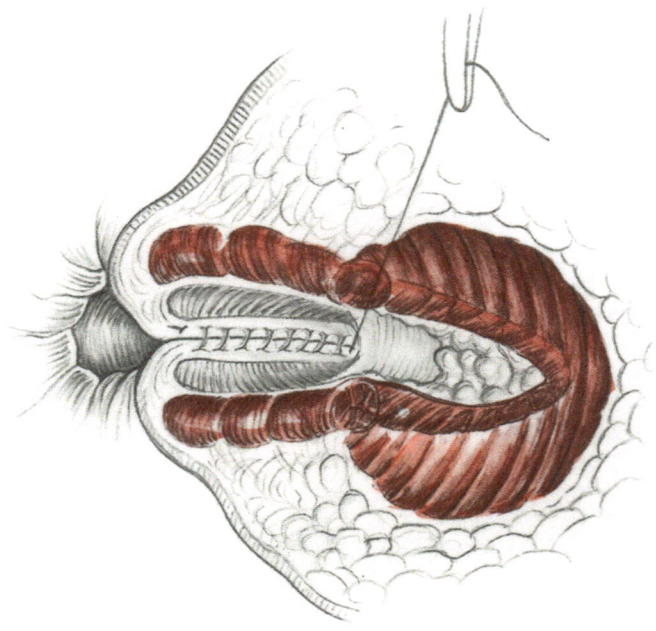

Fig. 10.2. Whenever possible, as a first stage the mucosal lining of the gut tube is closed with a continuous layer of 000 chromic catgut.

tion. With experience it is usually possible to correct even a major injury, so long as there is not excessive tissue loss. If muscle loss is great then it is wise simply to dress the wound with gauze swabs, soaked in sodium hypochlorite solution and laid in its base and to perform a defunctioning colostomy. At a later date, definitive reconstruction (possibly involving a muscle transfer) may be undertaken. It is a great advantage to label the injured muscle groups that have been divided by marking them with different non-absorbable sutures. This helps with later repair by facilitating the accurate union of important layers. As discussed earlier, the general physical condition of the patient must be considered, and the degree of associated injury, before undertaking a complex sphincter and pelvic floor repair either primarily or after wound sepsis has subsided. If necessary, a colostomy is made which need not be closed until after sphincter reconstruction and the patient is fit.

The first stage of the reconstruction is to repair the defect in the mucosal lining of the gut tube. In high and extensive injury of the bowel wall, this may be impossible, but if the injury is low and involves only the lower rectum or anal canal, the mucosal layers on each side of the wound should be freed and closed with fine continuous (000) chromic catgut stitches (Fig. 10.2).

The muscles should now be examined. If possible all the levator muscle should be repaired, but in practice, except in patients with minimal injury, close approximation of the divided edges of iliococcygeus is difficult, and in the majority of cases all that can be achieved is to narrow the muscle defect using interrupted stitches of 0 Vicryl (Fig. 10.3). The most important part of the levator ani muscle complex is the lowest (puborectalis) which combines with the external anal sphincter and is the major component of sphincter competence. This must be identified, and can virtually always be repaired with deep, horizontal mattress stitches of No. 1 Prolene (Fig. 10.4). The repair continues with union of the external anal sphincter using an "0" Prolene suture. After the initial injury the external anal sphincter muscles always retract leaving at least a one – and usually a two – quadrant defect. Cautious mobilisation to achieve

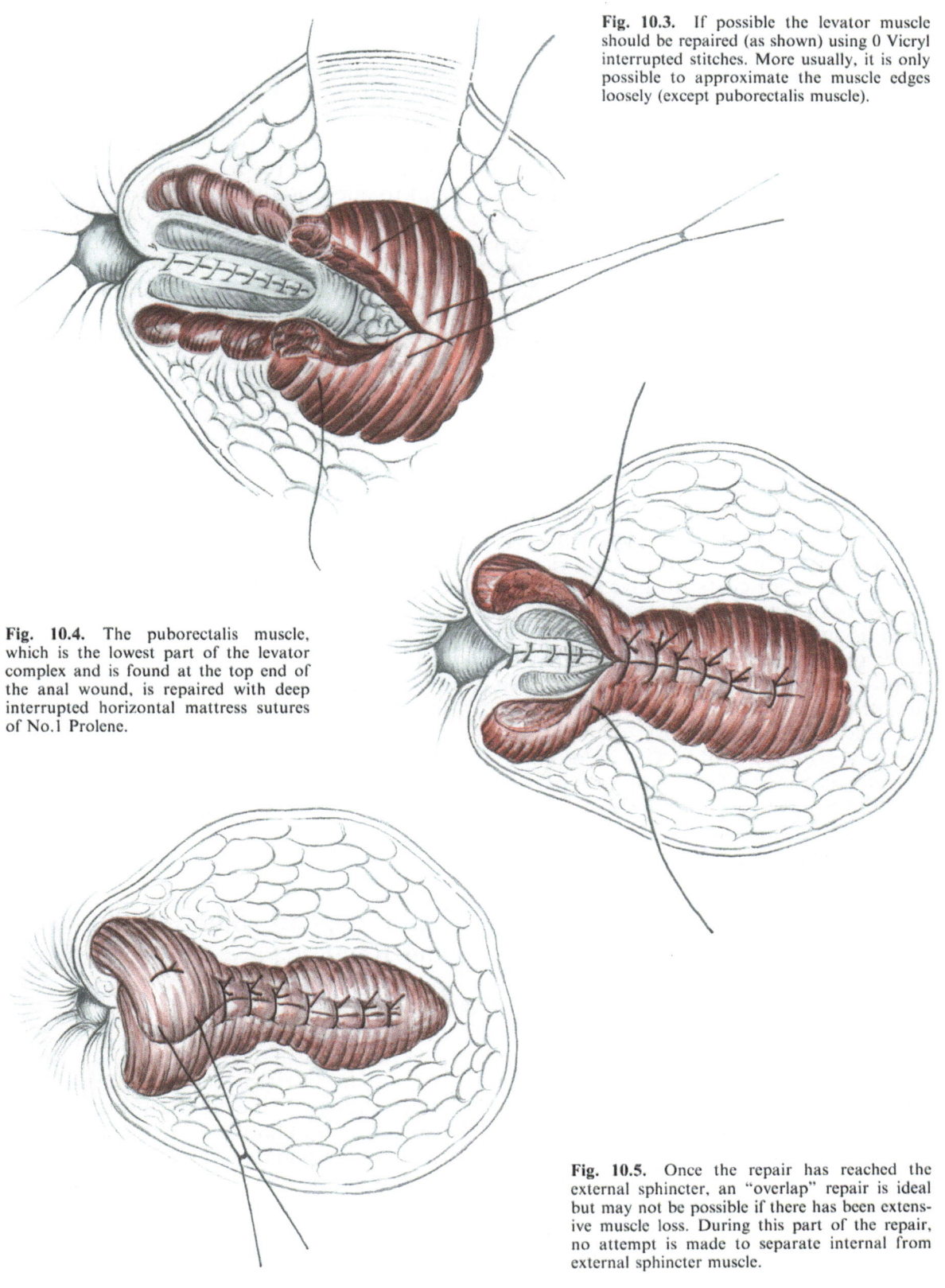

Fig. 10.3. If possible the levator muscle should be repaired (as shown) using 0 Vicryl interrupted stitches. More usually, it is only possible to approximate the muscle edges loosely (except puborectalis muscle).

Fig. 10.4. The puborectalis muscle, which is the lowest part of the levator complex and is found at the top end of the anal wound, is repaired with deep interrupted horizontal mattress sutures of No.1 Prolene.

Fig. 10.5. Once the repair has reached the external sphincter, an "overlap" repair is ideal but may not be possible if there has been extensive muscle loss. During this part of the repair, no attempt is made to separate internal from external sphincter muscle.

apposition (Fig. 10.5) is always necessary. An overlap repair is advantageous and the surgeon should not be worried about seemingly excessive narrowing of the anal sphincter at this stage. A tight anal sphincter can easily be dilated at a later date, whereas a lax sphincter is difficult to alter. It is useless to search for the internal sphincter muscle separately from the external sphincter and they are repaired as one layer, but deep enough bites into the external sphincter will include the internal layer of muscle. The ischiorectal fossa is left open and lightly packed with gauze swabs soaked in sodium hypochlorite solution. Skin cover is not critical and it is better to leave the wound open to allow free drainage, and prevent pocketing of pus or blood. Later cover by rotation skin flaps or skin grafts can be used if necessary, but in most cases the skin heals well by granulation. It is important, however, that any intact skin of the perineum and anus should be preserved at all costs, to give support to the repair and to provide a scaffold for fibrous tissue to develop on.

After the layered repair is completed the surgeon must decide if a colostomy is necessary. If the injury is complex and involves either excessive tissue loss or a suprasphincteric injury into the rectum, a colostomy is mandatory. This is especially true if the repair has unduly narrowed the lumen. With simple low sphincteric injury, a primary repair can be performed in safety without a covering stoma. *If, however, there is any doubt at all it is wiser to perform a temporary defunctioning colostomy rather than to risk disruption of the repair.*

Post-operative Management

If the injury has been one of a straightforward sphincter division and repair, the post-operative management follows the lines set down in Chap. 8. With a complex injury (e.g. high-velocity missile), involving extensive muscle loss, post-operative management is more difficult and relies on creating the best circumstances for healing of the wound by controlled, secondary intention. The initial dressings should be left undisturbed for 24 to 48 hours, after which they should be soaked off. If the wound is extensive it is necessary on the first or second occasion to change the dressings under anaesthetic to avoid excessive pain and to allow additional debridement if indicated. Thereafter, the dressings should be changed twice daily, or more frequently if there is copious discharge of pus and blood. If there is much infection or slough, the wound should be irrigated daily with hydrogen peroxide solution (0.5% available chlorine). After a complex muscle repair it is wise to examine the patient under anaesthetic 7–10 days after the initial injury: the wound can then be re-assessed and further steps planned.

With a complex repair, healing may take up to 3 months to become established and further evaluations under anaesthetic may be necessary during this period. Assessment of function is only possible after the wound has healed, at which time the surgeon decides when the colostomy can be closed. It is usually necessary to dilate a narrowed anal canal in gradual stages before restoring faecal continuity, and if the surgeon is doubtful about the integrity of the repaired sphincter, it is wise to carry out follow-up electromyographic studies before any decision is made to close the colostomy.

Trans-vaginal Injury to the Anus and Rectum

Introduction

In civilian practice the commonest traumatic injury to the anal sphincter is that which follows childbirth accompanied by a third degree tear or a too deep episiotomy. If forceps are used (nowadays rare) they can also severely injure the anal sphincter. Such injuries result in acute trans-vaginal injury to the anus and rectum.

Primary repair is frequently performed for these by the attending obstetrician who may not be experienced, and the results may often be less than perfect, particularly so if there is subsequent infection and wound breakdown. A late repair is often the optimum treatment after the primary wound has healed; it is fortunate that in most instances it is possible to perform sphincter reconstruction in these patients without a covering colostomy.

Third degree tears of the perineal body and anal sphincters after obstructed delivery, or division of the sphincter by misplaced episiotomy, do not always result in anal incontinence, the degree of incontinence depending very much on the severity of the injury. The injury is best classified as being high or low according to whether the muscle division extends above the puborectalis muscle. The majority of childbirth injuries are low perineal tears, which do not extend high up the posterior of the vaginal wall and spare the puborectalis and upper sphincter [3,6,7].

High injuries are rare and are usually caused not by mechanical tearing but by pressure necrosis from an impacted head. They often have associated injuries to bladder and urethra. Such injuries require an immediate defunctioning colostomy and a secondary repair after a suitable interval. The later management of these injuries is discussed in the chapter dealing with recto-vaginal fistulas (pp. 161–179).

Most low perineal tears are repaired at once by the attending obstetrician and, despite all that has been said, good functional results are usual. If, however, sepsis occurs, the wound heals with excessive fibrous tissue. Although the bowel wall may seem to heal well, the external sphincter muscle retracts, leaving a large anterior defect. Despite this, many patients retain continence unless stressed by an attack of diarrhoea. A number, however, present later in life (when their anal sphincter tone diminishes) with progressively poor control and require formal sphincter repair. In these patients there is often considerable distortion of tissue, with scarring which

contracts the lower end of the rectum and anus, drawing it towards the vagina with guttering or key-hole deformation of the anal canal. The mucosa of the rectum may prolapse, and persistent mucus leakage can cause intense pruritis.

Two techniques are available for the repair of such obstetric injuries. First, an immediate layered closure of the injury, and second, a late repair for correction of delayed incontinence resulting from faulty previous management.

Immediate Repair of Acute Transvaginal Injury [3,6,7]

The majority of obstetric injuries cause a low perineal tear which extends a variable distance up the posterior vaginal wall, disrupts the external anal sphincter muscle and perineal body, and opens the anterior wall of the rectum and anus. The injury should be fully assessed with the patient in the lithotomy position under general anaesthetic. The passage of a urinary catheter will help post-operative management.

Operative Technique

The rectal and anal mucosa should be repaired first. The edges of the torn mucosa must be raised and trimmed and then sutured with a continuous 00 chromic catgut stitch (Fig. 10.6). The external sphincter muscle should be identified and there will always be more retraction of the torn edges than is expected. As with all sphincter repairs, the internal anal sphincter is repaired synchronous with the external sphincter muscle, treating both as one unit with no attempt to separate the two muscles into layers. The divided external anal sphincter should be brought together with interrupted horizontal mattress sutures of 00 Prolene (polypropylene) and the authors do not recommend "overlap" in an

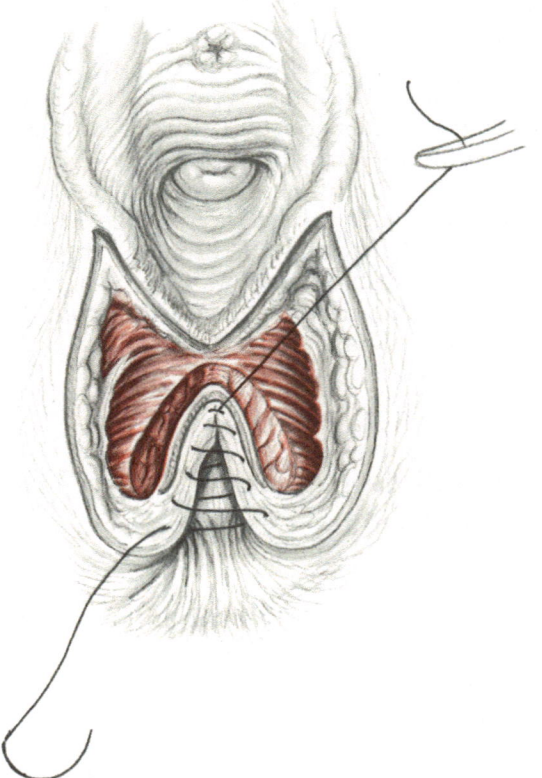

Fig. 10.6. The first stage of the repair of a trans-vaginal tear is preparation and suturing of the ano-rectal mucosal lining by a continuous 00 chromic catgut suture.

acute repair (Fig. 10.7). With the muscle repaired (Fig. 10.8) the posterior vaginal wall is now closed using 00 chromic continuous catgut stitch (Fig. 10.9). If the wound is ragged or there is contamination, it is best to leave the perineal skin open, and allow healing of the wound by secondary intention. If the repair is treated acutely, however, primary closure of the subcutaneous tissue and skin can be always achieved using interrupted stitches of catgut and nylon respectively. In any situation of skin shortage an "s-anoplasty" or "rotation" technique will always allow skin cover to be achieved (see Fig. 10.10 a–e).

Post-operative Management

Post-operative management of the wound is straightforward, and merely requires daily cleaning and application of a flat gauze dressing. As after all sphincter repairs, the bowels should be kept working freely and the patient may require aperients and regular stool softeners to achieve unobstructed evacuation without straining. The urinary catheter can be removed as soon as the patient is mobilised. Excessively early

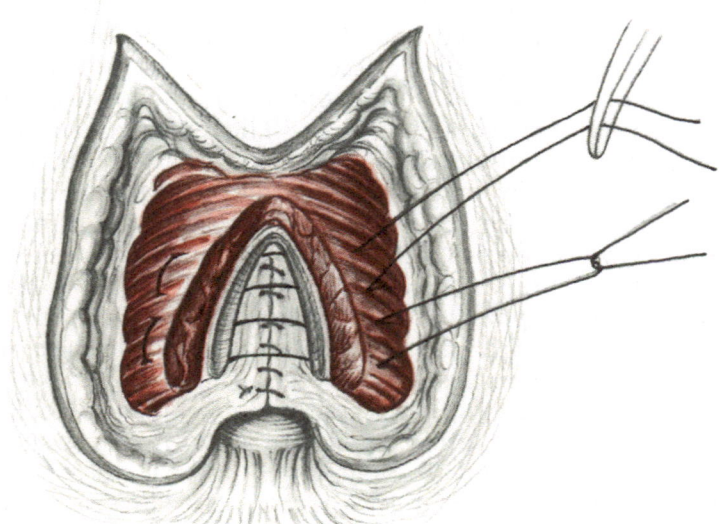

Fig. 10.7. The next stage of the repair of a trans-vaginal tear. The external sphincter muscle is repaired with horizontal mattress sutures of 00 Prolene. No attempt is made to repair the internal sphincter muscle as a separate layer: both muscles are treated and joined as a single unit.

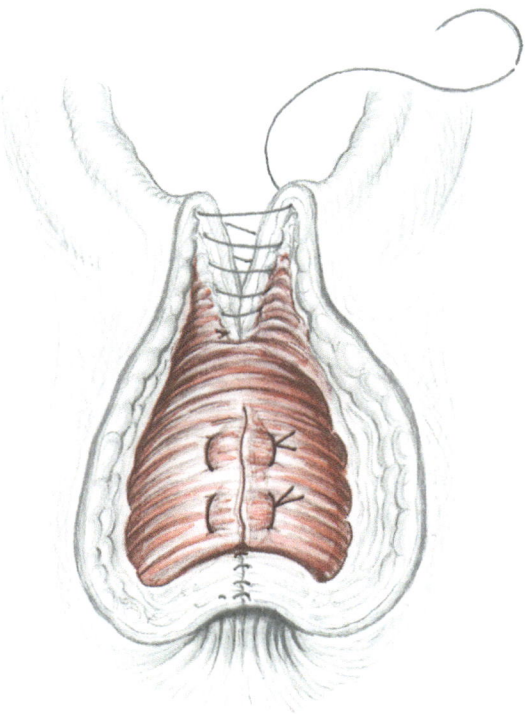

Fig. 10.8. After the muscle repairs are complete, the vaginal epithelium is closed with a continuous 00 chromic catgut stitch.

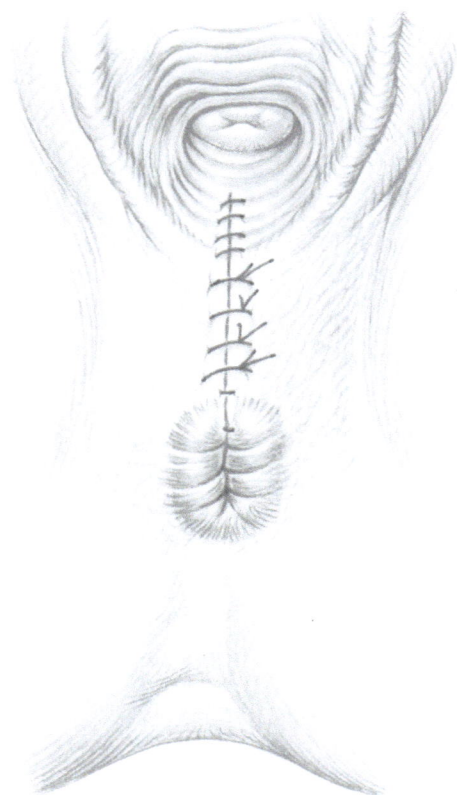

Fig. 10.9. The final situation in the repair of a trans-vaginal tear. No drain is shown because one is not usually required, but occasionally a fine suction line (e.g. Redivac) can be helpful to remove immediate losses of sero-sanguineous fluid.

mobilisation should be avoided as the wound needs to heal undisturbed in the early stages, and excessive buttock movement can cause additional strain on the suture lines.

Delayed Repair of Chronic Unhealed Recto-vaginal Septal Defect [2,3,4,8,9]

If an acute trans-vaginal injury to the anus and rectum is not recognised or repair is delayed for any reason, the wound heals with considerable distortion of tissues. Contraction of the scar tissue causes the lower anterior end of the anal canal to become puckered and drawn into the vagina. The line of union between the posterior vaginal wall and the bowel mucosa is thin and forms an arc of tight but brittle fibrous tissue. This distortion and scarring makes repair difficult, but good results are obtainable in experienced hands. Such wounds are sometimes difficult to close without tension.

Preparation

The lower bowel must be emptied with enemas or oral aperients. A defunctioning colostomy is not usually present, and is unnecessary for the repair of low recto-vaginal septal defects. Pre-operative and post-operative antibiotics are recommended (metronidazole and a cephalosporin). The

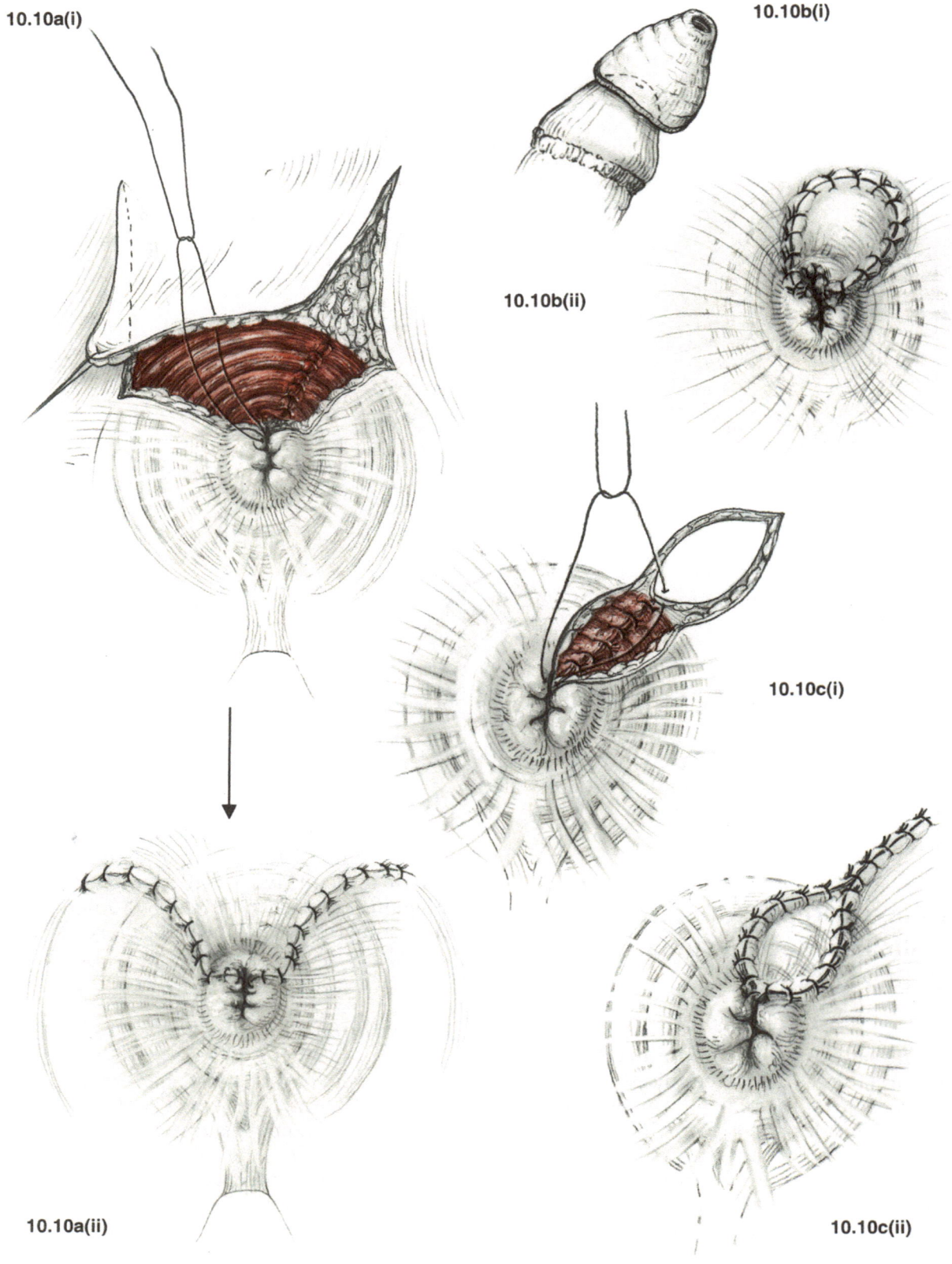

10.10a(i)

10.10b(i)

10.10b(ii)

10.10c(i)

10.10a(ii)

10.10c(ii)

10.10d(i)

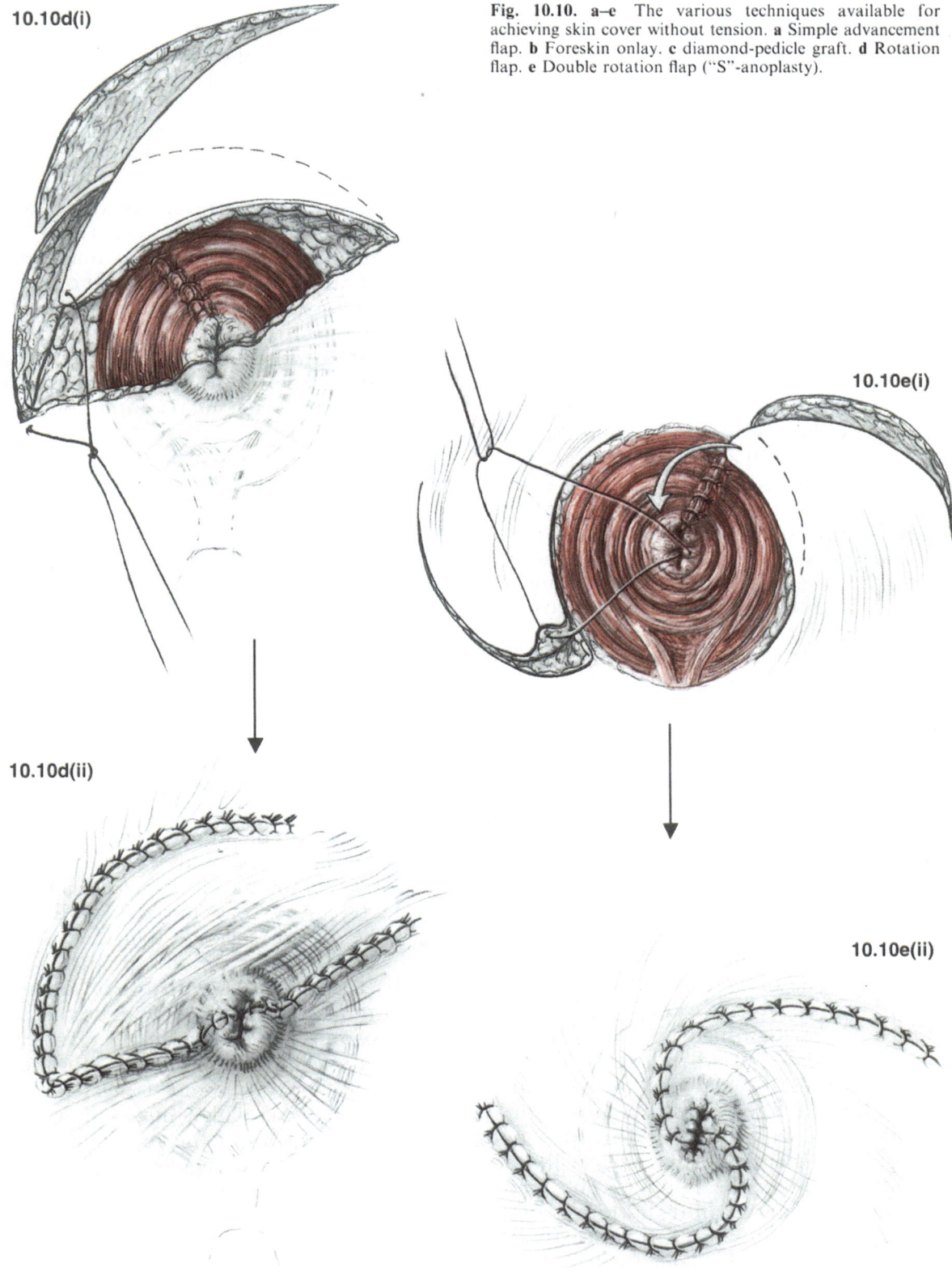

Fig. 10.10. a–e The various techniques available for achieving skin cover without tension. **a** Simple advancement flap. **b** Foreskin onlay. **c** diamond-pedicle graft. **d** Rotation flap. **e** Double rotation flap ("S"-anoplasty).

10.10e(i)

10.10d(ii)

10.10e(ii)

vagina should be cleansed pre-operatively with local bactericidal solutions, e.g. povidone-iodine.

Operative Technique

With the patient in the lithotomy position and under a general anaesthetic the extent of the wound can be assessed. Very often the external sphincter has retracted posteriorly and is tethered laterally by the fibrous tissue mass that has also replaced the perineal body. An infiltration of the tissues with a weak solution of adrenaline (1:300 000 in physiological saline) aids dissection. The first stage in the procedure is to cut away the fibrous tissue from the posterior vaginal wall and to separate this from the scarred attenuated mucosa of the anus and rectum. Tissue forceps are next placed at the apex of the vaginal wound and sharp dissection made on either side to expose the edges of the retracted sphincter. By further knife dissection the mucosa of the posterior vaginal wall is freed and lifted. As the mucosa is raised it is possible to find the fibres of the puborectalis sling in the superior lateral depths of the wound. Next the mucosal lining of the anus and rectum must be elevated and this requires careful dissection with the knife in the submucosal plane, freeing the delicate mucosa from the underlying fibrous tissue which binds down the retracted external sphincter muscle. Once the mucosa edges have been mobilised to provide a generous 1.0 cm margin they should be trimmed and closed with a continuous 00 chromic catgut stitch (Fig. 10.1). The divided edges of the external sphincter muscle and puborectalis should now be identified by further dissection. They are buried in dense fibrous tissue, and must be elevated by sharp dissection. The divided muscle edges should be grasped with tissue forceps and mobilised sufficiently so that they will meet without tension in the midline. The repair starts with the muscle fibres of puborectalis and the levator ani which are approximated with interrupted 0 Prolene sutures (Figs.

10.3, 10.4). This drawing together of the puborectalis and lower parts of levator ani aids considerably the repair of the external anal sphincter which is brought towards the midline as the stitches are tightened. Once the levator muscles and puborectalis have been brought soundly together, the external anal sphincter muscle is directly in view and is repaired using interrupted horizontal mattress sutures of 00 Prolene (Fig. 10.2). Some overlap is desirable but may not be possible in all cases. Lastly, the vaginal epithelium is closed with interrupted catgut stitches (Fig. 10.3). If the skin over the perineum is insufficient for closure without tension it is better to leave it open as it heals quickly by secondary intention, but if the gap is wide, cover can be achieved by an advancement flap or one of the other techniques available (Fig. 10.10 a–e).

Post-operative Management

Post-operative management is straightforward and is similar to that of any sphincter repair. Accurate anatomical apposition of the external anal sphincter invariably closes the canal quite tightly. If the patient has a defunctioning colostomy (which simplifies the post-operative management) such a stenosis is of little consequence, as it can easily be dilated at a later date. If the patient has no colostomy then it is wise to prescribe laxatives and ensure that the patient does not develop faecal impaction. If the repair is very narrow, a diversion must be given serious consideration: if there is any doubt on this point, a diversion is necessary. As with other situations, if you think about a diversion, a colostomy (or ileostomy) is indicated. Careful rectal examination must be performed on the 5th or 6th post-operative day to test for possible anal stenosis which may require intermittent dilation until the repair has healed and all fibrous tissue has matured.

References and Further Reading

1. Abcarian H, Lowe R (1978) Colon and rectal trauma. Surg Clin North Am 58: 519
2. Corman ML, Veidenheimer MC, Coller JA (1976) Anoplasty for anal stricture. Surg Clin North Am 56: 727
3. Corman ML (1985) Anal incontinence following obstetrical injury. Dis Colon Rectum 28: 86
4. Fergusson JA (1959) Repair of "Whitehead" deformity of the anus. Surg Gynecol Obstet 108: 115
5. Hass PA, Fox FA (1979) Civilian injuries of the rectum and anus. Dis Colon Rectum 22: 17
6. Hawkins J, Hudson CN (1983) Shaw's Textbook of operative gynaecology, 5th edn. Churchill Livingstone, Edinburgh, pp 375–378
7. Lawson J (1972) Recto-vaginal fistula following difficult labour. Proc R Soc Med 65: 283
8. Oh C, Zinberg J (1982) Anoplasty for anal stricture. Dis Colon Rectum 25: 809
9. Parks AG, McPartlin JF (1971) Late repair of injuries of the anal sphincter. Proc R Soc Med 64: 1187
10. Snooks SJ, Setchell M, Swash M, Henry MM (1984) Injury to innervation of pelvic floor sphincter musculature in childbirth. Lancet ii: 546

CHAPTER 11

Techniques for Repair of Recto-vaginal Fistula

PART I
Low Recto-vaginal Fistula Repairs

General Introduction

Acquired recto-vaginal fistulas usually develop as a consequence of trauma, malignancy, inflammatory disease or tissue necrosis. The treatment of the fistula depends, therefore, on the underlying pathology. Recto-vaginal fistula due to carcinoma of the rectum, vagina or cervix clearly requires radical surgical treatment for the carcinoma and if this is not possible, a defunctioning colostomy to save the patient from the distressing consequence of uncontrollable leakage of faeces per vaginam. The treatment of fistulas due to an inflammatory bowel disease (usually Crohn's disease) must be also directed mainly at the primary pathology. If there is untreated active disease attempts at conservative repair of any associated recto-vaginal fistula are almost always doomed to failure. It is a good general rule that if the primary inflammatory pathology is Crohn's disease even the most innocent-looking fistula should always be left alone until the primary bowel disease has been controlled [18]. Diverticular disease is the commonest cause of colo-vaginal fistula and follows the rupture of a peri-colic abscess into the posterior fornix of the vagina. Again, treatment must be directed at the underlying bowel pathology, and repair of the fistula regarded as a secondary consideration.

Recto-vaginal fistula is one unfortunate consequence of high-dose irradiation treatment of patients with cancer of the cervix and body of the uterus [1,2,5,15]. If associated with continuing active malignant disease then urgent radical surgery will be indicated. Often, however, the fistula develops as a late result of tissue necrosis in patients who are cancer-free. There is evidence that the incidence of irradiation-caused fistulas is increasing [1]. Special techniques are required to deal with such fistulas, especially if the defect is high and large. A colo-anal anastomosis gives good results in such cases [2,16] (see pp. 175–180). A further cause of recto-vaginal fistula is obstetric injury. Many of these are small, low and due to incomplete or partial healing of a third degree tear (see pp. 163–166). High fistulas after childbirth are fortunately rare and follow prolonged obstructed labour [12]. They are almost always associated with urogenital damage and the patient is then incontinent of both faeces and urine (for which major complex multi-stage reconstructive surgery is required). Other traumatic recto-vaginal fistulas are iatrogenic and follow pelvic operations carried out per vaginam, per rectum or trans-abdominally: again their treatment depends greatly on the location of the lesion and any underlying pathology.

Recto-vaginal fistulas may be considered as being high (i.e. above the puborectalis and involving the upper vagina) or low (i.e. involving the inferior half of the vagina). If traumatic in origin there may be associated sphincteric injury. In general, high fistulas require trans-abdominal surgery, but a few selected cases can be dealt with per vaginam or per anum [12].

Indications and Selection of Patients

The results of surgical correction of a traumatic, low recto-vaginal fistula by an experienced surgeon are very rewarding. Unless the patient is too frail to withstand an anaesthetic, reconstruction should be undertaken in all cases. If injury to the recto-vaginal septum or upper sphincter complex is recognised during a surgical procedure or after the birth of a baby, immediate repair has many advantages. Transfer of the patient to a specialised unit may be neces-

sary and a delay for this reason of 12–24 hours does not jeopardise the result of an expert primary repair. Sadly, many recto-vaginal fistulas come late to the proctological specialist because they are not recognised until faeces start to leak and in these circumstances reconstruction should be delayed until the wound is clean, fibrous tissue has matured and local sepsis has been eliminated.

Fistulas associated with active distal inflammatory bowel disease present multiple unique problems. For patients with Crohn's disease, even in the absence of obvious local inflammation of the rectum and anus, direct surgical treatment must be avoided unless the surgeon is certain the disease is quiescent: attempts to repair the fistula in the presence of *active* disease lead in most cases to breakdown of the wound with increased local sepsis, and extension of the inflammatory process [3,7,8,11,18]. Progression of extensive local Crohn's disease has often been precipitated by apparently minimal surgery for a fistula. Urgent surgery for a recto-vaginal fistula in these circumstances should be confined to the drainage of sepsis and curetting of any inflammatory tracts. Diversion by colostomy or ileostomy is commonly necessary. If the clinician can be sure the cause of an inflammatory fistula is ulcerative colitis rather than Crohn's disease, early surgery may be successful but medical measures to control the colitis must be in place before operative treatment is instituted. Care must be taken, however, to avoid any surgical risk to sphincter muscle, as sacrifice of any strength of the sphincter may be critical in a patient suffering from persistent diarrhoea due to chronic colitis or proximal bowel resection. Fistulas secondary to local malignant disease obviously require radical surgical excision, and are beyond the scope of this work; reconstruction in these circumstances is usually inappropriate. For patients with a colo- or recto-vaginal fistula due to underlying diverticulitis, removal of the diseased length of bowel is obligatory: if this is carried out successfully, and the suture-line of the bowel anastomosis is adequately separated from the fistula's orifice either by a sheet of omentum or by its distant situation, self-closure of the fistula will follow: a temporary colostomy is not necessary unless a large abscess cavity or "inflammatory nest" has been encountered.

Preparation

The patient should be fit to withstand a general anaesthetic, although the procedures described can be performed if necessary under a spinal anaesthetic or regional block. Adequate exposure is important and the patient will need to be placed in the lithotomy position with the hips well flexed. In the young patient with a narrow perineum and/or muscular buttocks, exposure can be difficult unless the patient is relaxed by a general anaesthetic.

It is difficult to eradicate bacterial contamination of the vagina in a patient with a recto-vaginal fistula, but pre-operative cleansing with twice daily Povidone-iodine vaginal douches is recommended. The lower bowel should be emptied pre-operatively with disposable enemas and the perineum and vagina cleaned with a bactericidal douche of povidone-iodine or aqueous chlorhexidine (1:200). Pre-operative antibiotics are not required for repair of simple fistulas, but may be advisable if surgery needs to be more extensive.

Excision and Repair of Low Juxtasphincteric Fistula

Introduction

If the fistula lies through the sphincter and well below the puborectalis muscle a simple lay-open technique [13,14,17], such as for a trans-sphincteric fistula in ano, can be used. However, it is the authors' view that this is

usually followed by some degree of incontinence and that it is better to perform a repair. If the fistula lies below the puborectalis muscle, the most popular method is to excise the fistula from below, in the process dividing the sphincteric complex and perineal body and then to perform an immediate layered sphincter repair [14,17]. This is also the authors' choice for all low fistulas.

Operative Technique

The technique closely resembles that used for acute low post-traumatic trans-vaginal repairs (pp. 153–155). The patient is placed

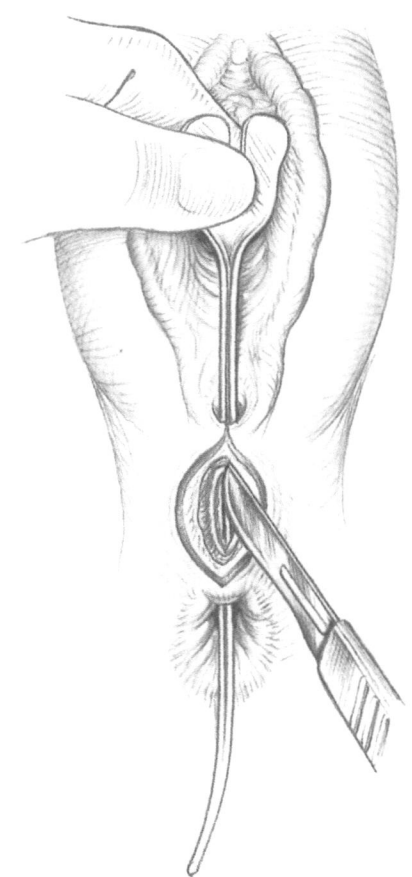

Fig. 11.1. After a probe has been passed through the low track from the vaginal opening into the lower rectum, the tissues external to the probe are laid open with a knife.

Fig. 11.2. All fibrotic and damaged tissues are removed from the surface of the wound and the edges freshened.

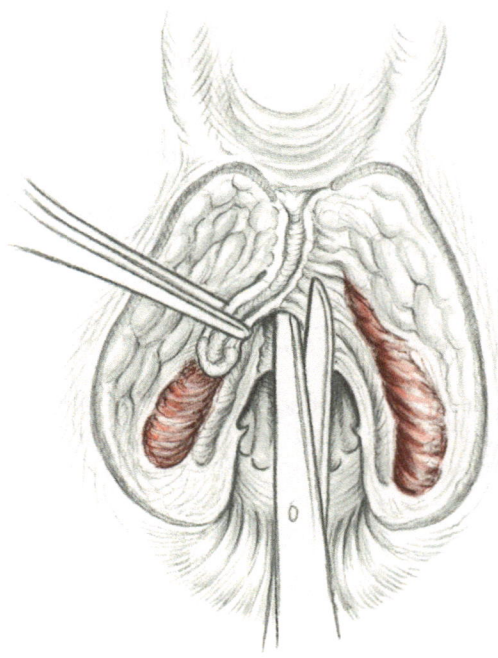

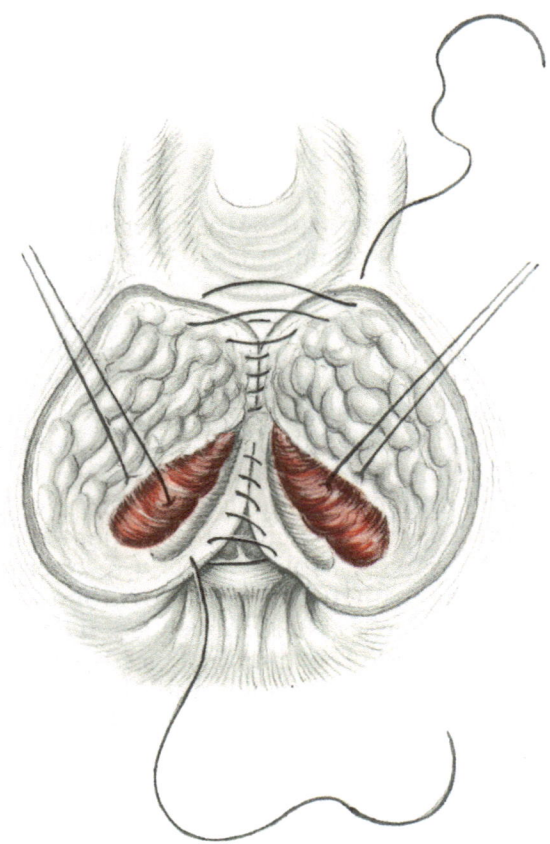

Fig. 11.3. After the tissues have been cleaned, the external sphincter muscle is marked (as shown) with long stitches which are held by the assistant, and the ano-rectal mucosal layer is closed with a continuous 00 chromic catgut suture.

in the lithotomy position and the perineum and vagina cleaned with povidone-iodine solution (Betadine, Napp). The fistula is identified and a probe passed from the vagina into the low rectum or anal canal (Fig. 11.1). The fistula is now laid open, dividing skin, perineal body and external sphincter muscle (Fig. 11.1). The external anal sphincter muscle should be identified and marked with stay stitches as it is revealed. The fistula track is now circumferentially excised down to fresh, clean tissue removing all fibrous scar (Fig. 11.2). The mucosa of the rectum and anus is first repaired with continuous 00 chromic catgut sutures (Fig. 11.3). The edges of the exter-

nal anal sphincter are mobilised sufficiently so that they can be brought together using horizontal interrupted mattress sutures of 00 polypropylene (Prolene) (Fig. 11.4). Once the sphincter muscle is approximated, the anterior vaginal wall can be closed using an absorbable suture (00 chromic catgut) (Fig. 11.5). The perineal skin is now repaired with interrupted nylon stitches.

Post-operative Management

The post-operative management of these cases follows the lines laid down for post-traumatic primary sphincter repair (p. 154).

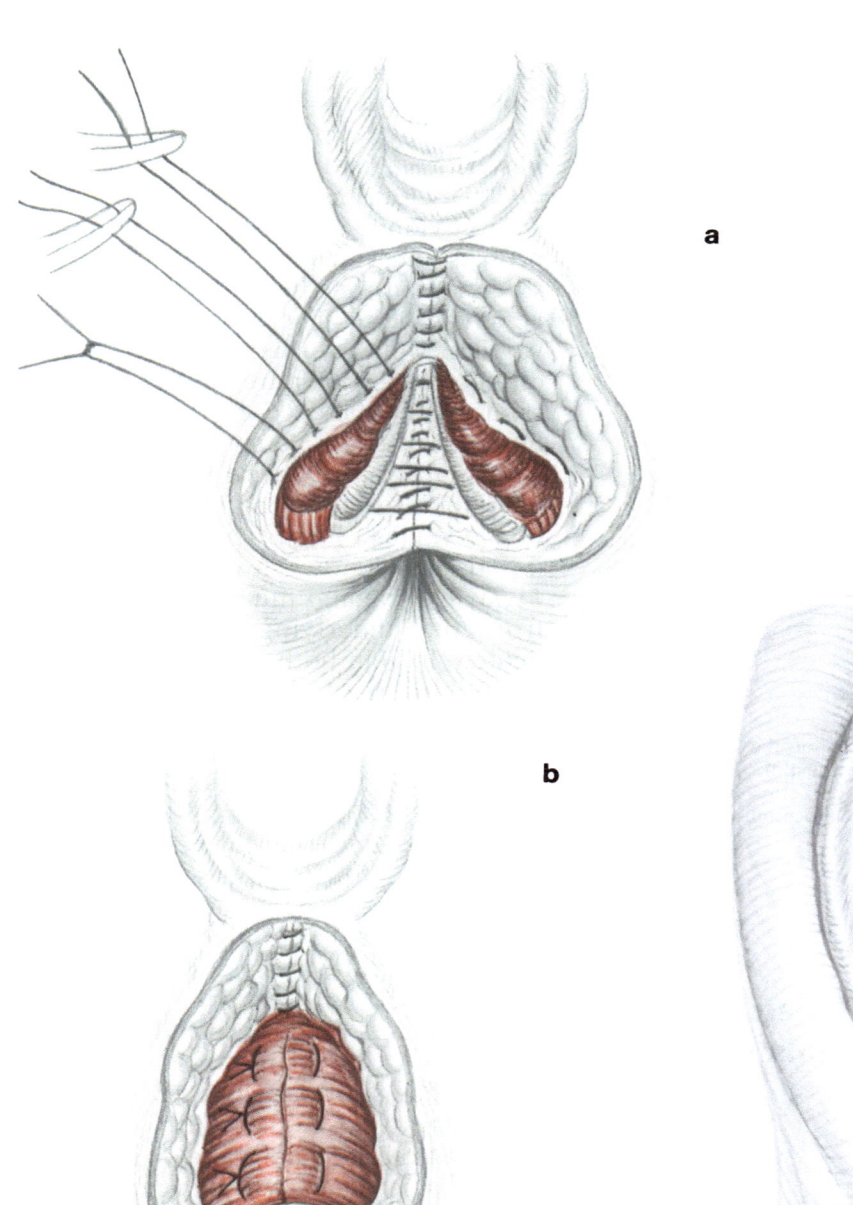

a

b

Fig. 11.4. a,b. The external sphincter mass (which also includes the adherent internal anal sphincter) is carefully repaired with 00 Prolene horizontally inserted mattress sutures. The insertion of the individual stitches is made away from the edge of the divided muscle. The muscle edges are apposed when the stitches are tied.

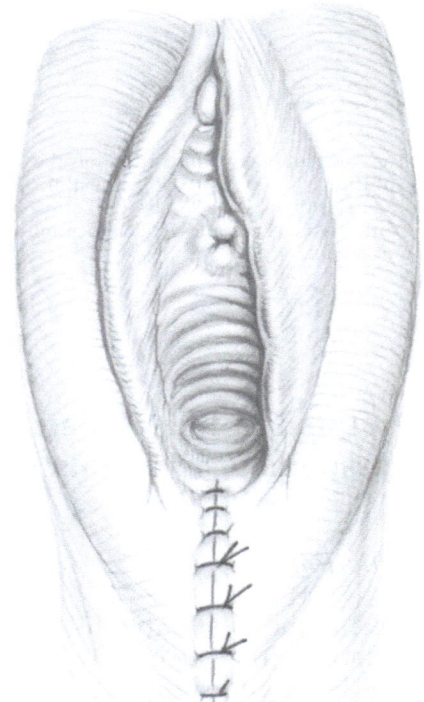

Fig. 11.5. Finally the vaginal epithelium is closed with continuous 00 chromic catgut. No drains are used.

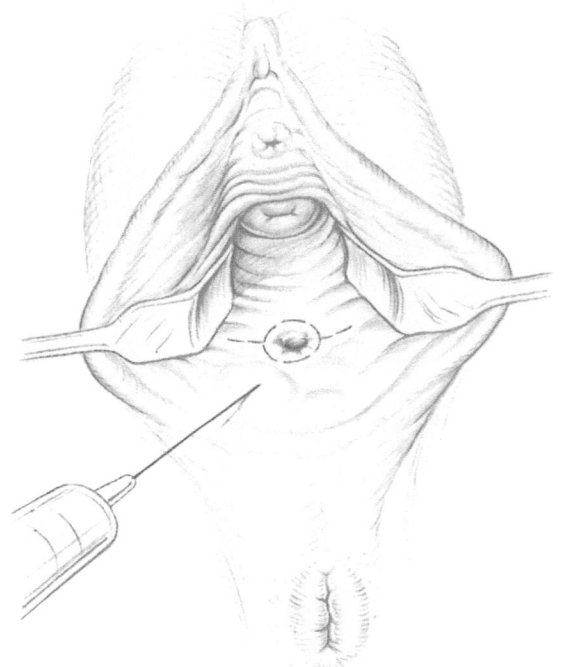

Fig. 11.6. Preliminary infiltration of the tissues with a weak solution (1:300 000) of adrenaline (ephedrine) in physiological saline greatly aids dissection of the scarred and fibrotic tissues, and allows identification of normal and abnormal layers.

Per-vaginal Direct Repair of Low Supra-sphincteric Fistula [9,13]

Introduction

This technique is suitable for the repair of small fistulas that definitely lie above the perineal body and sphincter muscle, but are still easily accessible from below. These fistulas have a track that is below the muscular floor of the pelvis.

Operative Technique

The patient is placed in the lithotomy position with the hips well flexed. Assistance will be needed to maintain exposure and

good illumination is essential, for which purpose a headlight is an advantage. A modified reverse Trendelenburg position may improve exposure of and access to the posterior vaginal wall.

After cleaning the vagina and perineum with povidone-iodine solution, the fistula is probed and can be marked by a through-stitch (seton) or alternatively the probe can be left in place. The tissues of the posterior vaginal wall are next infiltrated with a dilute solution of adrenaline (ephedrine) in saline (1:300 000) (Fig. 11.6). An elliptical horizontal (transverse) incision is made which circumscribes the fistula and extends laterally into the normal tissues at the sides of the vagina. The track with its surrounding tissue is now slowly cored out (Fig. 11.7). The vaginal mucosa is separated next from the underlying rectum for approximately 1–2 cm both proximally and distally throughout the full extent of the transverse incision. This part of the dissection is made easier by the adrenaline infiltration, but the surgeon will need to use careful sharp dissection (with either a small-bladed knife, or scissors) to find the correct planes to free the tissues. Haemostasis is achieved by using diathermy coagulation or underrunning individual blood vessels with fine chromic catgut stitches. The defect in the rectal muscle is delineated, and its edges freshened and then accurately closed with interrupted vertical mattress sutures of 000 Vicryl. The suture technique is designed to invert the closed edges into the lumen of the rectum after being tied (Fig. 11.8). The vaginal defect is closed with interrupted 000 or 00 Vicryl stitches, placed as horizontal mattress sutures, so everting the mucosal closure into the vaginal lumen (Fig. 11.9). Haemostasis is rarely a problem and the tissues can be closed without drainage. A vaginal pack should not be used.

Post-operative Management

Post-operative management is usually straightforward. The vagina should be cleaned by twice daily saline baths or irri-

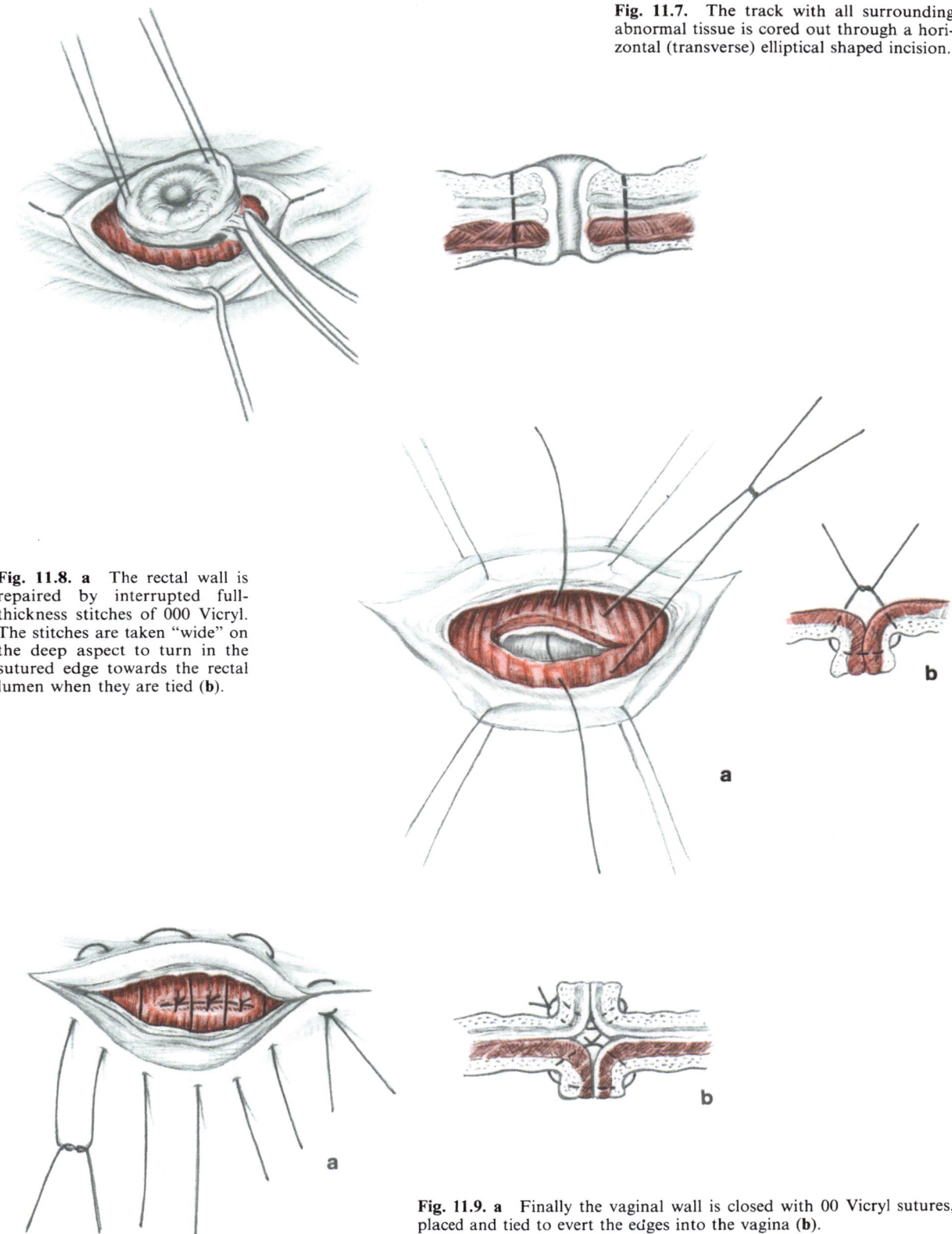

Fig. 11.7. The track with all surrounding abnormal tissue is cored out through a horizontal (transverse) elliptical shaped incision.

Fig. 11.8. a The rectal wall is repaired by interrupted full-thickness stitches of 000 Vicryl. The stitches are taken "wide" on the deep aspect to turn in the sutured edge towards the rectal lumen when they are tied (**b**).

Fig. 11.9. a Finally the vaginal wall is closed with 00 Vicryl sutures, placed and tied to evert the edges into the vagina (**b**).

gated with physiological saline. A laxative should be prescribed to ensure semi-liquid stools for several weeks and a cautious digital rectal examination is performed on the fifth or sixth day to assess rectal emptying. The patient should be mobilised freely the day after the operation and prophylaxis against thrombo-embolism is seldom required except in previously identified high risk patients.

Results

Despite excellent technical closure, it is well-recognised that a direct repair may fail and the fistula reform. For this reason the "advancement flap" procedure was developed (pp. 168–170).

Per-anal Closure of Low Suprasphincteric Fistula by Advancement Flap [16]

Introduction

As with per-vaginal direct closure (pp. 166–168) this technique is suitable for accessible low fistulas situated above the sphincter, but within 3–4 cm of the ano-rectal junction.

Operative Technique

It may be easier to operate with the patient placed in prone jack-knife position which gives the best exposure of the anterior rectal wall. For convenience the following illustrations are shown with the patient in the lithotomy position. The anus and lower rectum are opened out by using an Eisenhammer or Parks anal speculum, as well as vaginal wall and anal retractors held by an assistant (Landon or Ferguson retractors). Good illumination is needed and a headlight is recommended.

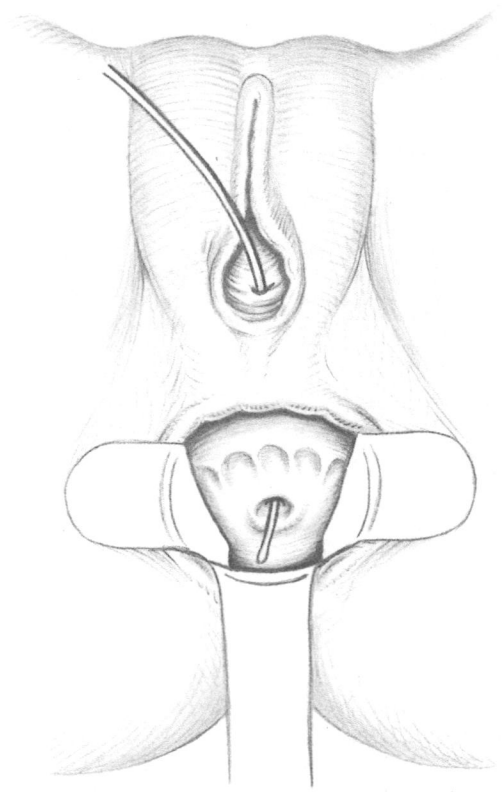

Fig. 11.10. The track is identified and marked by a probe in the usual way.

The fistula is probed and identified in the usual way (Fig. 11.10). The dissection of the fistula is facilitated by preliminary infiltration of the fistula and surrounding tissues with a weak solution of adrenaline (ephedrine) in saline (1:300 000). An incision is made in the rectal wall below the fistula as an opened "U" and deepened through mucosa and muscle into the rectovaginal septum (Fig. 11.11). The limbs of the "U" are extended laterally and cranially for approximately 1–2 cm. A full thickness flap of the rectal muscle tube and mucosa which encloses the fistula is now raised by sharp dissection (Fig. 11.12). This dissection is continued cranially for approximately 2 cm beyond the fistula and the fistula with all abnormal tissue is next

Fig. 11.11. A "U"-shaped incision is made through all layers of the rectal wall. The margin of clearance of the fistula should be enough to ensure that the incision is made in normal tissues.

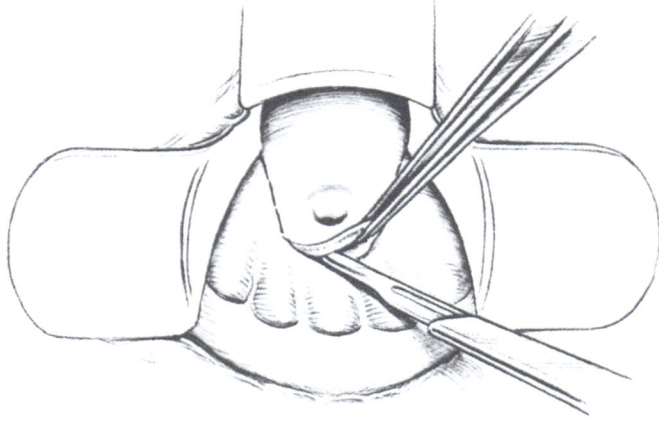

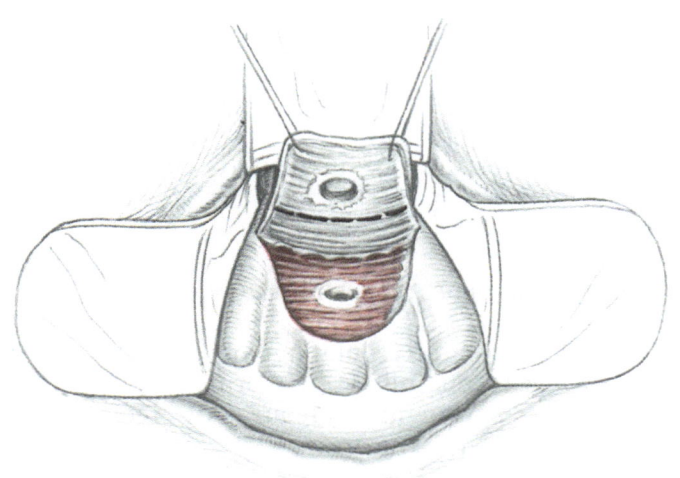

Fig. 11.12. After the flap is raised, leaving only the vaginal epithelium in the base of the wound, the distal end of the flap is cut away (---).

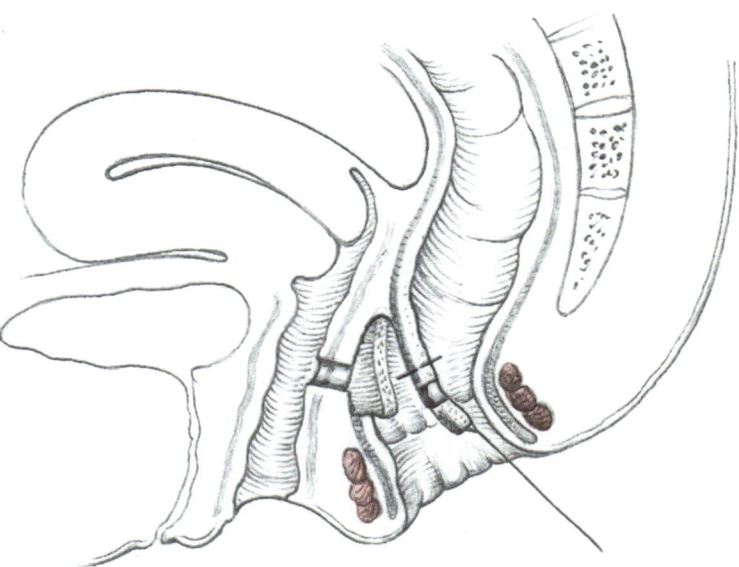

Fig. 11.13. Sagittal view of the raised flap being trimmed to leave only normal tissue.

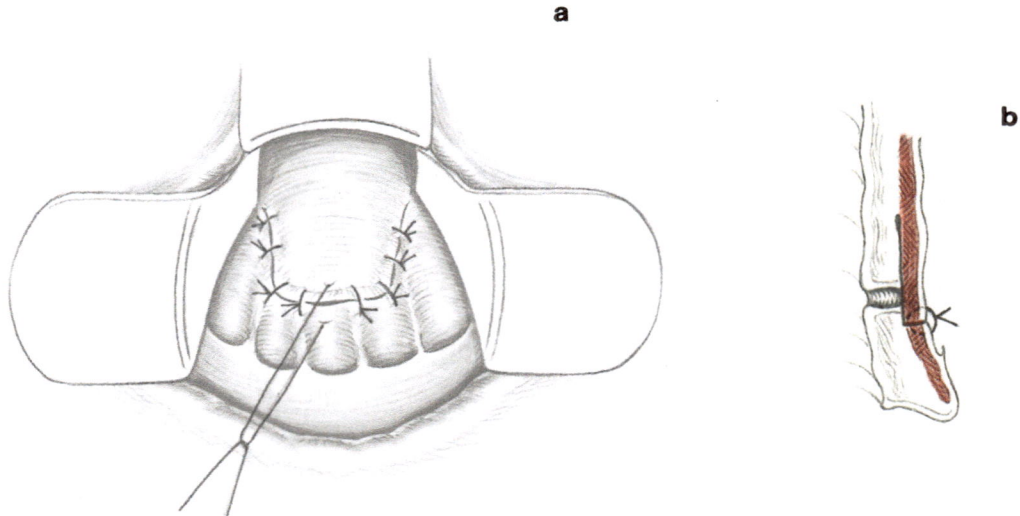

Fig. 11.14. a Finally, the flap is advanced to close the defect (**b**). The flap is stitched in place by solid full-thickness bites of tissue using 00 Vicryl.

trimmed from the muscle flap (Fig. 11.13). Haemostasis is achieved by diathermy coagulation or by underrunning blood vessels with chromic catgut. The rectal muscle flap is now advanced over the vaginal defect and is firmly secured to the distal rectal muscle wall by interrupted stitches of 00 Vicryl. A "J"-shaped needle (Ethicon) is useful to ensure appropriately deep bites of tissue distal to the fistula. The sutures are tied in turn to close the fistula defect (Fig. 11.14).

Post-operative Management

Post-operative management is straightforward and follows the principles laid down for per-vaginal closure of recto-vaginal fistulas (p. 166).

PART II
High Recto-vaginal (Supralevator) Fistula Repairs

General Introduction

Most surgeons (which includes the authors) recommend an abdominal approach for the treatment of high recto-vaginal fistulas which are definitely above the muscular diaphragm of the pelvis, and would consider this approach mandatory when the fistula is secondary to malignant disease or diverticulitis. Gynaecologists, however, report successful treatment of "benign" fistulas by a per-vaginal but intra-peritoneal operation deliberately opening the Pouch of Douglas to separate the fistula from the rectum and allow direct closure of the defect in the bowel [12]. We have no experience of this technique.

The authors prefer an abdominal approach whenever the vaginal opening of the fistula lies above the lower two-thirds of the vagina. For irradiation fistulas, in which normal tissue must be used for any successful technique of closure, an abdominal approach is also necessary even when the fistula is low down.

In the relatively rare case of a "benign" fistula (usually post-traumatic), in which the bowel is not primarily involved by a pathological process, the fistula may be divided and the rectum closed by primary suture reinforced with an omental graft. In patients with malignant disease or an inflammatory process arising from the bowel (such as irradiation, or inflammatory bowel disease) the affected segment of bowel must be resected en-bloc with the fistula. Restorative anastomosis may be possible by either a low anterior resection, or a colo-anal anastomosis. This last technique is especially recommended for post-irradiation recto-vaginal fistulas [2,16]. Here the rectum is always involved in the inflammatory process and the resultant fibrosis often causes a coincidental stricture in both vagina and rectum. The stenosed rectum requires removal "en bloc" with the fistula and then a restorative anastomosis is performed. Many surgeons recommend re-anastomosis by a sleeved colo-anal anastomosis preserving the last 2–3 cm of the muscle coat of the rectum, hopefully to improve rectal sensation and to avoid dissecting in peri-rectal irradiated tissue. However a direct end-to-end colo-anal anastomosis is also satisfactory: either stapled or manually performed. The anastomosis should always be between normal (i.e. transverse) colon and normal anal canal.

In many patients with malignant disease, radical surgery in combination with high-dose irradiation generally precludes restorative anastomosis; but in a few selected cases this may still be attempted. This is particularly so if there is evidence of a poor prognosis when the surgeon will wish to avoid a stoma in an incurable patient.

Surgical techniques required for the radical treatment of malignant disease of the pelvis are outside the scope of this text. Details will be found in standard surgical works devoted to surgery of malignant disease of the pelvis. Two techniques for repair of high recto-vaginal fistulas are described here: (i) direct closure of the fistula using an isolating omental graft or (ii) treatment by colo-rectal resection with restoration of continuity by colo-anal anastomosis, which is the procedure of choice for a post-irradiation fistula.

Indications and Selection of Patients

Reconstruction of a high recto-vaginal fistula requires major pelvic surgery and the patient must be fit to withstand such a procedure. A temporary protective stoma is nearly always required after colo-anal reconstruction and if the patient is unwell and the fistula associated with intra-abdominal sepsis, the patient is best served by a preliminary colostomy or ileostomy followed by elective fistula closure at a later date. Before attempting formal repair, it is often wise to examine the patient under anaesthetic to establish the anatomy of the fistula. Only then can the true extent and nature of the fistula be established and the best decision made whether to proceed to primary repair or whether it is better to start with a temporary defunctioning colostomy or ileostomy.

In those patients who are too frail to withstand major pelvic reconstruction, a permanent colostomy or ileostomy is the only alternative.

Preparation

Pre-operative preparation of the patient is that required for any major endo-pelvic bowel surgery. The patient may be old and frail and will require careful management of the cardiovascular and respiratory systems. Pre-operative physiotherapy may be required in some cases. The large bowel should be completely emptied pre-operatively by purgatives (Picolax) supplemented by enemas and washouts. Prophylactic antibiotics should be given and the authors recommend the use of metronidazole (500 mg iv) and a cephalosporin (Cephradine G1.0 iv) administered on induction of the anaesthetic and two further follow-up doses given intravenously at eight hourly intervals after surgery. Unless contraindicated, it is wise to use prophylaxis against thrombo-embolic complications with subcutaneous heparin and graduated compression stockings.

Direct Closure Using Interposed Omental Graft [8]

Introduction

This technique is suitable for non-malignant fistulas when resection of the rectum is not required, and the fistula track is simple and unassociated with active sepsis or extensive tissue damage.

Operative Technique

The patient is placed on the operating table in the Lloyd-Davies position and a catheter passed into the bladder. After skin cleansing and draping, the abdomen is opened in the usual fashion and after satisfactory completion of the initial laparotomy, the small bowel packed into the upper abdomen. The patient is now tipped into a steep Trendelenburg position and the sigmoid colon mobilised from the left, dividing the congenital peritoneal adhesions. Both ureters must be seen and preserved at this early stage of the dissection. If the uterus is

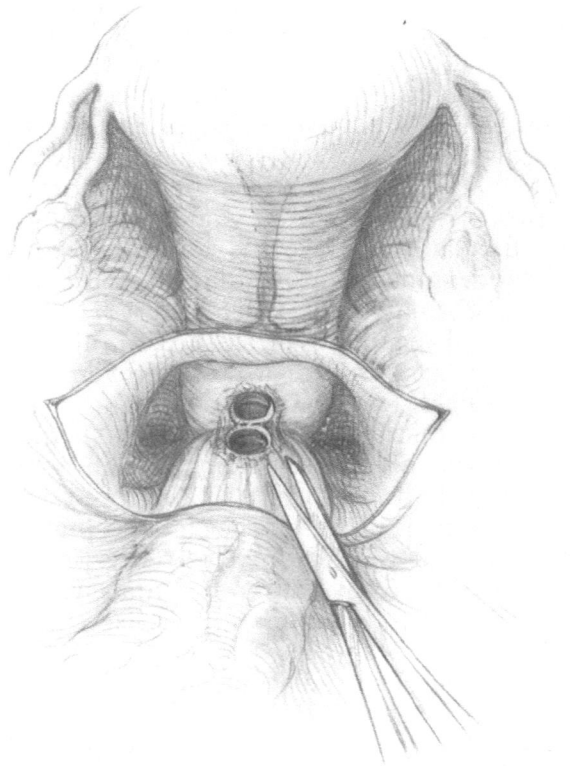

Fig. 11.15. The peritoneum over the anterior rectum is incised and with sharp dissection the fistula divided. The dissection is continued downward and laterally to separate widely the rectum from the posterior vaginal wall.

present, it should be lifted out of the pelvis and it is useful to stitch it to the lowermost part of the incision to aid retraction. The peritoneum over the anterior part of the rectum is incised, and the dissection continued downwards behind the cervix (or the site of the vaginal closure in the case of previous hysterectomy). Sharp dissection will be required of all the dense fibrous tissue which surrounds the fistula. Using sharp dissection the fistula is now divided across and the rectum widely separated from the posterior vaginal wall (Fig. 11.15). Once the fistula has been transected, the dissection is continued downwards into the lower layers of the recto-vaginal septum; here the tissues are normal and the separation of the layers more straightforward. Closure of the fistula is often easier if the

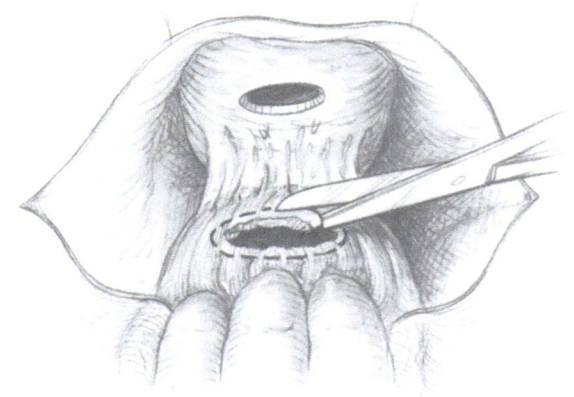

Fig. 11.16. The rectal opening is trimmed back to healthy, pliant tissue.

rectum is freed posteriorly and fully raised from the sacral hollow and the uppermost parts of the lateral ligaments divided. The rectal defect must always be trimmed back to pliant healthy tissues before repair can be performed safely (Fig. 11.16). The defect is closed with interrupted full thickness sutures of 000 Vicryl (Fig. 11.17). The tissues surrounding the vaginal defect should be freshened by sharp dissection with curettage to remove all débris and dead tissue but it is not necessary to close the vaginal defect.

The great omentum should now be freed from the transverse colon and greater curve of the stomach. The left gastro-epiploic vessels are ligated and divided well to the left and the line of omental mobilisation carried far to the right by dividing the vessels close to the greater curvature of the stomach. The greater omentum is now on a pedicle with its blood supply from the right gastro-epiploic artery. The omentum can now be swung down into the pelvis and it is often found that it descends most directly and easily down the right paracolic gutter. The omentum is secured with catgut stitches into the depths of the recto-vaginal fossa and is applied to the front of the

Fig. 11.17. The rectal defect is now closed with interrupted full-thickness sutures of 000 Vicryl. A vertical mattress suture helps to invert the edges of the fistula.

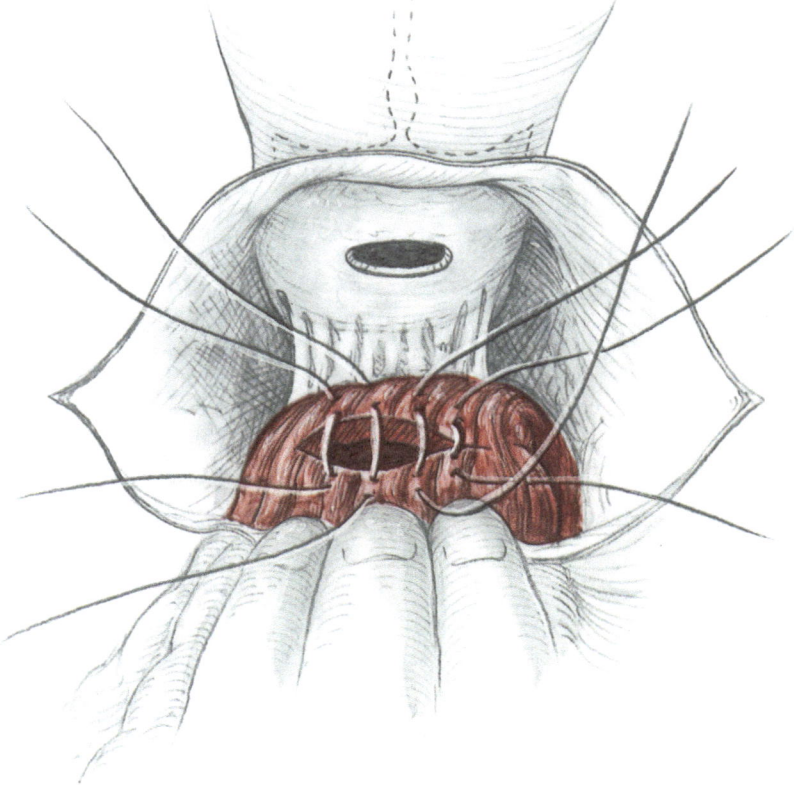

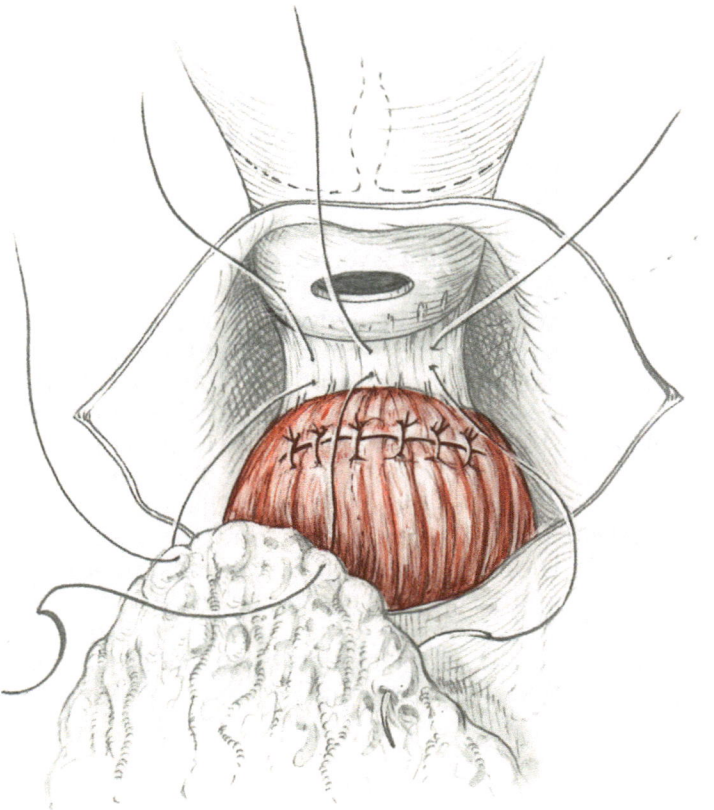

Fig. 11.18. An omental graft is prepared and secured into the depths of the recto-vaginal fossa.

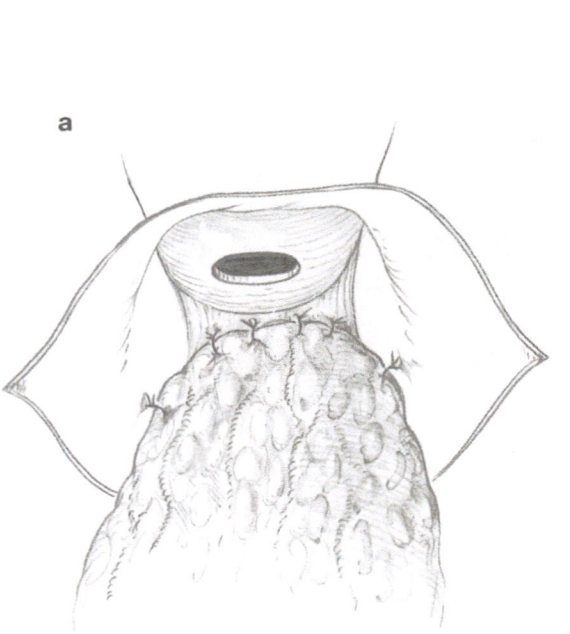

a

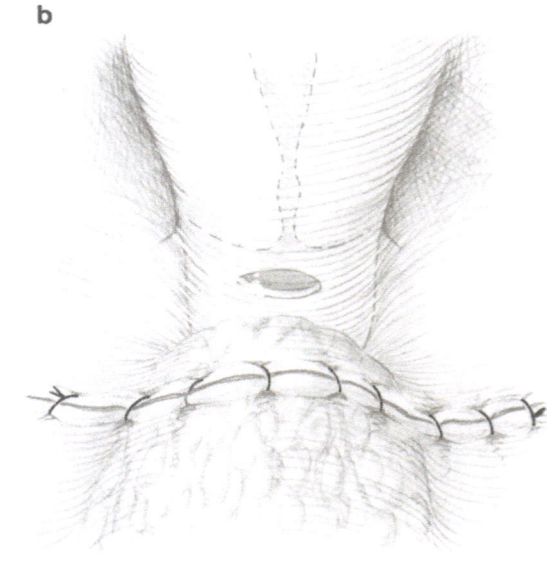

b

Fig. 11.19. a,b The omental graft fills the base of the (open) vaginal defect, completely separating it from the rectal suture line. Finally, the peritoneum is closed over the omental graft using catgut stitches.

stitches closing the rectal defect. Omentum also fills the base of the (open) vaginal defect, which is thus completely separated from the rectal suture line (Figs. 11.18 and 11.19 a,b).

At this stage the surgeon should consider if a defunctioning colostomy or ileostomy is required; if there is any doubt it is always wise to "play safe". A small suction cannula may be passed into the pelvis if the operation has been unusually moist and the abdomen is closed in the usual fashion. It is not necessary to pack the vagina, but it may be worth having a small absorbent dressing on the perineum to control any sero-sanguineous exudate from the vagina. The suction drain should not remain for more than 48 hours.

Post-operative Management

The post-operative management is that which follows any major pelvic procedure.

Extended Resection with Colo-anal Anastomosis [2,16]

Introduction

This technique is particularly useful for the repair of recto-vaginal fistulas that follow irradiation treatment for carcinoma of the cervix or body of the uterus. The fistula usually lies at the vault of the vagina and is associated with considerable tissue fibrosis. There is usually a stenosis of the rectum at this level. It is necessary, therefore, not only to divide the fistula but also to resect the narrow fibrosed rectum as part of the cure. Restoration of continuity is difficult and early experience with direct anastomosis showed an unsatisfactory number of complications, with numerous anastomotic leaks and recurrence of the fistula. These failures can be directly attributed to the use of irradiated tissues for the repair. Such

experiences led surgeons to develop the technique of colo-anal anastomosis which brings down normal proximal bowel behind the vaginal opening. Since the sigmoid colon is often subjected to irradiation, normal proximal colon cannot be secured with complete certainty below the level of the splenic flexure.

Operative Technique

The patient is placed in the Lloyd-Davies position and a urinary catheter passed into the bladder. After skin cleaning and draping, the abdomen is opened in the usual fashion. After initial laparotomy the splenic flexure is mobilised as a first step by dividing the congenital adhesions of the descending colon and separating the greater omentum from the left transverse colon and splenic fixture. The sigmoid colon is also mobilised and the ureters seen and preserved.

The surgeon now turns his attention to the pelvis and rectum. In the majority of cases total hysterectomy will have been performed, and the fistula will be found to lie at the vault of the vagina within dense fibrous tissue. The post-rectal space is entered and the rectum mobilised posteriorly down to the pelvic floor. The peritoneum is now incised over the lateral and anterior surface of the rectum and, with sharp dissection, the rectum is separated from the back of the bladder and vagina. At this point the surgeon will encounter the dense fibrous tissue at the site of the fistula and the rectum must be separated by careful sharp dissection from the posterior vaginal wall. The fistula is divided during this process but the dissection must be continued for several centimetres beyond the fistula (Fig. 11.20). The rectum is now amputated well below the fistula and the edge of the opening in the vagina freshened and trimmed (Fig. 11.21). The rectum and lower sigmoid are now raised from the pelvis, the inferior mesenteric and left colic vessels having been divided. The rectum apart from the last 2–3 cm, and much of

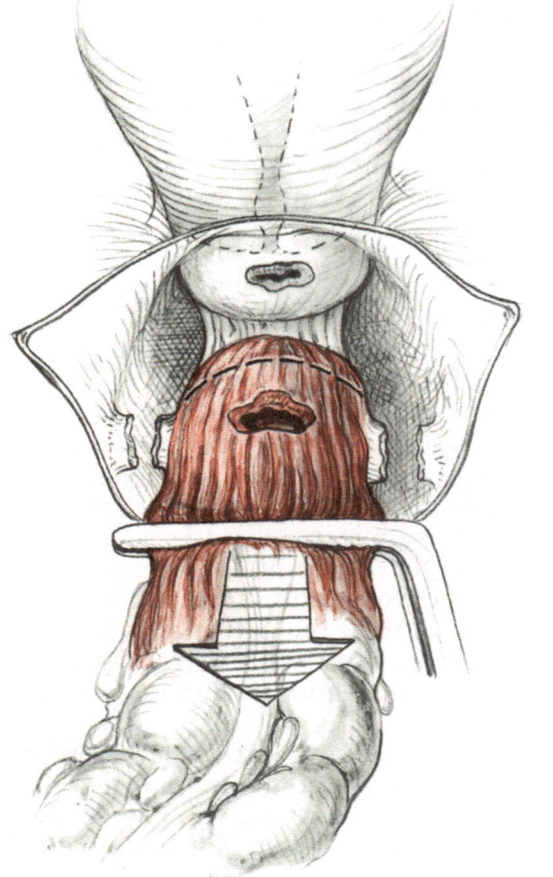

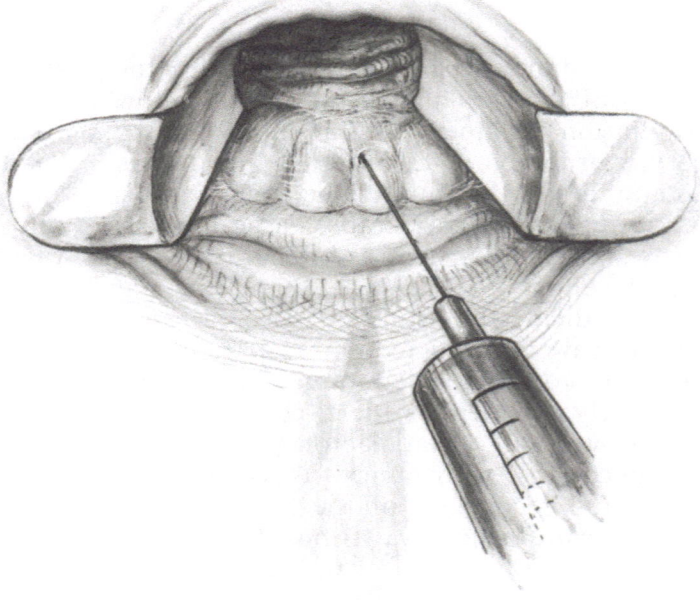

Fig. 11.21. The rectum is amputated well below the fistula.

the left colon are usually sacrificed at this stage of the procedure to ensure that the proximal bowel required for anastomosis is free from effects of radiation. The blood supply to the descending colon is examined critically to ensure that viable bowel will now reach to the level of the anus, and whenever possible the left end of the transverse colon is used for the anastomosis to ensure freedom from irradiation effects.

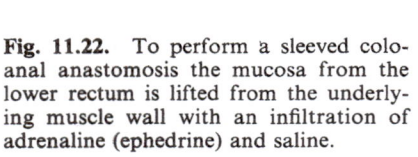

Fig. 11.20. The peritoneum over the anterior and lateral surface of the rectum is incised and by sharp dissection the rectum is separated from the back of the vagina to reveal the fistula. The dissection is continued for several centimetres below the fistula and the rectum mobilised laterally and posteriorly down to the pelvic floor.

Fig. 11.22. To perform a sleeved colo-anal anastomosis the mucosa from the lower rectum is lifted from the underlying muscle wall with an infiltration of adrenaline (ephedrine) and saline.

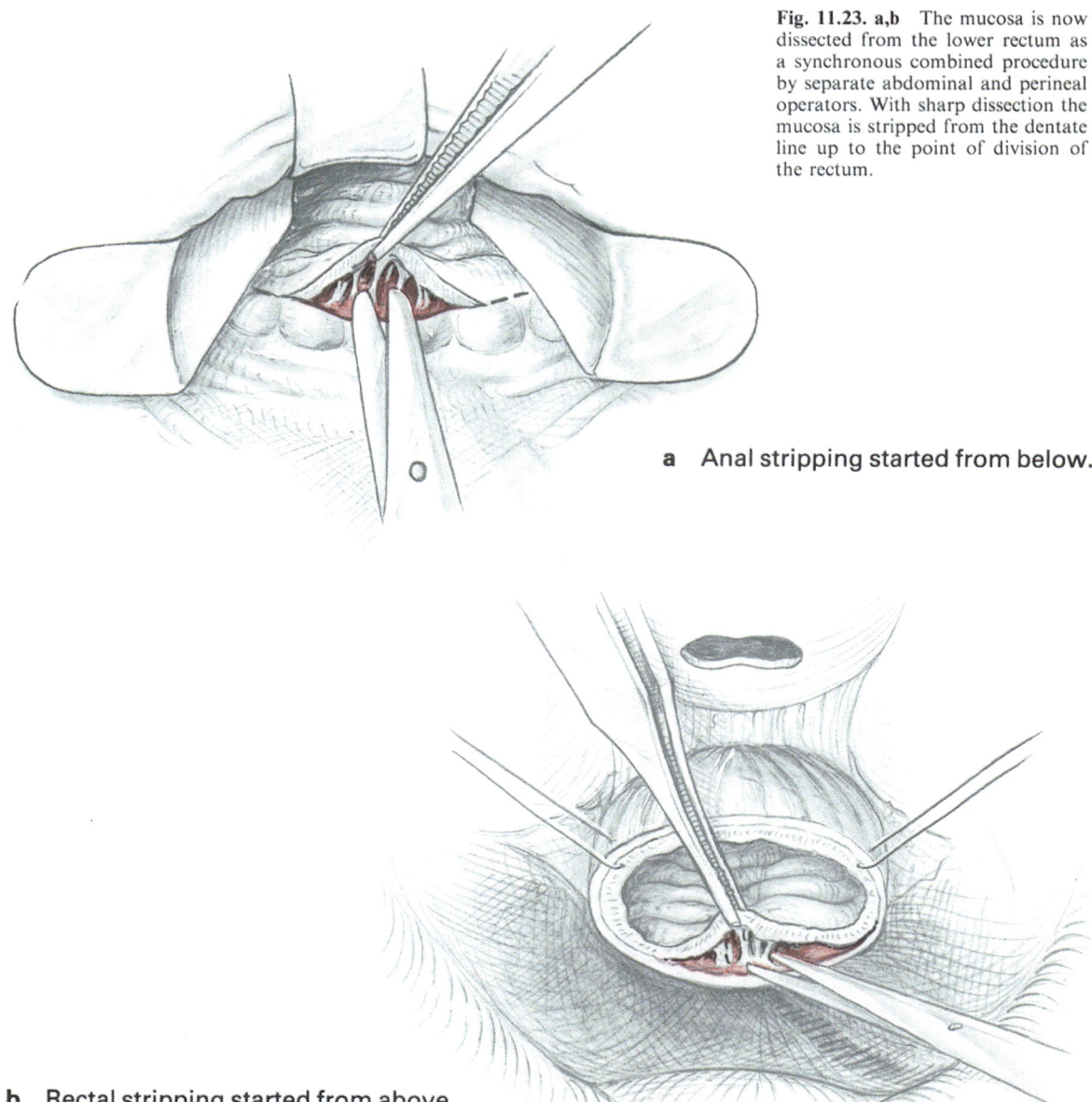

Fig. 11.23. a,b The mucosa is now dissected from the lower rectum as a synchronous combined procedure by separate abdominal and perineal operators. With sharp dissection the mucosa is stripped from the dentate line up to the point of division of the rectum.

a Anal stripping started from below.

b Rectal stripping started from above.

The mucosa is now dissected from the lining of the lower rectum. This is done as a synchronous combined procedure by separate abdominal and perineal operators. Infiltration from above and below with adrenaline (ephedrine 1:300 000 in physiological saline) solution in the submucosal space lifts the mucosa from the underlying muscle wall (Fig. 11.22). With sharp dissection the mucosa is stripped from the level of the dentate line up to the point of division of the rectum (Fig. 11.23 a,b). Small blood vessels may need to be underrun or coagulated with diathermy. Eventually the whole rectal stump for 2–3 cm above the dentate line is denuded of mucosa and the proximal colon is brought down through this denuded muscle tube to reach the anal

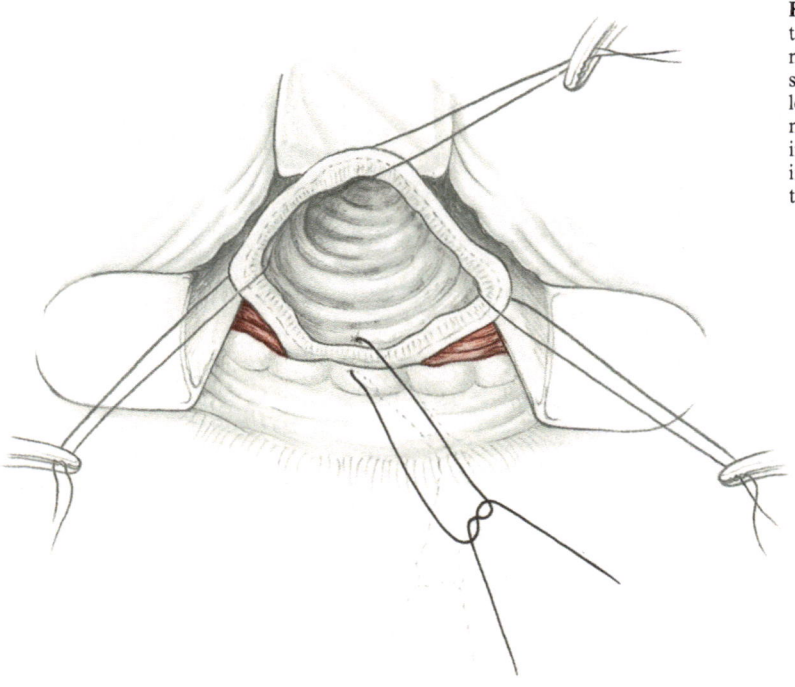

Fig. 11.24. The proximal colon is delivered to the perineal operator through the rectal muscle tube. There must be no doubt in the surgeon's mind that there is both adequate length and good blood supply to the proximal colon. With an anal speculum in place, interrupted stitches of 00 Vicryl are placed in all four quadrants taking deep bites of the underlying ano-rectal muscle.

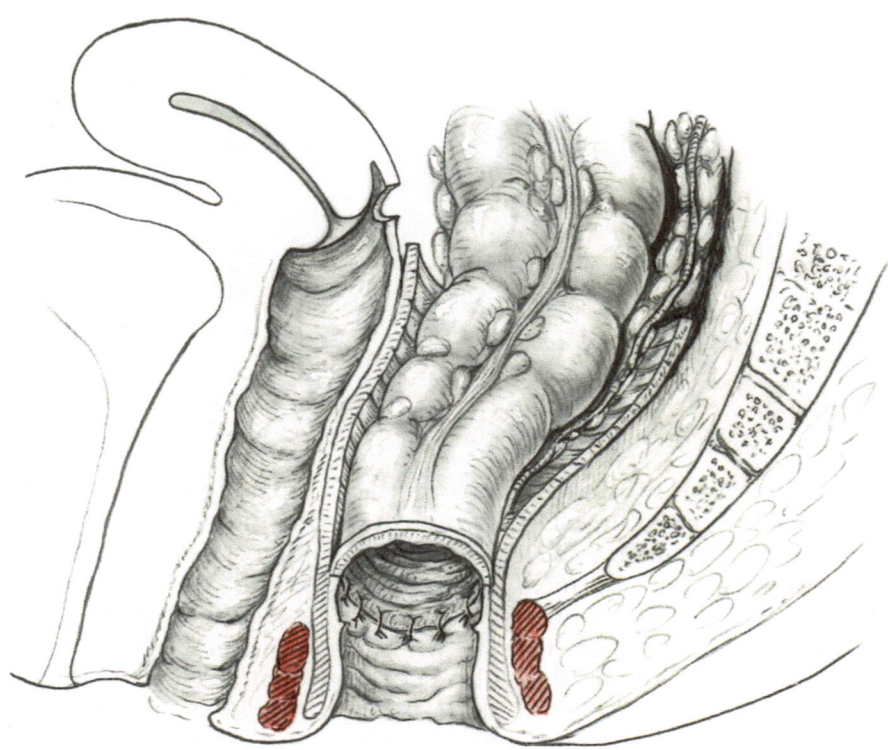

Fig. 11.25. The completed colo-anal sleeved anastomosis.

Fig. 11.26. The upper limit of the rectal muscle cuff is sutured to the proximal colon. An omental graft is prepared and brought down to lie between the unclosed vaginal opening of the fistula and the anterior wall of the rectum. A suction drain may be placed in the pelvis and the peritoneum closed.

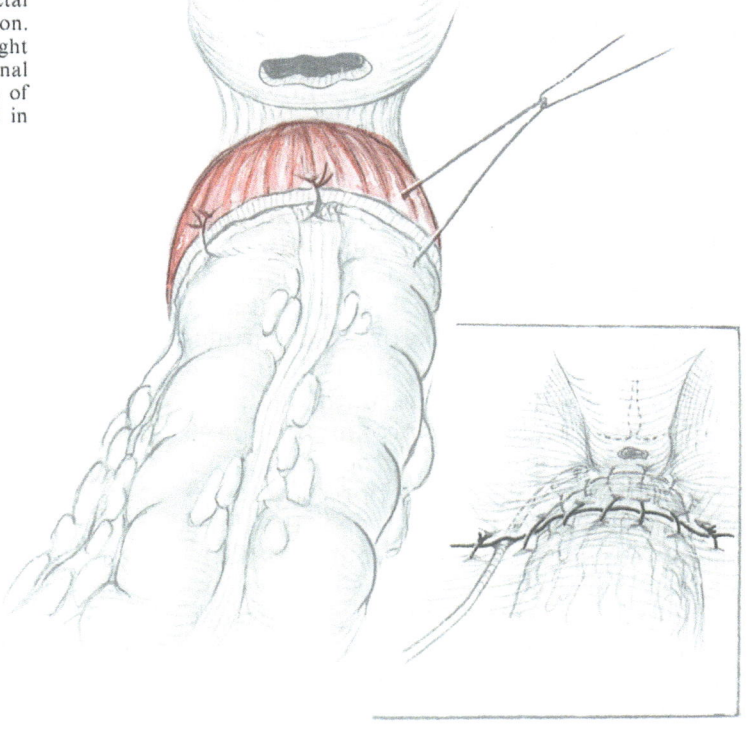

canal. The length of the colon and its blood supply is critical and there must be no doubt in the surgeon's mind that there is both adequate length and good blood supply before the anastomosis is performed. The rectum is cross-clamped and amputated at the lowest point that is well below the fistula and any abnormal tissue.

The perineal operator now carries out stapled or open manual anastomosis of colon to anus with interrupted 00 Vicryl sutures. For manual per-anal anastomosis a suture mounted on a "J"-shaped fishhook needle (Ethicon) is ideal. An Eisenhammer anal speculum gives excellent vision and facilitates anastomosis as long as there is adequate colon length and no tension. Interrupted stay stitches are placed in all four quadrants (Fig. 11.24). By "quadrant-by-quadrant" rotation of the Eisenhammer further stitches are put into each quadrant between the stay sutures (Fig. 11.25) to complete the anastomosis. If the surgeon is

not using a sleeve and chooses a direct end-to-end anastomosis of colon to anus, stapling is easiest and best for the anastomosis. A "double-stapling" technique is ideal in these cases [6,10]. A length of greater omentum is prepared as a final step as previously described (p. 172), and brought down to surround the rectum and lie between the unclosed vaginal opening of the fistula and the anterior wall of the bowel which has been brought down into the pelvis (Fig. 11.26). A suction drain may be placed in the pelvis and a defunctioning stoma now performed, either by loop colostomy or loop ileostomy. The abdomen is closed in the usual fashion.

Post-operative Management

Post-operative management is straightforward and involves the usual care of a patient who has undergone major abdominal surgery. The anal wound needs little attention as there is usually very little discharge unless sepsis supervenes or there is tissue necrosis. The patient is allowed to take oral fluids as soon as there are signs of intestinal activity and the ileostomy or colostomy has functioned.

The anastomosis should be examined carefully between the 10th and 14th days after surgery. Narrowing is not unusual and this development must be detected as it may require dilatation before the defunctioning stoma is closed. Such dilatation should be delayed, however, until the anastomosis has healed (approximately 4–6 weeks post-operation). The colostomy or ileostomy is usually closed approximately 3 months after surgery, provided the anal anastomosis has healed without complications. The anastomosis can easily be examined digitally or with a narrow proctoscope to check its integrity prior to closure.

Recent experience has shown that in a small number of cases stenosis at the level of the divided rectal wall can occur. This complication is common if a sleeve of denuded rectal stump of more than 2–3 cm is left. In these circumstances, unsatisfactory function with obstructed defecation occurs. Because of this problem many surgeons now advocate stapling or manual direct colo-anal manual anastomosis without retaining any rectal stump.

References and Further Reading

1. Allen-Mersh TG, Wilson EJ, Hope-Stone HF, Mann CV (1986) Has the incidence of radiation induced bowel damage following treatment of uterine carcinoma changed in the last 20 years? J R Soc Med 79: 387
2. Allen-Mersh TG, Wilson EJ, Hope-Stone HF, Mann CV (1987) The management of late radiation induced rectal injury after treatment of carcinoma of the uterus. Surg Gynecol obstet 164: 521
3. Alexander-Williams J, Buchmann P (1980) Peri-anal Crohn's disease. World J Surg 4: 203
4. Bentley RJ (1973) Abdominal repair of high recto-vaginal fistula. J Obstet Gynecol Br Common W 80: 364
5. Bricker EM, Johnston WD (1979) Repair of post-irradation recto-vaginal fistula and stricture. Surg Gynecol Obstet 148: 499
6. Cohen Z, Myers E, langer B et al. (1983) Double-stapling technique for low anterior resection. Dis Colon Rectum 26: 231
7. Fielding JF (1972) Perianal lesions in Crohn's disease. J R Coll Surg Edinb 17: 32
8. Goldberg SM (1980) Recto-vaginal fistula. In: Essentials of ano-rectal surgery. Lippincott, Philadelphia, pp 316–332
9. Greenwald JC, Hoexter B (1978) Repair of recto-vaginal fistulas. Surg Gynecol Obstet 146: 443
10. Griffin FD, Knight CD (1984) Stapling technique for primary and secondary rectal anastomoses. Surg Clin North Am 64: 579
11. Hobbis JH, Schofield PF (1982) Management of perianal Crohn's disease. J R Soc Med 75: 414
11. Lawson J (1972) Recto-vaginal fistulae following difficult labour. Proc R Soc Med 65: 283
13. Lescher TC, Pratt JH (1967) Vaginal repair of the simple recto-vaginal fistula. Surg Gynecol Obstet 124: 1317
14. Macleod D, Hawkins J (1964) Bonney's Gynaecological surgery, 7th edn. Ballière Tindall and Cassell, London
15. Palmer JA, Bush RS (1976) Radiation injuries to the bowel associated with treatment of carcinoma of the cervix and uterus. Surgery 80: 458
16. Parks AG, Allen CL, Frank JD, McPartlin JF (1978) A method of treating post-irradiation recto-vaginal fistula. Br J Surg 65: 417
17. Russell TR, Gallagher DM 91977) Low recto-vaginal fistulas: approach and treatment. Am J Surg 134: 13
18. Wolff BG, Culp CE, Beart LW (Jr) et al. 91985) Ano-rectal Crohn's disease. A long-term perspective. Dis Colon Rectum 28: 709

CHAPTER 12

Salvage Procedures

General Introduction

Despite the many procedures available for treating patients with faecal incontinence, a few remain incurable. The main reasons that account for such cases are patients whose mental or physical state constitutes a contraindication to a definitive attempt at surgical cure or a small residue of cases in whom surgery has failed. Many such "incurable" cases are residents of long-stay facilities for the elderly, and these form a constant pool of incontinent patients for whom a satisfactory cure of their incontinence problem has not been devised. It has been estimated that 17% of nursing home residents suffer from a significant incontinence problem [12]. For such cases a salvage procedure is often the only practical solution, especially when there is a serious degree of incontinence in a patient whose life expectancy is measured in years rather than months.

Three different approaches are available for treating such patients, which are collectively grouped as *salvage procedures* [4].

The first type of procedure is one that is simple, quick, minimally traumatic and requires no specialist surgical expertise. A good example is *silastic sling encirclement* of the anal canal.

The second type of procedure is of intermediate severity but requires specialist colo-proctological surgeons to perform it. The best example of this type is the *inflatable anal prosthesis*.

The third type of procedure is the most severe and consists of *faecal diversion by a stoma* (colostomy, ileostomy). Although the infliction of a permanent stoma is repugnant to both patients and surgeons, it is the most reliable in its results.

Each of these procedures will be considered separately.

Silastic Sling Encirclement [3]

Despite the well founded criticisms of the Thiersch procedure previously enumerated (Chapter 6, pp. 79–82), it can be attended with success in some cases. It has considerable advantages for an elderly infirm patient because it is simple to perform; can be done with a minimum of anaesthesia; involves only a very short stay in hospital; and can be easily reversed if problems arise. The procedure can be repeated if necessary.

Many of the complications associated with the Thiersch procedure derive from the rigidity of the materials which have been used to encircle the anal canal (wire, nylon). These problems can be reduced by using a material with some degree of elasticity, and silastic ribbon has been employed for this reason. By using silastic ribbon, problems of faecal impaction and cutting out have been reduced, but not entirely eliminated. The main complication associated with the use of silastic is persisting sepsis requiring removal of the sling.

Because of its safety and simplicity, a silastic sling operation can be performed by surgeons who do not have special colo-proctological experience. The procedure can also be done as a day-case, and under caudal anaesthesia if this is indicated by the poor state of health of the patient.

The complication of wound sepsis can be reduced by emptying the colon and rectum pre-operatively by enemas and rectal wash-outs, and by per-operative antibiotic cover against both aerobic and anaerobic organisms. Cutting out of the material can be minimised by making deep incisions into the ischiorectal fossae on each side of the anal canal; by inserting the ribbon around the upper third of the anal canal; and by taking great care that the ribbon is inserted outside the external sphincter muscle. Faecal impaction can be averted to a large extent by ensuring that the ribbon is tightened to the correct degree (i.e. does not narrow the canal too much) by using a finger (or a Hegar dilator of the correct size) to check the size of the lumen as the ribbon is tightened. The silastic ribbon, when it has been threaded through the peri-anal tunnel created by blunt dissection, and has been tightened to the appropriate degree, has its ends joined either by overlapping unabsorbable sutures or by staples, and any surplus ribbon is discarded. In order to lessen the possibility of wound sepsis, extreme care should be taken to avoid faecal contamination of the wounds, which should be closed in layers without drainage. Before closure the wounds should be irrigated with an antiseptic solution (e.g. Povidone–iodine).

Post-operatively it is imperative to ensure that faecal impaction is prevented by suitable precautions to obtain adequate rectal evacuation from the first post-operation day onward. A supervised programme of laxatives and enemas must be instituted and the state of the rectum must be checked frequently by digital examinations; unless this is carried out by reliable nursing and medical attendants, the chances of a successful result will be negated.

Inflatable Anal Prosthesis [2,4,8]

An artificial anal prosthesis has been developed (American Medical Systems – AMS 800) which is a modification of a similar device for controlling urinary incontinence. The device uses an inflatable silastic balloon cuff to occlude the anal canal which can be deflated to allow rectal evacuation when required. The device is illustrated in Fig. 12.1, and consists of three parts, the inflatable *perianal cuff*, a *balloon reservoir* and a manually operated *pump*. The system is fluid-filled and the various parts are connected by fine silastic tubes. The system is implanted by two surgeons working simultaneously, a *perineal surgeon* who inserts the perianal balloon and an *abdominal surgeon* who puts in the reservoir and the pump. During the operation the

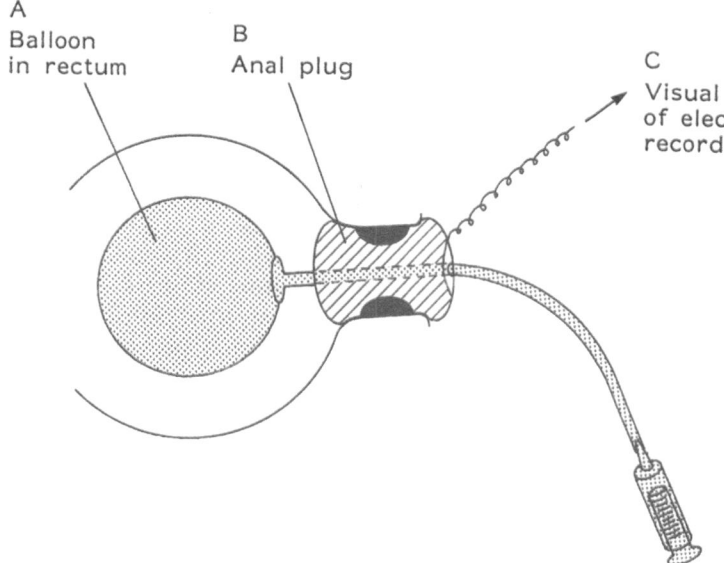

A
Balloon
in rectum

B
Anal plug

C
Visual display unit
of electromyometer
recordings

Fig. 12.1. The patient is trained to recognise the distension of the balloon in the rectum (A) and to respond by a voluntary anal contraction. The strength of the anal sphincter response is registered by an anal plug fitted with electrodes (B), which is connected to a visual display unit (C) which shows the strength of the muscle contraction recorded by an electromyometer (not shown).

amount of fluid in the system requires careful calibration to ensure that the quantity is *exactly* that required to achieve gentle occlusion of the anal canal when the perianal cuff is inflated *and no more*. If too much fluid is introduced and the pressure in the cuff rises above what is required, the risk of post-operative necrosis of the anal and perianal tissues is substantial. It is also necessary to cover the operation with full precautions against septic complications by emptying the colon pre-operatively, and by full perioperative antibiotic cover against aerobic and anaerobic bacteria. It is also advisable to ascertain by discussion the best side for the patient to have the reservoir and pump inserted, with particularly enquiry as to whether the patient is left handed. *Because the system requires delicate manometry to calibrate, and achieves its best results by careful post-operative training in correct use of the device, the inflatable prosthesis system should be put in by colo-proctological surgeons working in a specialist centre with full back-up by laboratory facilities.*

The perianal cuff is placed in a deep perianal tunnel around the upper part of the anal canal and its ends fastened by a press-stud system at the point where the cuff fits snugly around the anal canal. The balloon reservoir is put into the retropubic space of Retzius through a small Pfannensteil incision by the abdominal surgeon, who also places the pump in the scrotal sac (or labia majora) on the appropriate side. The tubing connecting the reservoir–pump elements to the perianal cuff is passed through a subcutaneous tunnel which descends through the pre-pubic, inner thigh and ischiorectal regions to the perianal cuff. The tunnel is formed by blunt dissection from above and below by the two surgeons co-operating. Once the system is connected, the amount of fluid is calibrated by the perineal operator. The system incorporates a valve system which allows fluid to be pumped between the reservoir and the balloon cuff, which can be emptied when rectal evacuation is desired.

Sepsis is the main complication of the procedure and it is desirable that *all patients should have faecal diversion by a defunctioning colostomy before the prosthesis is inserted.* The wounds should be closed in layers without drainage and the patient should be confined to bed for a few days while the wounds consolidate.

Six weeks after the operation, when all the wounds have healed soundly, the patient is readmitted to hospital for training in the use of the device. Only when the patient has complete familiarity with the use of the scrotal pump to deflate–inflate the perianal cuff should the colostomy be closed.

Providing there has been good patient selection for the procedure, and the requisite degree of surgical and laboratory expertise has been available, good results have been achieved. The procedure is particularly suitable for patients with *extensive damage to spinal and pelvic nerves*; *severe destruction of ano-rectal tissues*; and *failed previous incontinence procedures* (e.g. after an unsuccessful stimulated graciloplasty [1,10,13], described in Chapter 6, pp. 95–100).

Faecal Diversion by a Stoma

The number of patients who need to be treated by a permanent stoma is small and is still falling, especially since the development of muscle transfer procedures, and in particular the stimulated graciloplasty operation. However, there will always exist a small residuum of cases who are either unsuitable for a definitive incontinence procedure or, sadly, who have remained incontinent despite one or more attempts at surgical correction; for these patients a permanent stoma may be the only practical answer. *An important indication for treatment by a stoma is inability of patients to cooperate in the social and nursing measures required to keep their problem under reasonable control because of mental or physical disabilities, often combined.* In such circumstances, control of the excreta by means of a well fitting disposable appliance of modern design fitted to a well constructed colostomy is a boon to both patients and their carers. It is important that the use of a colostomy is seen as a constructive answer to an insuperable difficulty and not as failure.

In order to maximise the benefit from a colostomy, several criteria should be satisfied. *First*, the stoma should be sited in the best position with due consideration to the problems of the whole patient. *Second*, the technique used for constructing the stoma should be meticulous [6] and *involve senior surgical staff*. *Third*, whenever possible, the patient should be an active and willing participant in the management of their condition, and particularly the use of the appliances. *Fourth*, the appliances should be well chosen and any problem associated with availability and disposal anticipated and minimised. *Fifth*, a sympathetic and experienced professional adviser or stoma nurse should be available to whom the patient can turn for prompt advice and practical assistance. *Sixth*, the family (and others when indicated) should know what is involved in stoma care. *Seventh*, surgical complications arising from the stoma should be diagnosed and treated expeditiously. *Eighth*, instruction should be given in the effects of diet and drugs on the frequency and nature of the faecal discharges. *Ninth*, the patients must have confidence that their surgical team constantly reviews the treatments that are available for treating incontinence, and remains willing to consider closure of the stoma if a new procedure that offers them hope for closing the stoma becomes available. *Tenth*, all concerned with the patients' management should have the attitude that the presence of a stoma is fully compatible with a normal life. These are the *ten commandments* for successful management of faecal incontinence by a stoma. Although the stoma employed is usually a colostomy, a few patients may prefer an ileostomy [5] because of its comparative lack of odour; the ileostomy can be of the continent type (Kock ileostomy [7]).

Because the faecal stream needs to be completely diverted, an "end-stoma" is recommended, and this is accomplished best by a standard trans-abdominal approach. *Although laparoscopic techniques are described for making a colostomy these do not provide the best conditions for a "guaranteed" success.* The authors recommend that the colostomy should be constructed at a site low in the sigmoid colon, and that following division of the colon, any distal colon should be removed and the rectal stump closed off intraperitonally just above the recto-sigmoid junction. The proximal end of the colon should be brought out through the lateral edge of the rectus sheath low in the left iliac fossa. This distal Hartmann-style procedure gives a faecal discharge that is solid or semi-solid; a colostomy that works only once or twice a day; and an inconspicuous site for the attachment of the bag. By reducing the length of distal bowel that remains, the problem of mucus leakage from the anus is minimised. The colostomy opening must be well away from the anterior iliac spine in order that the bag can be attached securely; in a cadaverous patient this may indicate a higher site for the stoma than is usual, and in a massively obese patient an umbilical site is preferred. In all cases the stoma must *not* be constructed at a site where skin folds could interfere with a water tight seal between the appliance and the skin. For a very frail patient it may be necessary to accept a less than "ideal" solution and a loop colostomy can be performed through a simple trephine abdominal opening without the need for a laparotomy (or laparoscopy).

A troublesome complication of a permanent colostomy that is seen in some patients is the condition known as *"disuse (defunctioned) proctitis"*. This is a non-specific inflammation of the rectal mucosa associated with a friable haemorrhagic epithelium exhibiting superficial ulceration, inflammatory pseudopolyps and fibrosis in long-term cases. There may be stricturing of the rectal wall with stenosis of the lumen in some late cases. The condition may be associated with profuse mucus discharge and some loss of blood P.R. The cause of the condition is thought to be loss to the colonocytes of the epithelium of essential nutrients produced by bacterial action, principally short-chain fatty acids, which leads to impaired mucosal resistance, reduced absorption and inflammatory changes of colitis type [9]. Treatment can be given by topical administration of short chain fatty acids or by instillation of faeces into the rectum; this last treatment is understand-ably unpopular with both staff and patients!

Before a patient is selected for treatment by a permanent colostomy, especially when there has been a prior failed attempt at surgical cure, it is imperative that all supportive (non-surgical) treatments should have been tried; these are described in Chapter 13, pp. 188–189. Biofeedback treatment is recommended by the authors as an essential preliminary when it is apparent that a patient is beyond help by any surgical procedure other than a colostomy. A surgeon should refer the patient for biofeedback training in a spirit of optimism rather than despair as psychological factors play a part in the success of this therapy; if the surgeon indicates that he has little faith in the response, it is not surprising that this should be unfavourable. It is doubly important that this treatment should be used when it is indicated, for there is nothing more destructive to the relationship between patients and their surgeons than the discovery that a potentially successful non-surgical treatment had not been given a chance before their stoma was made.

References and Further Reading

1. Baeten C, Spaans F, Fluks A (1988) An implanted neuromuscular stimulator for faecal continence following previously implanted gracilis muscle. Dis Colon Rectum 31: 134
2. Christiansen J, Lorentzen M (1987) Implantation of artifical sphincter for anal incontinence. Lancet. 2 (8553): 244
3. Guillemot F, Columbel JF, Neut C et al. (1991) Treatment of diversion colitis by short-chain fatty acids: prospective and double blind study. Dis Colon Rectum 24: 861
4. Williams JG, Rothenberger DA (1993) Faecal incontinence: an American perspective. In Modern Coloproctology (Philips R, Northover J: eds). Edward Arnold p 140
5. Oakley JR, Fazio VW (1993) Ileostomy. In Rob and Smith's Operative Surgery, 5th Edn. Alimentary Tract 3. Colon, Rectum and Anus. (Fielding LP, Goldberg SM: eds) Butterworth–Heinemann. p 243
6. Philips RKS, Thompson JPS (1993) Colostomy. In Rob and Smith's Operative Surgery, 5th Edn. Alimentary Tract 3. Colon, Rectum and Anus (Fielding LP, Goldberg SM: eds) Butterworth–Heinemann. p 274

7. Kewenter JK, Brevinge H (1993) Continent (Kock) Ileostomy. In Rob and Smith's Operative Surgery, 5th Edn. Alimentary Tract 3. Colon, Rectum and Anus (Fielding LP, Goldberg SM: eds) Butterworth-Heinemann. p 592

8. Wong WD, Rothenberger DA (1993) Artificial Anal Sphincter. In Rob and Smith's Operative Surgery, 5th Edn. Alimentary Tract 3. Colon, Rectum and Anus (Fielding LP, Goldberg SM: eds) Butterworth-Heinemann. p 773

9. Roediger WEW (1990) The starved colon-diminished mucosal nutrition, diminished absorption and colitis. Dis Colon Rectum 33: 858

10. Salmons SS, Hendriksson J (1981) The adaptive response of skeletal muscle to increased use. Muscle Nerve 4: 94

11. Stricker JW Schoetz DJ, Clooer JA, Veidenheimer MC (1988) Surgical correction of anal incontinence. Dis Colon Rectum 31: 533

12. Thomas TM, Ruff C, Karran O et al. (1987) Study of the prevalence and management of patients with faecal incontinence in old people's homes. Community Med 9: 232

13. Williams NS, Hallan RI, Koeze TH et al. (1990) Construction of a neoanal sphincter by transposition of the gracilis muscle and prolonged neuromuscular stimulation for the treatment of faecal incontinence. Ann Roy Coll Surg (Engl) 72: 108

CHAPTER 13

General Supportive Measures

General Introduction

The anal sphincters are dependent on several factors for optimal function. They must be able to respond to stimuli from the rectum, (and in particular to *rectal distention*) by alterations in tone (e.g. the recto–anal reflex); they must respond to gas, liquid and solid signals mediated by anal sampling with an appropriate response; they must be able to maintain "watertight" closure by a constant plateau of anal tone, reinforced by a voluntary contraction when needed; they must be able to participate by suitable relaxation–contraction responses in the neuromuscular mechanisms of defaecation, and these responses must be properly coordinated. When the sphincters are damaged, these subtle and delicate functions are likely to suffer, and sphincteric responses may never return to complete normality.

Surgical operations are primarily concerned with restoration of normal anatomical structure, with recovery of physiological function a subsidiary aim. While they can buttress and support weak anal muscles and increase the length of the anal canal, they are unable to replace lost muscle or to repair damaged sensory and motor nerves, although it is often observed that neuromuscular function improves following a good anatomical reconstruction and that anal tone increases after many procedures (e.g. after abdominal rectopexy for prolapse). Nevertheless the surgeon must accept that the final result of his reparative efforts depends to a considerable extent on the pre-surgical functional competence of the anal sphincter mechanism.

Both before and after surgery on the anal sphincters it is possible in many cases to enhance the performance of the anal sphincters. This can be done in many ways, and maximum effect is often achieved by combining several methods. The principal methods that are employed are:

1. Enhancement of sphincter responses to sensory stimuli

2. Improvement of anal sphincter tone and reactivity

3. Enhancement of the efficiency of rectal emptying
4. Alteration of the physical nature of the stools
5. Reduction of colonic motor activity
6. Promotion of increased patient awareness and cooperation

By selective employment of these measures it is possible to improve a patient's incontinence score (p. 2), and in some cases it may be possible to restore anal continence to normal. It must also be emphasised that due regard to these supportive measures can not only improve the results of surgery but may even abolish the need to operate at all. Each method is considered in turn below.

Enhancement of Sphincter Responses to Sensory Stimuli by Biofeedback

Control of defaecation is established during infancy by the development of sophisticated relationships between the central (cortical) and peripheral (pelvic) nerves. The peripheral nerves involved are both somatic and autonomic, and their relays may either be cholinergic or adrenergic, with lumbo–sacral reflex arcs playing an important role in the maintenance of anal tone. In clinical practise, many cases of incontinence are initiated or aggravated by diminished awareness of rectal filling or by inability to respond to rectal filling by sphincter augmentation. Incontinence can be caused by loss of sensory awareness either by allowing uncontrolled escape of faeces or by promoting faecal impaction with "overflow" leaking of excessive liquefied faecal content. Common causes of these problems include psychic disturbance, senile dementia, peripheral neuropathy (including diabetic neuropathy), childbirth injury (especially extended labour), cerebro–vascular accidents and trauma to the sacrum and pelvis. In some cases the nerve deficit is accompanied by diminished mass of the pelvic and anal muscles, whose weakness aggravates the reduction of anal

sphincter tone and reactivity. The importance of childbirth injury, particularly prolonged labour, as a cause of pudendal nerve damage is now recognised as a prime factor in promoting incontinence in otherwise healthy young women.

Biofeedback [1–5] was developed as a means of enhancing or restoring normal function of the anal sphincters by a programme of retraining the sphincteric responses to rectal distention. The method is illustrated in Fig. 13.1. If successful, biofeedback leads to heightened responsiveness of the anal sphincters to rectal distention and strengthening of the sub-cortical reflex mechanisms which maintain anal tone. Biofeedback achieves its best results when the incontinence is not severe, and it is particularly effective for minor degrees of soiling in post-surgical and post-obstetric cases; it is also helpful for radiation damage and has an important role in correcting minor leakage problems after sphincter repair. The greater the degree of neuropathic damage, the lesser the response to biofeedback, and the method is ineffective for the treatment of total incontinence from any cause [1].

Although the results of biofeedback have been good when practised in special units staffed by experts and backed up by enthusiastic laboratory and paramedical auxilliaries (Table 13.1), surgeons outside special centers have little experience of the technique. However, they should be aware of its possibilities and be prepared to refer patients for treatment when a suitable indi-

Table 13.1 Biofeedback treatment of faecal soiling*

Reported by	Number of patients	Success (%)
1. Cerulli et al. 1979	50	72
2. Goldenberg et al. 1980	12	83
3. MacCleod 1987	113	63
4. Jensen and Lowry 1991	31	90

* Biofeedback achieves its best results for minor degrees of faecal incontinence, as these results reported for soiling show. Ideally, the patients who are selected for treatment should be intelligent, well motivated, co-operative and retain both rectal sensibility (distention) and some power of voluntary anal contractility.

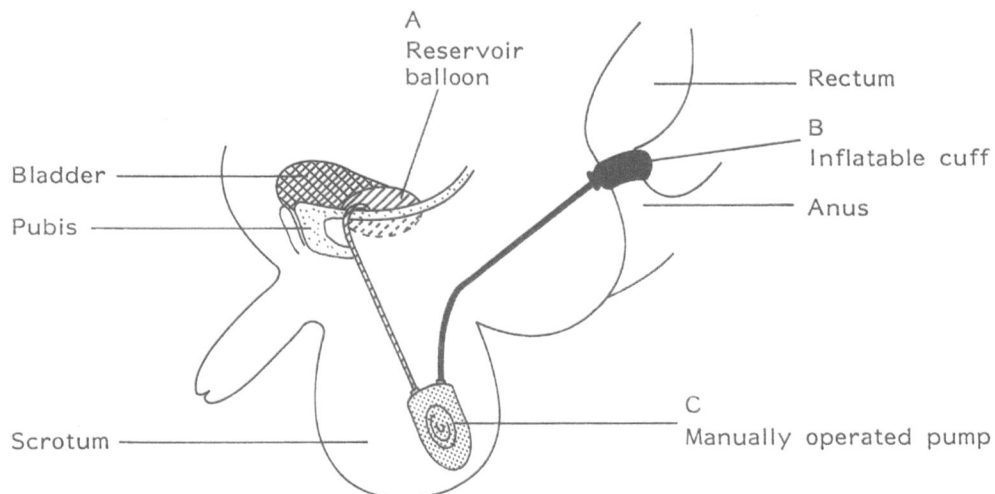

Fig. 13.1. The apparatus consists of a fluid filled system linked by fine tubing to its three parts – A a reservoir balloon placed in the cave of Retzius, B an inflatable cuff around the anus, and C a manually operated pump in the scrotum or labia majora.

cation is apparent. Patients who have a mild problem of soiling, especially in a young age group, benefit greatly from this method.

Another group in which biofeedback should always be considered are patients who have a post-surgical leakage problem, as after a fistula operation or surgical repair of a torn sphincter. Biofeedback is ineffective in restoring tone to a patulous sphincter associated with rectal prolapse.

One factor that limits the applicability of the technique is that it requires frequent visits to hospital over a long period (months) to achieve its best results, and there is evidence that a period of further retraining may be required every three or four years. This means that the method is limited to patients who reside mainly in large conurbations and are close to a treatment facility.

The success of biofeedbcak management for incontinence depends upon careful selection of patients and the expertise with which the technique is given.

Improvement of Anal Sphincter Tone and Reactivity

The tone of the sphincter ani externus and its ability to exert an effective voluntary squeeze can be improved by a course of anal sphincter exercises supervised by a physiotherapist. The strength of the abdominal and pelvic floor muscles can also be increased by suitable exercises, which include prone lifts and leg raising elements. Such exercises can be important in restoring tone to a flaccid sphincter, as after childbirth or severe illness (including major trauma). Where suitable facilities are available, electrical stimulation of the external sphincter can also be used, and both physiotherapy and electrotherapy can be used alongside biofeedback (v.s).

The general health and nutritional status of the patient, especially their total body protein mass, should be taken into account when a weak anal sphincter is causing incontinence because this may be part of a more general problem of muscle wasting. The anal sphincters are subject to the same catabolic processes as the rest of the body's musculature and may require similar attention to the correction of nutritional or endocrine deficiencies. Unless such deficiencies are eliminated, the response of the anal sphincters to exercises (and other methods of stimulation) will be impaired, and a high protein intake is recommended when a course of anal sphincter exercises is being carried out.

Enhancement of the Efficiency of Rectal Emptying

Some patients are incontinent, not because of a primary problem with their anal sphincters, but because they are unable to empty their rectum properly at defaecation. If a significant faecal residue remains at completion of defaecation this can be a cause of leakage between defaecations. This problem is made much more severe if faecal impaction develops or if the anal sphincter also is weak for any reason. If the anus is patulous, any faeces present in the rectum can escape and the leakage is often particularly profuse at night or during activity, and is aggravated by liquid stools or mucus. Patients with widespread neurological damage (multiple sclerosis, spinal injuries) or autonomic neuropathy (diabetes) are especially prone to problems of rectal retention combined with anal sphincter weakness. In patients who have multiple sclerosis or a paraplegia, their inability to contract their abdominal muscles to supplement rectal emptying by abdominal straining is a major contribution to build-up of faeces in the rectum.

Many of these patients can have their incontinence problem alleviated, and even in some cases, cured, by improving rectal evacuation, leaving a clean empty rectum. Judicious use of suppositories (*glycerine*, *bisacodyl*), laxatives (*magnesium sulphate*, *sodium picosulphate*), and enemas can be effective for achieving satisfactory rectal emptying. Enemas can be particularly useful for patients with motility problems, especially bed-ridden cases. Enemas may be stimulant (*Fletcher's enemette* containing dioctyl sodium succinate, *Micralax* contain-

ing sodium citrate) or passive (wash-outs administered by staff).

In some instances a patient can be kept clean by a regular programme of intermittent colonic irrigations, the number judged according to the individual's needs. Such a programme is best suited to patients who retain some degree of anal tone (so that they can retain the irrigating fluid and minimise post-irrigation leakage of wash-out fluid). It can be used for patients who would be considered otherwise suitable for a colostomy which they refuse for religious or psychological reasons.

Alteration of the Consistency of the Stools

It is stating the obvious to say that a weakened anal sphincter is able to control dry hard stools much better than liquid faeces, mucus or gas. Constipating drugs (*codeine phosphate*) can be used to harden the stools, and oral intake of fluid should be reduced. Intake of beer or wine should be strictly controlled. The diet should be regulated to avoid excessive bulk and it may be necessary to reduce the fibre content of the food. It is important to enquire about the intake of bran, vegetables and cellulose products because many patients have been persuaded by health food "experts" that a healthy diet is linked to excessive use of such products.

There is little practical help that can be offered for problems of excess gas or mucus. Air swallowing must be curbed, especially if there is a psychological cause, such as anxiety. Mucus seapage can be minimised by a cotton wool tampon tucked into the anal orifice but the problem of mucus leakage is primarily related to mucosal prolapse (rectocele, anterior mucosal prolapse, third-degree haemorrhoids) and is handled by the appropriate surgical operation. Some patients with inflammatory bowel diseases present as mucus incontinence ("mucus colitis"), and should be treated by the appropriate drugs (e.g. *salazopyrine*, *steroids*); once their colitis is controlled, the problem of excessive mucus production is reduced.

Reduction of Colonic Motor Activity

Fast transit of faeces through the intestines, and especially through the large bowel, can lead to rapid rectal filling and incontinence. Even a sphincter of normal tone is unable to withstand problems caused by severe diarrhoea, and a weak sphincter is correspondingly worse at controlling frequent sools, especially so if these are semi-solid or liquid. In any patient with a problem of faecal incontinence, measures should be taken to control or reduce colonic transit time and to treat any tendency to colonic overactivity ("irritable colon" syndrome). This can be done by using drugs that inhibit colonic motor activity. A desirable side effect of iatrogenic diminished colonic activity is that the increase in transit time allows more water to be extracted from the luminal contents, thus hardening the stools i.e. drugs that are used to slow intestinal transit are also constipating.

Opioids reduce intestinal motility and both *codeine phophate* and *diphenoxylate hydrochloride* (Lomotil) can be used for short-term treatment but are contraindicated for long-term use because of the danger of addiction. For long-term use, *loperamide hydrochloride* (Imodium) is the preferred drug as it has low risk of dependency. If the patient suffers from anxiety-induced bowel frequency, or has the "irritable bowel" syndrome, in addition to loperamide a tranquilising agent such as *nitrazepam* can be useful, but here, again, the possibility of dependence associated with long-term use should be remembered and long-term chronic use is not recommended. When stress is an obvious case of bowel frequency, beta-blockers can be used in exceptional situations where any loss of control would be disastrous (e.g. during a public speech).

When consideration is given to the use of drugs to assist in continence control it is always wise to scrutinise the patient's use of drugs for other reasons. The obvious pitfall is to fail to spot the patient whose incontinence is due to excessive use of laxatives ("laxative abuse" syndrome). Many drugs in common use (e.g. metaclopramide for reflux oesophagitis) have a stimulatory action on intestinal motor activity. It is also important to eliminate any possibility that food allergy or a malabsorption problem is contributing to the incontinence by promoting intestinal hurry.

Promotion of Increased Patient Awareness and Co-operation

If a patient is encouraged to understand the basis of their incontinence and how it can be handled, the results of treatment can be improved. Given suitable information and instruction the patient becomes an active partner in their therapy. To obtain the best results from supportive measures such as diet, exercises, biofeedback and drugs the cooperation of the patient is essential. To gain the patient's cooperation takes time and patience on the part of the incontinence team, who must remain flexible and encouraging throughout the course of treatment. If a good result is achieved, the gratitude of the patient is great, and more than repays the effort involved.

References

1. Cerulli MA, Nikoomanesh P, Schuster MM (1979) Progress in biofeedback conditioning for faecal incontinence. Gastroenterology 76: 742
2. Goldenberg DA, Hodges K, Hersh T, Jinich H (1980) Biofeedback therapy for faecal incontinence. Am J Gastroenterology 74: 342
3. Jensen LL, Lowry AC (1991) Biofeedback: a variable treatment option for anal incontinence. Dis Colon Rectum 34: 6
4. MacCleod JH (1987) Management of anal incontinence by Biofeedback. Gastroenterology 93: 291
5. Miner PB, Donnelly TC, Read NW (1990) Investigation of mode of action of biofeedback in treatment of faecal incontinence. Dig Dis Sci 35: 1291

SUBJECT INDEX